A GUIDE TO

physical examination
Second Edition

Barbara Bates, M.D., SENIOR DOCENT AND PROFESSOR OF MEDICINE
UNIVERSITY OF MISSOURI-KANSAS CITY

With a Section on the Pediatric Examination

BY

Robert A. Hoekelman, M.D., PROFESSOR AND ASSOCIATE CHAIRMAN,
DEPARTMENT OF PEDIATRICS
UNIVERSITY OF ROCHESTER SCHOOL OF MEDICINE
AND DENTISTRY

AND

PROFESSOR OF NURSING, UNIVERSITY OF ROCHESTER
SCHOOL OF NURSING

ILLUSTRATIONS BY ROBERT WABNITZ AND STAFF
OF THE MEDICAL ILLUSTRATION UNIT
DIVISION OF MEDICAL EDUCATION AND COMMUNICATION
UNIVERSITY OF ROCHESTER SCHOOL OF MEDICINE AND DENTISTRY

J. B. LIPPINCOTT COMPANY: Philadelphia Toronto

ISBN 0-397-54224-0

Library of Congress Catalog Card Number 78-21634

Printed in the United States of America

7 9 8

Library of Congress Cataloging in Publication Data

Bates, Barbara.

  A guide to physical examination.

  Bibliography: p. 427

  Includes index.
  1. Physical diagnosis. I. Hoekelman, Robert A.
II. Title.
RC76.B37 1979   616.07'54   78-21634
ISBN 0-397-54224-0

TABLE OF CONTENTS

TABLE OF CONTENTS _____

LIST OF TABLES

LIST OF TABLES

ACKNOWLEDGMENTS

For their suggestions, advice and help we would like to thank numerous colleagues and students in both medicine and nursing at the University of Rochester and the University of Missouri–Kansas City. Others have written to us with ideas and suggestions which we also appreciate. We have been gratified to hear from our readers, although we may neither share the same classroom nor stand at the same bedside. We hope they can detect the fruits of their advice in our Second Edition.

Special thanks go to Mark Funk, B.A., B.S., M.A., Clinical Medical Librarian, who helped in searching the literature and tracking down the answers to many questions. The sources of even "well-known facts" can be remarkably obscure.

For the original illustrations that have been included in the Second Edition we again thank Robert Wabnitz and the staff of the Medical Illustration Unit, Division of Medical Education and Communication, University of Rochester School of Medicine and Dentistry. These include Diane E. Bellinger, Marilyn J. Wilbur and Richard D. Howe. New illustrations have been created by Pamela Rowles, medical illustrator; the photographs for the adult sections of the book are by William L. Chisholm, senior medical photographer, both of the Office of Educational Resources, University of Missouri–Kansas City School of Medicine.

Jean Graeff, Anne Donahue, Mary Helen Doran and Rebecca Jones prepared the manuscript in its several revisions.

Barbara Bates, M.D.
Robert A. Hoekelman, M.D.

INTRODUCTION

A GUIDE TO PHYSICAL EXAMINATION is designed as a text for beginning practitioners in health care who are learning to talk with and examine patients. This group includes students of medicine, students of nursing and members of other health professions whose scope of responsibility now includes these fields. The *GUIDE* has a second important function, confirmed by our own experience and by reports from others. It serves as a working reference for patient care, providing guidance in specific techniques, in assessment of health status, and in the differentiation of abnormal findings.

The Second Edition

Two new chapters have been added in the Second Edition of the *GUIDE:* one on Interviewing and the Health History, and the other on Recording the History.

Few changes have been made in the basic organization of the remaining text. The chapter on Recording the Physical Examination has been moved forward so that it now follows the Overview and is close to the section on Recording the History. Other chapters, however, remain intact, with their original tripartite structure.

The text has been updated, new examples have been included, further clarifications have been made in difficult areas, illustrations have been improved and photographs added. There are several new sections and tables dealing, for example, with the patient in coma, and the section on the cardiac examination has been expanded.

Use of the Text

The basic philosophy of the book has not changed. Although we have assumed that the learners have had basic courses in human anatomy and physiology, we recognize the need for a bridge between these classic basic sciences and their application to examining patients. Accordingly, most chapters start with sections on anatomy and physiology that are intended to fill this gap.

The sections on techniques are intentionally quite detailed. They are presented systematically and without interruption to be suitable guides to practice, both in a student laboratory and at the bedside. Although usually only one method of examination is described, the learner should be aware that there are other methods. Other instructors may prefer or even insist upon alternatives. Learners should not despair in the face of conflicting advice but ask instead about their instructors' rationale. In the end, each person can weigh the evidence and make up his or her own mind.

Abnormalities have been selected primarily because of their estimated frequency or importance. An occasional physical sign has been included despite its rarity because it enjoys a solid niche in classic physical diagnosis. We have tried *not* to present an encyclopedic array of abnormalities, but have attempted instead to guide the learner toward the common and important in contrast to the infrequent or esoteric.

These abnormalities are presented in two places: parallel to the techniques and in tabular form at the end of each region or system. (In developing the latter, we acknowledge that the idea originated in the Roger Tory Peterson Field Guide Series.) While learning the techniques of examination, it is suggested that the student survey quickly some of these abnormalities so that they may guide his observations. However, he should not try to memorize them. The best time to learn from this section is when a patient presents with an abnormality. Confronted by a clinical problem, the student can then analyze it with the help of the *GUIDE* and subsequently pursue the problem further in textbooks of medicine, pediatrics or other specialties.

In designing the text, we have assumed that practitioners will learn their examination skills by first practicing on other adults. Most of the anatomy and physiology, some of the techniques and many of the abnormalities are common to both adults and children. Dr. Hoekelman's chapter on The Pediatric Physical Examination describes variations as they occur in the younger age groups and those that are unique to them.

The *GUIDE* is intended to present a fairly comprehensive approach to examining patients. There is, however, no clearly defined "complete physical examination." What one includes depends upon the age and sex of the patient, the patient's symptoms, other physical findings or laboratory data, the purpose of the examination and the specialty of the practitioner. For each body region or system described, further detail could have been presented. On the other hand, in examining an average healthy person, the practitioner will probably not be as thorough as the text suggests. One approach to the full examination is described in Chapter 3. Chapter 4 suggests a method of recording the findings and includes one written example.

A Visual Guide to Physical Examination

A series of 12 sound motion pictures based upon this text provides the student with a model of the techniques, special procedures and sequencing of the physical examination. The VISUAL GUIDE is available from J.B. Lippincott Co.

Approach to the Patient

The patient almost always brings to the examination some or even a great deal of anxiety about his illness or about the examination itself.

The practioner must be aware of these feelings. His demeanor should demonstrate self-confidence, patience, courtesy, consideration and gentleness. All procedures should be explained. Surprise, alarm, worry, distaste or annoyance easily steal across one's face but should be avoided. At times it may be necessary to cause the patient some discomfort or pain in order to assess his condition accurately. The practitioner must be willing and able to do this, too, without undue anxiety or guilt and with matter-of-fact dispatch.

To cooperate with the examiner, the patient should be as physically relaxed as possible. It is also important for the examiner to be relaxed since awkward positioning impairs perceptions. Good lighting and a quiet environment are important, although sometimes remarkably difficult to achieve.

Equipment

Equipment necessary for a physical examination includes the following:
1. An otoscope and ophthalmoscope. If the otoscope does not include a short wide speculum, a separate nasal speculum is required.
2. A flashlight
3. Tongue depressors
4. A ruler and flexible tape measure, preferably marked in centimeters
5. A thermometer
6. A watch with a second hand
7. A sphygmomanometer
8. A stethoscope. Ideal characteristics suggested by Hurst and Schlant* include:
    a. Snugly fitting and comfortable ear tips, achieved through properly sized tips, an angle that approximates that of the ear canal and an appropriately tight spring in the connecting metal band
    b. Thick-walled double tubes about 25 to 30 cm (10–12 inches) in length and 3 mm ($\frac{1}{8}$ inch) in internal diameter

---

*Hurst J. W. The Heart, Arteries and Veins. 4th Edition. New York: McGraw-Hill Book Co., 1978, p. 232.

    c. A trumpet-shaped bell about 2.5 cm (1 inch) in diameter

    d. A diaphragm about 3.7 cm (1½ inches) in diameter (2.5 cm or 1 inch in diameter for those specializing in pediatrics)

9. Gloves
10. Lubricant ⎱ For vaginal and rectal examination

11. Vaginal specula

12. A reflex hammer

13. Tuning forks, one of 128 cps and one of 512 or preferably 1024 cps

14. Safety pins

15. Cotton

16. Two test tubes (needed only for selected neurological examinations)

17. Paper and pen or pencil

A GUIDE TO PHYSICAL EXAMINATION

interviewing and the health history

by Barbara Bates, M.D., and Robert A. Hoekelman, M.D.

Talking with the patient and obtaining his health history are usually the first and often the most important parts of the health care process. Here you *gather the information* necessary to form a tentative diagnosis. You *begin a relationship* with the patient that will help him trust and confide in you. By talking with you *the patient may learn something about himself,* for example, how his illness relates to his life situation. You share in that learning. Finally both you and the patient can *start to define your therapeutic goals.* You have made an implicit contract.

The relative importance of these four goals varies, as do the time and effort they require. A patient with mild poison ivy is quite different from one with brittle diabetes. You must modify your interviewing style according to the needs of the patient as they unfold.

The Information Needed

No person can ever fully comprehend another, nor can any history be truly complete. Yet with practice, guidance and self-awareness, you can learn to talk with a patient and obtain the comprehensive, organized set of data that constitutes the traditional health history. You must know (1) what information to get and (2) how to get it, while building a relationship as you proceed.

On pages 2 to 4 are outlined the components of a *comprehensive history* suitable when an adult patient makes a first visit. Pages 5 to 7 give a suggested format for the comprehensive evaluation of a child. In most settings clerical staff have already collected the identifying patient data; in some settings printed forms or computerized systems help in gathering information. Since you may not always have such aids, however, you should become thoroughly familiar with each component of the history and be able to gather all the necessary information on your own.

The items listed in the outlines are neither mandatory nor all-inclusive. You need judgment in deciding when to limit or to expand your questions. Skilled clinicians may demonstrate a disconcerting ability to ask the one additional question that unlocks the door to understanding and to do so in a tenth of the time that you have spent. Let this be a stimulus rather than a discouragement!

COMPREHENSIVE HISTORY: ADULT PATIENT

Date of History

Identifying Data, including at least age, sex, race, place of birth, marital status, occupation and perhaps religion

Source of Referral, if any

Source of History, for example, the patient or relative or friend, together with the practitioner's judgment of the validity of his reporting. Other possible sources include the patient's medical record or a referral letter.

Chief Complaints, when possible in the patient's own words

Present Illness.   This is a clear, chronological narrative account of the problems for which the patient is seeking care. It should include the onset of the problem, the setting in which it developed, its manifestations, treatments, its impact upon the patient's life, and its meaning to the patient. The principal symptoms should be described in terms of their (1) location, (2) quality, (3) quantity or severity, (4) timing, i.e., onset, duration and frequency, (5) setting, (6) factors that have aggravated or relieved these symptoms and (7) associated manifestations. Relevant data from the patient's chart, for example, laboratory reports, also belong in the present illness, as do significant negatives, i.e., the absence of certain symptoms that will aid in differential diagnosis.

Past Medical History

General state of health

Childhood illnesses, for example, measles, German measles, mumps, whooping cough, chickenpox, rheumatic fever, scarlet fever, polio

Immunizations, for example, tetanus, pertussis, diphtheria, polio, measles, German measles, mumps

Adult illnesses

Psychiatric illnesses

Operations

Injuries

Hospitalizations, not already described

Current medications, including home remedies

Allergies

Habits, including dietary patterns, sleep patterns, exercise, use of coffee, alcohol, other drugs and tobacco

Family History

The age and health, or age and cause of death, of each immediate family member, i.e., parents, siblings, spouse and children. Data on grandparents or grandchildren may also be useful.

The occurrence within the family of any of the following conditions: diabetes, tuberculosis, heart disease, high blood pressure, stroke, kidney disease, cancer, arthritis, anemia, headaches, mental illness, or symptoms like those of the patient.

Psychosocial History

This is an outline or narrative description that captures the important and relevant information about the patient as a person

His lifestyle, home situation, significant others
A typical day—how he spends his time from when he gets up to when he goes to bed
Important experiences, including upbringing, schooling, military service, job history, financial situation, marriage, recreation, retirement
Religious beliefs relevant to perceptions of health, illness and treatment
His view of the present and outlook for the future

Review of Systems

General: usual weight, recent weight change, weakness, fatigue, fever

Skin: rashes, lumps, itching, dryness, color change, changes in hair or nails

Head: headache, head injury

Eyes: vision, glasses or contact lenses, last eye examination, pain, redness, excessive tearing, double vision, glaucoma, cataracts

Ears: hearing, tinnitus, vertigo, earaches, infection, discharge

Nose and sinuses: frequent colds, nasal stuffiness, hay fever, nosebleeds, sinus trouble

Mouth and throat: condition of teeth and gums, bleeding gums, last dental examination, sore tongue, frequent sore throats, hoarseness

Neck: lumps in neck, "swollen glands," goiter, pain in the neck

Breasts: lumps, pain, nipple discharge, self-examination

Respiratory: cough, sputum (color, quantity), hemoptysis, wheezing, asthma, bronchitis, emphysema, pneumonia, tuberculosis, pleurisy, tuberculin test; last chest X-ray film

Cardiac: heart trouble, high blood pressure, rheumatic fever, heart murmurs; dyspnea, orthopnea, paroxysmal nocturnal dyspnea, edema; chest pain, palpitations; past electrocardiogram or other heart tests

Gastrointestinal: trouble swallowing, heartburn, appetite, nausea, vomiting, vomiting of blood, indigestion, frequency of bowel movements, change in bowel habits, rectal bleeding or black tarry stools, constipation, diarrhea; abdominal pain, food intolerance, excessive belching or passing of gas, hemorrhoids; jaundice, liver or gall bladder trouble, hepatitis

Urinary: frequency of urination, polyuria, nocturia, dysuria, hematuria, urgency, hesitancy, incontinence; urinary infections, stones

Genito-reproductive:
Male: discharge from or sores on penis, history of venereal disease and its treatment, hernias, testicular pain or masses; frequency of intercourse, libido, sexual difficulties

Female: age at menarche; regularity, frequency and duration of periods; amount of bleeding, bleeding between periods or after intercourse, last menstrual period; dysmenorrhea; age of menopause, menopausal symptoms, post-menopausal bleeding. Discharge, itching, venereal disease and its treatment; last Pap smear. Number of pregnancies, number of deliveries, number of abortions (spontaneous and induced); complications of pregnancy; birth control methods; frequency of intercourse, libido, sexual difficulties

Musculoskeletal: joint pains or stiffness, arthritis, gout, backache. If present, describe location and symptoms (for example, swelling, redness, pain, stiffness, weakness, limitation of motion or activity). Muscle pains or cramps.

Peripheral vascular: intermittent claudication, cramps, varicose veins, thrombophlebitis

Neurological: fainting, blackouts, seizures, paralysis, local weakness, numbness, tingling, tremors, memory

Psychiatric: nervousness, tension, mood, depression

Endocrine: thyroid trouble, heat or cold intolerance, excessive sweating, diabetes, excessive thirst, hunger or urination

Hematologic: anemia, easy bruising or bleeding, past transfusions and possible reactions

COMPREHENSIVE HISTORY: CHILD PATIENT

In addition to the obvious age-related differences between histories obtained on children and adults, there are present and past historical data specifically pertinent to the assessment of infants, children and adolescents. These relate particularly to the patient's chronological age and stage of development. The pediatric history, then, follows the same outline as the adult's history, with certain additions which are presented here.

Identifying Data. Date of birth for patients less than 3 years of age. Nickname particularly for those between 2 and 10 years of age. First names of parents (and last name of each, if different) and where they may be reached during work hours.

Chief Complaints. It should be made clear whether these are concerns of the patient, the parent(s) or both. In some instances, it may be a third party, such as a schoolteacher, who has expressed concerns about the child.

Present Illness. Should include how each member of the family responds to the patient's symptoms, their concerns about them, and whether the patient achieves any secondary gains from his illness.

Past Medical History

Birth History: Particularly important during the first 2 years of life and for neurological and developmental problems. Hospital records should be reviewed if preliminary information from the parent(s) indicates significant difficulties before, during or after delivery.

Prenatal. Maternal health before and during pregnancy including nutrition and specific illnesses related to or complicated by pregnancy; doses and duration of all drugs taken during pregnancy; weight gain; vaginal bleeding; duration of pregnancy; parental attitudes concerning the pregnancy and parenthood in general and for this child in particular.

Natal. Nature of labor and delivery, including degree of difficulty, analgesia used and complications encountered; birth order if a multiple birth; birth weight.

Neonatal. Onset of respirations; resuscitation efforts; Apgar scores and estimation of gestational age; specific problems with feeding, respiratory distress, cyanosis, jaundice, anemia, convulsions, congenital anomalies or infection; mother's health postpartum; separation of mother and infant and reasons for; initial maternal reaction to her baby and the nature of bonding; patterns of crying and sleeping, and of urination and defecation.

Feeding History: Particularly important during the first 2 years of life and in dealing with problems of under and overnutrition.

Infancy. *Breast feeding*—frequency and duration of feeds; use of complementary or supplementary artificial feedings; difficulties encountered; timing and method of weaning. *Artificial feeding*—type, concentration, amount, and frequency of feeds; difficulties (regurgitation, colic, diarrhea) encountered; timing and method of weaning. *Vitamin and iron supplements*—type, amount given, frequency, and duration. *Solid foods*—types and amounts of baby foods given; when introduced; infant's response; introduction of junior and table foods; self-feeding; maternal and infant responses to feeding process

Childhood. *Eating habits*—likes and dislikes; specific types and amounts of food eaten; parental attitudes toward eating in general and toward this child's under- or overeating; parental response to feeding problems (if present). A *diet diary* kept over a 7 to 14-day period may be required for an accurate assessment of food intake in childhood feeding problems.

Growth and Developmental History: Particularly important during infancy and childhood and in dealing with problems of delayed physical growth, psychomotor and intellectual retardation, and behavioral disturbances.

Physical Growth. Actual (or approximate) weight and height at birth and at 1, 2, 5 and 10 years; history of any slow or rapid gains or losses; tooth eruption and loss pattern.

Developmental Milestones. Ages at which patient held up head while in a prone position; rolled over from front to back and back to front; sat with support and alone; said first word, combinations of words and sentences; tied own shoes; dressed without help.

Social Development. *Sleep*—amount and patterns during day and at night; bedtime routines; type of bed and its location; nightmares, terrors and somnambulation. *Toileting*—methods of training used; when bladder and bowel control attained; occurrence of accidents or of enuresis or encopresis; parental attitudes; terms used within the family for urination and defecation (important to know when a young child is admitted to hospital). *Speech*—hesitation; stuttering; baby talk; lisping; estimate of number of words in vocabulary. *Habits*—bed rocking, head banging, tics, thumb sucking, nailbiting, pica, ritualistic behavior. *Discipline*—parental assessment of child's temperament and response to discipline; methods used; success or failure; negativism; temper tantrums; withdrawal; aggressive behavior. *Schooling*—experience with day care, nursery school and kindergarten; age and adjustment upon entry; current parental and child satisfaction; academic achievement; school's concerns. *Sexuality*—relations with members of opposite sex; inquisitiveness regarding conception, pregnancy and girl-boy differences; parental responses to child's questions and the sex education they have offered regarding masturbation, menstruation, nocturnal emissions, development of secondary sexual characteristics and sexual urges; dating patterns. *Personality*—degree of independence; relationship with parents, siblings and peers; group and independent activities and interests; congeniality; special friends (real or imaginary); major assets and skills; self-image.

Childhood Illnesses: Mention of any recent exposures to childhood illnesses should be made here.

Immunizations: Specific dates of administration of each vaccine should be recorded so that an ongoing booster program can be maintained throughout childhood and adolescence. Any untoward reactions to specific vaccines should also be recorded.

Screening Procedures: The dates and results of any screening tests performed should be recorded. For example, vision, hearing, tuberculin, urinalysis, hematocrit, sickle cell, blood lead, phenylketonuria, galactosemia and other genetic-metabolic disorders, alpha$_1$ antitrypsin deficiency and others that may be indicated for certain high-risk populations.

Operations
Injuries   The reactions of the child and his parents to these
Hospitalizations   events should be ascertained.

Allergies: Particular attention should be given to those allergies that are more prevalent during infancy and childhood—eczema, urticaria, perennial allergic rhinitis and insect hypersensitivity.

Family History.
The education attained, job history, emotional health and family background of each parent or parent substitute; the family socioeconomic circumstances, including income, type of dwelling and neighborhood in which they live; parental work schedules; family cohesiveness and interdependence; support available from relatives, friends and neighbors; the ethnic and cultural milieu in which they live; parental expectations of the patient and attitudes toward him in relation to his siblings. (All or portions of this information may be recorded in the Present Illness, if pertinent to it, or under Psychosocial History.) Consanguinity of the parents should be ascertained (by inquiring if they are "related by blood").

Some patients may not need a comprehensive evaluation or you may lack the time to do one. Under these circumstances you should obtain a short history appropriate to a *limited visit*. In addition to the routine identifying data, a history of the present illness is usually all that is indicated. You must remain alert, however, to the need for a somewhat broader line of inquiry. When seeing a patient with an acute sore throat, for example, you may need to inquire about similar illnesses in the family, past rheumatic fever or possible penicillin allergy.

Still another pattern of history is appropriate to a *follow-up* visit. Here you need to find out how the patient thinks he is doing, how his symptoms have changed, what he understands about his condition and treatment, and what therapeutic measures he has taken or perhaps not taken.

You can enhance your understanding of the patient's concerns on any visit if you keep in mind three questions: why he has come ("I have a pain in my stomach"), what is worrying him ("I think I may have appendicitis"), and why that is a worry ("My Uncle Charlie died of a ruptured appendix"). The answers to these questions must be determined directly or indirectly at some point during the visit, since the patient is not likely to be satisfied if they are not addressed. Patients often need to know what they do *not* have as much or more than what they *do* have, especially if they believe they may be suffering from a serious or potentially fatal disease.

Once you know what information to get, it is time, paradoxically, to lay that knowledge temporarily aside, lest it come between you and the patient, for the course of the interview should be guided primarily by what the patient says and does. At least at the start you should be following his cues, not the printed form.

Setting the Stage for the Interview

Reviewing the Chart. Before seeing the patient, quickly review his chart. Note the identifying data. His age, sex, race, marital status, address, occupation and religion give you important glimpses into his likely life experiences and may even guide your diagnostic hypotheses. If the patient has been referred from elsewhere, you should know both the source and goals of referral. Reviewing the medical chart will give you invaluable information about past diagnoses and treatments, although it should not so bias you as to preclude new approaches or ideas. In a complex medical setting this review might even remind you that you have seen the patient before and help to avoid an awkward interaction.

The Environment. Although you may have to talk with the patient under difficult circumstances, for example, in a four-bed room or in the corridor of a busy emergency department, a proper environment will improve communication. Your relationship with the patient may begin with his first telephone call to clinic or office. If the response projects courtesy, interest and a desire to be helpful, if he can be seen reasonably promptly, if you are punctual for his appointment, you are setting the stage for a trusting relationship.

These early stages in the patient-provider communication, including the proper use of names (Mrs. Jones instead of Mary), are the critical determinants of the patient's "reflexive self-concept" (what he thinks you think of him). If this is high, the patient is more likely to be satisfied and more likely to be compliant with your diagnostic and therapeutic recommendations. If it is low, it may not matter what you say or do later in the visit in terms of gaining the patient's trust and cooperation.

The environment itself tells the patient something about your interest in him. Is it quiet? Does it afford privacy? Are you free from interruptions? There should be places where both you and the patient can sit down in clear view of each other, preferably at eye level. Leaning against the far wall, inching toward the door or shifting around uncomfortably from foot to foot discourage the patient's attempts at communication. Greeting a woman and taking a short history while she is lying supine positioned for a pelvic examination scarcely help either. Your distance from the patient should probably be several feet, not so close as to be uncomfortably intimate nor too distant for easy conversation. Patients may be able to talk with you more easily when sitting next to your desk rather than peering over it, as if over a barrier. When patients prefer greater social distance, they are telling you something about themselves, psychologically or perhaps culturally. Lighting also makes a difference. Beware of sitting between the patient and a bright light or window. Although you can see him well, he must squint uncomfortably toward your silhouette. You unwittingly conduct an interrogation, not a helping interview.

Finally, your clothing may also affect the ease with which you establish a relationship. There are few rules here except that you should be clean, reasonably neat and dressed appropriately to the patients you wish to serve. Conservative dress and white coat, for example, are suitable for most adults whereas casual dress without uniform may be preferable when dealing with children or young people. You may feel that you should dress so as to express yourself rather than to respond to the wishes of others. You should be aware of the effects of your own appearance, however, and not blame the patient for adverse consequences. Compromises are usually possible.

Approach to the Present Illness

Greeting the Patient. You are now ready to approach the patient, greet him by name and give him your undivided attention. Shake hands if you feel comfortable doing so. Unless you are talking with a child or adolescent or unless you already know the patient well, use the appropriate title, for example, Mr. O'Neill or Mrs. Washington. Use of first names or terms of endearment for unfamiliar adults, use of "Granny" for an aged woman or "Mother" for a child's parent tend to depersonalize and demean. Introduce yourself by name; and if there is any ambiguity in your role, for example, if you are a student, explain your relation to the patient's care.

The Patient's Comfort. Be alert to the patient's comfort. In office or clinic, there should be a place for his coat and belongings other than his own lap. In the hospital inquire how the patient is feeling and whether it is convenient for him to see you now. Watch for signs of discomfort, for example, poor positioning, evidence of pain or anxiety, or the need to urinate. An improved position in bed, a short delay so that he can say goodbye to his family or make a trip to the bathroom may be the shortest route to a good history.

Opening Questions. Now you are ready to find out why the patient is here—his chief complaints, if any, and the present illness. (Occasionally a patient may come for a checkup or may wish to discuss a health-related matter without having either complaint or illness.) Begin your interview with a general question that allows full freedom of response, for example, "What brings you here?" or "What seems to be the trouble?" After he answers, inquire again, or even several times, "Anything else?" When he has finished, encourage him to amplify by saying "Tell me about it," or, if there seems to be more than one problem, ask about one of them: "Tell me about the headaches" or ". . . about what bothers you most." As he answers, you pick up the thread of his history and follow wherever it leads.

Following the Patient's Leads. Not all histories are complicated. Many patients want help with relatively straightforward medical problems. Others, however, have illnesses with complex psychosocial and pathophysiologic causes; they have complicated feelings about themselves, their illnesses, potential treatments and those who are trying to help them. At the start you cannot tell one kind of patient from another. In order to do so your interviewing technique must allow each patient to recount his own story spontaneously. If you intervene verbally too soon, if you ask specific questions prematurely, you risk trampling on the very evidence you are seeking. Your role, however, is not a passive one. You should listen actively and watch for clues to important symptoms, emotions, events and relationships. You can then guide the patient into telling you more about these areas. Methods of helping and guiding the patient without diverting him from his own account include facilitation, reflection, clarification, empathic responses, confrontation, interpretation and questions that elicit feelings. Your demeanor throughout is also important.

Facilitation. You use facilitation when by posture, actions or words you encourage the patient to say more but do not specify his topic. Silence itself, when attentive yet relaxed, is facilitative. Leaning forward, making eye contact, saying "Mm-hmm" or "Go on" or "I'm listening" all help the patient to continue.

Reflection. Closely akin to facilitation is reflection, a repetition of the patient's words that encourages him to give you more details. Reflection may be useful in eliciting both facts and feelings, as in the following example.

> *Patient:* The pain got worse and began to spread. (Pause)
> *Response:* It spread?

Patient:	Yes, it went to my shoulder and down my left arm to the fingers. It was so bad that I thought I was going to die. (Pause)
Response:	You thought you were going to die?
Patient:	Yes. It was just like the pain my father had when he had his heart attack, and I was afraid the same thing was happening to me.

Here a reflective technique has helped to discover not only the location and severity of the patient's pain, but also its meaning to the patient. There was no risk of biasing the patient's story or interrupting his train of thought.

Clarification. Sometimes the patient's words are ambiguous or his associations are unclear. If you are to understand what he is saying, you must request clarification. For example, "Tell me what you meant by a 'cold'" or "You said you were behaving just like your mother. What did you mean?"

Empathic Responses. As a patient talks with you, he may express—with or without words—feelings about which he is embarrassed, ashamed or otherwise reticent. These feelings may well be crucial to understanding his illness or planning treatment. If you can recognize and respond to them in a way that shows understanding and acceptance, you show empathy for the patient, make him feel more secure and encourage him to continue. Empathic responses may be as simple as "I understand." Other examples include "You must have been very upset" or "That must have been very depressing for you." Empathic responses may also be nonverbal, for example, offering a tissue to a crying patient or gently placing your hand on his arm to convey understanding. In using an empathic response, be sure that you are responding correctly to what the patient has already expressed. If you have acknowledged how upset a patient must have been at the death of a parent when in fact he was relieved to be freed from a long-standing financial and emotional burden, you have seriously misunderstood your patient and probably blocked further communication on the subject.

Confrontation. While an empathic response acknowledges expressed feelings, confrontation points out to the patient something about his own words or behavior. If you observe clues of anger, anxiety or depression, for example, confrontation may help to bring these feelings out in the open. "Your hands are trembling whenever you talk about that," or "You say you don't care but there are tears in your eyes." Confrontation may also be useful when the patient's story has been inconsistent. "You say you don't know what brings on your stomach pains; yet whenever you've had them, you were feeling picked on."

Interpretation. Interpretation goes a step beyond confrontation. Here you make an inference, rather than a simple observation. "Nothing has been right for you today. You seem fed up with the hospital." "You are asking a lot of questions about the X-rays. Are you worried about them?" In interpreting a patient's words or behavior, you take some risk of making the wrong inference and impeding further communication. When used wisely, however, an interpretation can both demonstrate empathy and increase understanding.

Asking about Feelings. Rather than making an inference or reflecting a feeling, you may simply ask the patient how he feels, or felt, about something, for example, his symptoms or an event. Unless you let him know that you are interested in his feelings as well as facts, he may withhold them, and you may miss important insights.

Your General Demeanor. Just as you have been observing the patient throughout the early portions of the interview, so too has he been watching you. Consciously or not, you have been sending him messages through both your words and your behavior. You should be sensitive to those messages and control them insofar as you can. Posture, gestures, eye contact and words can all express interest, attention, acceptance and understanding. The skilled interviewer seems calm and unhurried, even when his time is limited. Reactions that betray disgust, disapproval, embarrassment, impatience or boredom block communication as do behaviors that condescend, stereotype or make sport of the patient. Be particularly aware of these harmful reactions when you are talking about the patient with colleagues or instructors, either at the bedside or within earshot of the patient.

Beginning practitioners may have special problems in dealing with their own limited knowledge; all practitioners confront this problem at least occasionally. When you do not know the answer to a patient's direct question, it is usually best to be honest about it and say so, but also add that you will try to find out the answer. Clearly acknowledging your status as a student may help you out of otherwise awkward situations.

Direct Questions. Using the nondirective techniques described thus far, you will usually be able to obtain a general idea of the patient's principal problems. You can encourage a chronological account by such questions as "What then?" or "What happened next?" Most of the time, however, you will need further specific information. Fill in the details with direct questions. If the patient's present illness involves pain, for example, you must determine the following: (1) Its location. Where is it? Does it radiate? (2) Its quality. What is it like? (3) Its quantity or severity. How bad is it? (4) Its timing. When did it start? How long does it last? How often does it come? (5) The setting in which it occurs. (6) Factors that make it better or worse. (7) Associated manifestations. Most other symptoms can be described in the same terms.

Several principles apply to the use of direct questions. They should proceed from the *general to the specific.* A possible sequence, for example, might be "What was your chest pain like? . . . Where did you feel it? . . . Show me . . . Did it stay right there or did it travel anywhere? . . . To which fingers?"

Direct questions *should not be leading questions.* If a patient says "yes" to "Did your stools look like tar?" you must always wonder if the description is his or yours. A better wording is "What color were your stools?" Leading questions often give misleading answers. A classic example: "Is everything all right at home?"

When possible ask questions that *require a graded response* rather than a yes or no answer. "How many stairs can you climb before stopping for breath?" is better than "Do you get short of breath climbing stairs?"

Sometimes patients seem quite unable to describe their symptoms without help. To minimize bias here, offer *multiple choice answers*. "Is your pain aching, sharp, pressing, burning, shooting or what?" Almost any specific question can have at least two choices. "Do you bring up any phlegm with your cough, or not?"

Ask *one question at a time*. "Any tuberculosis, pleurisy, asthma, bronchitis, pneumonia?" may lead to a negative answer out of sheer confusion.

Finally, *use language that is understandable and appropriate* to the patient. Although you might ask a trained health professional about dyspnea, the more customary term is shortness of breath. When talking with an Appalachian coal miner, on the other hand, it may help to use the colloquial "smothering spells." Words in the history outlines are not intended for verbatim use. They need appropriate translations.

The Rest of the Story

By now you should be able to synthesize a chronologic narrative of the patient's illness, using both his spontaneous account and his answers to direct questions. You are ready to proceed to past medical history, family history, psychosocial history and the review of systems. Except in the psychosocial history, specific questions will constitute your major technique. Stay alert, however, for important medical or emotional material and be prepared to revert to a nondirective style whenever indicated. While taking a family history, for example, you may learn of a parent's death or a child's illness. Here is a good opportunity to find out what it meant to the patient. "How was it for you then?" or "What were your feelings at the time?" The review of systems may also uncover material that requires as full an exploration as the present illness. Keep your technique flexible.

Two sections of history beyond the present illness seem particularly troublesome to many interviewers: the psychosocial and the sexual histories. These will be discussed in somewhat more detail.

The Psychosocial History. Earlier in the interview the patient may already have told you much of his psychosocial history. Some further clues, as yet unexplored, can be followed now. Try to use words or ideas that the patient himself has expressed before. At times you may still know relatively little about the patient and will be entering new territory. Open-ended questions can give you some leads.

Who lives at home with you?
What is a typical day like?
Where were you born? . . . raised? What was your childhood like?
How is it going for you in school?
What is your job like?
What do you think of your boss?
How is your financial situation? How much money do you have coming in now? How about expenses? Do you have any problems with your medical bills? . . . Any insurance? . . . Medicare? . . . Medicaid?
What do you do for recreation or fun?
What do you think about retirement?
What do you see for yourself in the future?

Sexual History. Like other parts of the history, a sexual history should be obtained where it seems most relevant, perhaps in the present illness or psychosocial history, but most probably in the review of systems. Because of our social taboos, both practitioner and patient may find this a difficult job. With a female patient, questions about sexual function follow naturally after the menstrual and obstetrical histories. Some useful questions to open the discussion:

Are you having sex, or intercourse, now?
About how often?
Is that more or less often than in previous years?
How often do you reach a climax (or have an orgasm)?
Do you have any pain or discomfort during intercourse?
Has your interest in sex changed recently?
How satisfied are you with your sex life as it is now?
How satisfied do you think your partner is?

For male patients, here is a similar group of questions:

Are you having intercourse now?
About how often?
Is that more or less often than in previous years?
Do you have any trouble getting an erection?
Do you have any trouble coming (ejaculating) too soon?
Has your interest in sex changed recently?
How satisfied are you with your sex life as it is now?
How satisfied do you think your partner is?

When approaching a sexual history, it may be helpful to make some introductory remarks that let the patient know that his experiences, feelings or problems are common, not rare, wrong or bizarre. For example:

Many teenagers are trying to figure out whether they should use birth control or when they should have sex. What are your thoughts about these things?

Most young people know that they can get VD but don't know what it's like or what to do about it. What has your experience been?

Not only may questions about sexual function give you important diagnostic insights; they also let patients know that they can discuss these problems with you in the future. Although occasional patients are unwilling to talk about this subject (and should not be pushed), most are willing and some quite relieved. As in other parts of the history, your demeanor is important: calm, unembarrassed, yet sensitive. Use words that the patient can understand, preferably his or her own, so long as both of you know what they mean. Further reading, discussion and interviewing experience will help you improve your skills and confidence in this area.

Transitions. As you move from one part of the history to another, it helps to orient the patient with brief transitional phrases. "Now I'd like to ask some questions about your past health," or ". . . about your family's health."

Closing. After you have completed your questions, return the initiative briefly to the patient: "Is there anything else we should talk about?" or "Have we omitted anything?" You may want to recapitulate part of the present illness to be sure of a common understanding. Finally, make clear to the patient what he is to do or what he is to expect next. "I will step out for a few minutes. Please get completely undressed and put on this gown. I would like to examine you."

Note-taking. Since no one can remember all the details of a comprehensive history, you need to take notes. Most patients are accustomed to note-taking but some may seem uncomfortable with it. If so, explore their concerns and explain your desire to make an accurate record. With practice you may be able to record most of the past medical history, family history and review of systems in final form as you talk with the patient, especially if you have the help of a written questionnaire. Note-taking should not divert your attention from the patient, however, nor should a written form prevent you from following a patient's leads. While eliciting the present illness, the psychosocial history or other complex portions of the patient's account, do not attempt to write your final report. Instead, jot down short phrases, words, dates, and so forth, that will aid your memory later. When the patient is talking about sensitive or disturbing material, it is best not to take notes at all.

Patients at Different Ages

As people develop, have families and age, they provide you with special opportunities and require certain adaptations in your interviewing style.

Talking with Parents. In obtaining histories regarding infants and children, for example, you gather all or at least part of your information from a third party, the parent(s) or legal guardian. Children under 5 years old usually add no relevant historical data. As children grow older, however, you can get information of increasing value and reliability by interviewing them directly. Special ways of enhancing your interviews with children and adolescents are described in subsequent sections. This section deals with parents. Here your techniques are basically the same as in interviewing adult patients, with some special modifications.

Parents, of course, are speaking about their children and describing what they have observed as well as what they perceive to be their child's symptoms. Although these observations and perceptions can generally be considered accurate, they are subject to parental biases and needs. This is especially true for the mother who, in our society, is usually responsible for the immediate care of the children. A mother includes her ability to keep her children well as part of her concept of adequate mothering. When you ask her questions concerning her child's health or ill health, you are in a sense testing her capabilities as a mother. Her responses to those questions may be accordingly biased. Mothers need health practitioners who are supportive rather than judgmental or critical. Comments like, "You mean you *didn't* give him aspirin for the fever?," "Why didn't you bring him in sooner?" or "Why, in heaven's name, did you do that?" will not improve your rapport with a worried and distraught mother whose infant or child is acutely ill.

Refer to the infant or child by his or her name rather than "him," "her" or "the baby." In situations where the mother's marital status is not immediately clear, you may avoid embarrassment in asking about the father by, "Is Jane's father in good health?" rather than, "Is your husband in good health?" Address the parents, like adult patients, as "Mr. or Mrs. Smith" rather than with their first names or, heaven forbid, "mother" or "father." First names may be used with permission when you have established a reasonably long-standing relationship. In this day and age, however, you should be prepared for the parent who calls you by your first name.

In interviewing parents, open-ended questions are usually more productive than direct questions. In the realm of psychosocial issues and problems, however, you must more often than not use explicit direct questions, since mothers rarely introduce these subjects spontaneously, even when given the opportunity with open-ended approaches. This is especially true for mothers of lower socioeconomic status.

Finally, you need to recognize that the chief complaint may not relate at all to the apparent reason the mother has brought the child to see you. The complaint may serve as a "ticket of admission" to care, where, if the circumstances are right, she may bring up another concern that, by itself, is not viewed as a "legitimate" reason for seeking care. Try to create an atmosphere that will allow the mother to express all of her concerns. If necessary, ask questions that will allow easier expression of those concerns.

Are there any other problems with Johnny that you would like to tell me about?

What did you hope that I would be able to do for you when you came today?

Is there anything special you would like me to explain to you about Jody?

Is there anything else bothering you about the other children, your husband or yourself that you'd like to talk about?

Talking with Children. For the most part, pediatric practitioners conduct interviews with both the parent and child present. This is a matter of convenience that presents some disadvantages as well as some distinct advantages. The history you obtain in the child's presence may be less accurate and couched in more limited terms than when you interview the parent(s) alone. When sensitive areas are not fully explored because the child is present, you will need to interview the parent at a later time (often at the end of the visit when the child has left the room) to clarify certain points or to fill in missing data.

The interview with the child present offers an opportunity to observe parent-child interactions and the child's ability to amuse himself while his mother is engaged in conversation. These observations may provide a clearer picture of the relationship between mother and child (or if the father is present, father and child and the parents themselves) than can the answers to any number of questions.

For the younger child, this interlude may help to dispel fears of the practitioner or of the visit and allow for a smooth transition from the interview to the examination.

The older child will be able to add significantly to his history and can describe more accurately the severity of his symptoms and his level of concern regarding them. You can sometimes improve the accuracy of your information by interviewing the child without the parent.

Take care to avoid "talking down" to children, for they are sensitive to affectations of speech and condescending behaviors.

Talking with Adolescents. Many adults find talking with adolescents difficult and frustrating because they cannot seem to get the adolescent to answer their questions except in a disdainful, laconic way, if at all. This need not be the case. The adolescent, like most other people, will respond positively to anyone who demonstrates a genuine interest in him, especially someone who wants to and shows promise of helping him. That interest, desire and promise must be established early and sustained if communication is to be effective.

Adolescents seek health care on their own advice or at the suggestion or insistence of their parents. They may come alone or with at least one parent. Whenever possible interview the adolescent alone. With his knowledge, you should also obtain additional information from the parents. You should share the nature of this information and the parental concerns with him, at least in general terms. Whenever possible, respect the wishes of the adolescent patient. If for his own sake, however, you must share information with the parents that he would like kept in confidence, so inform him.

Most adolescents will talk to someone they respect and accept when given the opportunity in a friendly, informal atmosphere. Acceptance is more likely for the professional who "plays it straight," acts his age and does not stretch too far in trying to bridge the generation gap.

Aging Patients. At the other end of the life cycle, aging patients also pose special opportunities and special problems. They run relatively high risks for a number of conditions, such as decreased vision and hearing, memory loss and depression. They often face chronic illness and diminishing control over their lives. Although you should be especially alert for cues to these problems, avoid stereotyping the aging patient. A personal empathic relationship has special value here. Find out your patient's priorities and goals. Learn how he has handled past crises. Since he may prefer similar adaptive patterns in the present situation, this knowledge will help you plan with him. Because aging patients have longer histories and may tell them more slowly, they often require extra time. Do not try to accomplish everything on one visit.

Many interviewers face special problems within themselves. They may feel helpless in curing the ills of the aged. Their views toward aging people may be distorted by their own feelings toward parents and grandparents. They fear their own old age and want to avoid reminders of it. Be alert to your own feelings.

Special Problems

Regardless of patient age, certain behaviors and special situations may particularly vex the practitioner.

Silence. Neophyte interviewers may grow uncomfortable during periods of silence, feeling somehow obligated to keep the conversation going. They need not feel so. Silences have many meanings and many uses. When recounting their present illnesses, patients frequently fall silent for short periods in order to collect their thoughts or remember details. An attentive silence on the interviewer's part is usually the best response here, sometimes followed by brief encouragement to continue. During periods of silence be particularly alert to nonverbal signs of distress. Patients may fall silent because they are having difficulty controlling their emotions. If so, these are almost invariably significant feelings that are best expressed. A gentle confrontation may help: "You seem to be having trouble talking about this." Depressed patients or those with organic brain syndrome may have lost their usual spontaneity of expression, give short answers to questions and fall silent quickly after each one. If you sense one of these problems, shift your inquiry to an exploratory mental status examination (see pp. 359–364).

At times, a patient's silence results from interviewer error or insensitivity. Are you asking too many direct questions in rapid sequence? The patient may simply have yielded the initiative to you and taken the passive role he thinks you expect. Have you offended the patient in any way, for example, by signs of disapproval or criticism? Have you failed to recognize an overwhelming symptom, for example, pain, nausea, dyspnea, the need to urinate or defecate? If so, you may need to abbreviate the interview considerably or return after the patient has been relieved.

Overtalkative Patients. The garrulous, rambling patient may be just as difficult as the silent one, possibly more so. Faced with limited time and the perceived need to "get the whole story," the interviewer may grow impatient, even exasperated. Although there are no perfect solutions for this problem, several techniques are helpful. First you may need to lower your own goals and accept less than a comprehensive history. It may be unobtainable. Second, give the patient free rein for the first 5 or 10 minutes of the interview. You will then have the chance to observe the patterns of his speech. Does he seem obsessively detailed or unduly anxious? Does he show a flight of ideas or the disorganized thought processes that suggest a psychotic disorder? Third, try to focus his account on what you judge to be most important. Show interest and ask questions in those areas. Facilitate sparingly. Interrupt if you must, but courteously. Finally, do not let your impatience show. If you have used up the allotted time, or more likely gone over it, explain it to the patient and arrange for a second meeting. Setting a time limit for the next appointment may be helpful. "I know we have much more to talk about. Can you come again next week? We will have a full half hour then."

Patients with Multiple Symptoms. Some patients seem to have every symptom that you mention. They have an "essentially positive review of systems." Although it is conceivable that such a patient has multiple organic illnesses, it is much more likely that he has serious emotional problems. If so, it will profit little to explore each symptom in detail. Guide the interview into a psychosocial assessment instead.

Anxious Patients. Anxiety is a frequent and natural reaction to sickness, to therapy and to the health care system itself. For some patients anxiety has importantly colored their reactions to life stress and may have contributed to their illnesses. Be sensitive to nonverbal and verbal clues.

For example, an anxious patient may sit tensely, fidgeting with his fingers or clothes. He may sigh frequently, lick his dry lips, sweat more than average or actually tremble. His carotid pulsations may betray a rapid heart rate. Some anxious patients fall silent, unable to speak freely or confide. Others try to cover their feelings with words, busily avoiding their own basic problems. When you sense an underlying anxiety, encourage the patient to talk about his feelings.

Reassurance. When you are talking with such a patient, it is tempting to reassure him: "Don't worry. Everything is going to be all right." This approach is usually counterproductive. Unless you and the patient have had a chance to explore fully what he is anxious about, you may well be reassuring him about the wrong thing. Moreover, premature reassurance blocks further communication. Since admitting anxiety exposes a weakness, it requires encouragement, not a coverup. The first step to effective reassurance involves identifying and accepting the patient's feelings. This helps him feel more secure. The final steps come much later in the health care process, after you have completed the interview, the physical examination and perhaps some laboratory studies. Then you can interpret for the patient what is happening and deal openly with his real concerns.

Anger and Hostility. Patients have reasons to be angry: they are ill, they have suffered loss, they lack their accustomed control over their own lives, they feel relatively powerless in the health care system. They may direct this anger toward you. It is possible that you have justly earned their hostility. Were you late for your appointment, inconsiderate, insensitive or angry yourself? If so, recognize the fact and try to make amends. More often, however, the patient is displacing his anger onto you as a symbol of all that is wrong. Allow him to get it off his chest. Accept his feelings without getting angry in return. Beware of joining the patient in his hostility toward another part of the clinic or hospital, even when you privately harbor similar feelings. After he has calmed down, you may be able to identify specific steps that will help in the future. Rational solutions to emotional problems are not always possible, however, and patients need time to resolve their angry feelings.

Crying. Like anger, crying is an important clue to emotions. Rarely should it be suppressed. If the patient seems on the verge of tears, gentle confrontation or an empathic response may allow him to cry. Quiet acceptance is then appropriate. Offer a tissue; wait for recovery; perhaps make a facilitating or supportive remark: "It's good to get it out." Most of the time the patient will soon compose himself and, if properly accepted, will feel better and capable of continuing the discussion.

Depression. Masquerading as fatigue, weight loss, insomnia, mysterious aches and pains, depression is one of the commonest problems in clinical medicine, and is commonly missed or ignored. Be alert for it, identify it, explore its manifestations. Be sure you know how bad it is. Just as you would evaluate the severity of angina pectoris, you must evaluate the severity of depression. Both are potentially lethal. You need not fear that asking about suicide will suggest it to the patient. A sequence of questions is useful, continued as far as the patient's responses warrant.

> Do you get pretty discouraged (or depressed or blue)?
> How low do you feel?
> What do you see for yourself in the future?
> Do you ever feel that life isn't worth living? Or that
>   you would just as soon be dead?
> Have you ever thought of doing away with yourself?

How did (do) you think you would do it?
What would happen after you were dead?

Sexually Attractive or Seductive Patients.   Practitioners of both sexes may occasionally find themselves attracted to their patients. If you become aware of such feelings, accept them as normal human responses, but prevent them from affecting your behavior. Keep your relationship with the patient within professional bounds.

Occasional patients, especially those with hysterical personalities or manic disorders, may be frankly seductive or may make sexual advances. Calmly but firmly, you should make clear that your relationship is professional, not personal. You may also wish to review your own image. Have you been overly warm with the patient? expressed your affection physically? sought his or her emotional support? Has your dress or demeanor been unconsciously seductive? Avoid this problem when you can.

Confusing Behaviors or Histories.   At times you may find yourself baffled, frustrated and confused in your interaction with the patient. His history is vague and difficult to understand, his ideas poorly related to one another, his language hard to follow. Even though you word your questions carefully, you seem unable to get clear answers. His manner of relating to you may also seem peculiar: distant, aloof, inappropriate or bizarre. Symptoms may be described in bizarre terms: "My fingernails feel too heavy" or "My stomach knots up like a snake." These characteristics should alert you to possible mental illnesses, such as, schizophrenia. With the usual nondirective techniques you may be able to get more information about the unusual qualities of the symptoms. You should also include in your interview an assessment of the patient's mental status with special attention to mood, thought processes and perceptions (see pp. 360–361).

Since drug therapy of schizophrenia and other psychotic disorders has become prevalent, many psychotic patients are functioning, with varying degrees of success, in the community. Such patients are frequently capable of telling you freely about their diagnosis, their symptoms, their hospitalizations and their current medications. You should feel comfortable inquiring about these without embarrassment or circumlocution.

Schizophrenia is not the only cause of confusing histories. Some patients have underlying disorders of cognitive function—disorders generally classified as organic brain syndromes, either acute (delirium) or chronic (dementia). Be particularly alert for the former when dealing with an acutely ill or intoxicated patient, for the latter when dealing with an elderly patient. These patients may be unable to give clear histories. They are vague and inconsistent about symptoms or events and unable to report when and how things happened. They may be inattentive to your questions and hesitant in their answers. Occasionally such a patient may confabulate, i.e., make up part of his history in order to fill in the gaps in his memory. When you suspect organic brain syndrome, do not spend too much time trying to get a detailed history. You will only tire and frustrate the patient. Switch your inquiry instead to an evaluation of his mental status, checking particularly on orientation, attention, concentration and memory (see pp. 361–362). You can work the initial questions smoothly into the interview. "When was your last appointment in the clinic? . . . Let's see, then, that was about how long ago?" "Your address now is? . . . And your phone number?" Responses can all be checked against the chart (presuming, of course, that the chart is accurate).

Patients with Limited Intelligence. Patients of moderately limited intelligence can usually give adequate histories. You may, in fact, overlook their limitations and thereby make mistakes, for example, omitting their dysfunction from a disability evaluation or giving instructions they cannot understand. If you suspect such a problem, pay special attention to the patient's schooling. How far did he go in school? Why did he drop out? How was he doing at the time? What kinds of courses is he taking? High school seniors of normal intelligence are not usually taking simple arithmetic. If your patient is, you can make a smooth transition into a mental status examination, including simple calculations, vocabulary, information and tests of abstract reasoning (see pp. 363–364).

Although it is not synonymous with intelligence, literacy should sometimes be assessed, especially before giving written instructions. Some patients who cannot read, because of a language barrier, learning disorder or poor vision, will admit it on direct questioning. Others, however, will deny it. You can check, as if testing their vision, by asking them to read some words or sentences for you.

When patients suffer from severe mental retardation you will have to obtain their history from family or friends. By showing interest in the patient himself, however, and by engaging him in simple conversation, try to establish a personal relationship.

Language Barriers. Nothing will more surely convince you that a history is essential than having to do without one. When you cannot communicate with your patient because you speak different languages, take every possible step to find a translator. A few broken words and gestures are no substitute. The ideal translator is a neutral, objective person who is familiar with both languages. When family members or friends try to help, they are more likely to distort meanings. They also present problems in confidentiality to both the patient and interviewer. Many translators try to speed up the process by telescoping a long communication into a few words. Try to make clear at the beginning that you need him to translate, not interpret or summarize. Make your questions clear and short. You can also help the translator by outlining the goals for each segment of your history.

When available, written bilingual questionnaires are invaluable, especially for the review of systems. Before using one, however, be sure the patient can read in his own language or can get help with it.

The Hard of Hearing and Deaf Mute. Communicating with the hard of hearing or deaf presents many of the same problems as does communicating with a patient who speaks a different language. Here again written questionnaires are a great help. Although very time-consuming, handwritten questions and answers may be the only solution. If a deaf mute patient knows sign language, make every effort to find a translator who speaks, hears and can use sign language. If the patient can read lips, face him directly, speak slowly, avoid covering your mouth and use gestures to reinforce your words. Since lip reading is never perfect, supplement instructions with writing. If the patient has a hearing aid, of course, he should use it.

Blind Patients. When talking with a blind patient, be especially careful to announce yourself and explain who and what you are. Taking his hand may help to establish contact and let him know where you are. If the room is unfamiliar to the patient, orient him to it, explain what is there and whether anyone else is present. Remember to respond vocally when he speaks. Facilitative postures and gestures will not work. At the same time guard against raising your voice unnecessarily.

Fatally Ill Patients. In communicating with fatally ill or dying patients, most interviewers face problems within themselves—their own discomforts, anxieties and desires to avoid the subject or even the patients themselves. With the help of reading and discussion, you will need to work through your own feelings. As in any clinical situation, it is helpful to know what reactions the patient is likely to have. Kübler-Ross has described five stages in the patient's response to his own impending death: denial and isolation, anger, bargaining, depression or preparatory grief, and acceptance. Regardless of the stage, your approach to the patient is basically the same. Be alert to the patient's feelings and to cues that he wants to talk about them. Help him to bring them out with nondirective techniques. Make openings for him to ask questions. "I wonder if you have any concerns about the operation? . . . your illness? . . . how it will be when you go home?" Explore these concerns and provide whatever information the patient is asking for. Be wary of inappropriate reassurance. If you can explore and accept the patient's feelings, if you can answer the patient's questions, if you can assure and demonstrate your ability to stay with the patient throughout his illness, reassurance will grow within the patient himself.

Talking with Families or Friends. Some patients are totally unable to give their own histories. Others may be unable to describe parts of them, for example, their behavior during a convulsion. Under these circumstances you must try to find a third person from whom to get the story. At times, although you may think you have a reasonably comprehensive knowledge of the patient, other sources may offer surprising and important information. A spouse, for example, may report significant family strains, depressive symptoms or drinking habits that the patient has denied. When you suspect such discrepancies, look for opportunities to get additional information from persons other than the patient.

When you decide to seek information from a third person, it is usually wise to get the patient's approval. Assure him that you will keep confidential what he has already told you, or get his permission to share certain information. Data from other persons must also be held in confidence.

The basic principles of interviewing apply to your conversations with relatives or friends. Find a private place to talk. Leaning against opposite sides of a hospital corridor is not conducive to good communication. Introduce yourself, state your purpose, inquire how the person is feeling under the circumstances, recognize and acknowledge his concerns. As you listen to his version of the history, be alert for clues as to the quality of his relationship with the patient. These may color his credibility or give you helpful ideas in planning the patient's care.

Responding to Patients' Questions. Patients' questions may seek simple factual information. More often, however, they express feelings or concerns. Try to elicit these feelings or delve further, lest you offer a misguided answer.

> *Patient:* What are the effects of this blood pressure
> medicine?
> *Response:* There are several effects. Why do you ask?
> *Patient:* (Pause) Well I was reading up on it in a friend's
> book. I read it could make me impotent.

Similar caution is indicated when patients seek advice for personal problems. Should the patient quit a stressful job, for example, or move to Arizona, or have an abortion? Before responding, find out what approaches he or she has considered, what pros and cons there might be to the possible solutions. A chance to talk through the problem with you is usually much more valuable than any possible answer you could give.

Finally, when the patient is asking for specific information about his diagnosis, progress or treatment plan, answer when you can but be careful that your responses do not conflict with those provided by others. When you are unsure of the answer, offer to find out if you can. Alternatively you can tell the patient that he should ask Dr. X since the latter knows more about his case or is making that decision. Beware, however, of using this approach to avoid a difficult issue. If you carry the primary patient responsibility yourself, share your opinions and plans and the patient's prognosis with other members of the health team so that they in turn can communicate with the patient most effectively.

A Final Note

This chapter is intended as a guide—to the information you need, to the ways of obtaining it and to the methods of establishing effective relationships with your patients. Its suggestions are not meant as ironclad rules fettering your every move or question. In the last analysis you are a sensitive, aware human being interacting with and trying to help another.

recording the health history

Writing a history has four goals. (1) You organize and record the patient's symptoms and the medical background that will help in formulating a diagnosis and developing a therapeutic plan. (2) You give to those who work with you or who will follow you a reasonable understanding of the patient's medical and psychosocial status. (3) You provide a recall mechanism for yourself. (4) You make a legal record of the patient's problems and care.

Recording a health history is more than just writing down what the patient has told you. You must review your data, organize them, evaluate the importance and relevance of each item, and construct a clear, concise, yet comprehensive story that will document the facts and guide you to the proper assessment.

If you are a beginner, determining what belongs in the present illness will constitute one of your most difficult problems, for you must cluster together the relevant data. Although the patient may do most of this for you, he may not recognize that some of his symptoms are, in fact, related to others. That muscular weakness, heat intolerance, excessive sweating, diarrhea, weight loss and palpitations all constitute a present illness will not be apparent to the patient or to the interviewer who is unfamiliar with the syndrome of hyperthyroidism. The quality of your histories depends on your clinical knowledge and will grow only as your reading and experience grow. Meanwhile, the seven key attributes of all principal symptoms, listed on page 2 will offer a helpful guide.

Regardless of your clinical experience, certain principles will help you write a good history. Order is imperative. Although there are modest variations in format, the subdivisions detailed in Chapter 1 not only help in obtaining a reasonably complete history, they also help future readers, including yourself, to find specific points of information. Make your headings clear, use indentations and spacing to accentuate your organization and asterisk or underline important points. The present illness should be presented in chronological order, starting with the current episode, but also filling in past relevant background. The terms in which you express time should be uniform, at least within the present illness. Avoid the confusion of this extreme example: "He has had three operations for this problem, the first at age 46, the second in 1974, and the third two years ago."

The amount of detail to be recorded poses a vexing problem. As you begin to write histories, be quite detailed, since doing so is the only way to build your descriptive skills, vocabulary and speed. Pressure of time will ultimately force some compromises, however. The following guidelines may be useful in deciding what to record and what to omit.

1. You should record all the data—both positive and negative—that contribute to your subsequent assessment or differential diagnosis.

2. Specifically describe negative information, i.e., the lack of a symptom, when other portions of the history or physical examination suggest that an abnormality might exist or develop in that area. For example, if the patient has rales, be sure to record whether he has cough, dyspnea or other cardiopulmonary symptoms.

3. Data not recorded are data lost. No matter how vivid your knowledge of them is today, you will probably not remember them in a few weeks or months.

4. In contrast, information can be buried in a mass of excessive detail, to be discovered by only the most persistent reader. Avoid long lists of relatively minor negative findings as well as repetitive introductory phrases such as: "The patient reports no . . ."

Be as objective as possible. This portion of the patient's record reflects primarily the patient's viewpoint. Your interpretations and assessments will come later. Nor is this the place for moralizing, expressions of social disapproval or disgust. These tell more about the writer than about the patient and furthermore might prove embarrassing in court.

Since charts are both scientific and legal documents, they should be understandable. Employ abbreviations and symbols only if they are commonly used. Some practitioners may wish to develop an elegant style and should certainly be encouraged to do so. Time is usually scarce, however, and style can be sacrificed in the effort to achieve both completeness and brevity. In the history that follows, for example, words and brief phrases have substituted for whole sentences. Legibility, of course, is always a virtue.

When should you write a history? As soon as possible, before it fades from your memory. In your initial attempts, you will probably prefer to take only notes when talking with a patient. As you gain experience, however, work toward recording in final form the past medical history, family history, and review of systems as you take them, leaving space to fill in the present illness and psychosocial history later. Always be prepared, however, to stop recording and give your undivided attention to listening.

What follows is an example of a history that is reasonably thorough but certainly does not include all possible information. Data from this patient's physical examination can be found in Chapter 4.

*   *   *

Mrs. Audrey N.   1463 Maple Blvd.   Born: Lake City
Capital City

12/13/78
Mrs. N. is a 54-year-old, widowed white saleswoman.

Referral. None

Source. Self, seems reliable

Chief Complaint. Headaches

Present Illness. For about 3 months Mrs. N. has been increasingly troubled by headaches: bifrontal, usually aching, occasionally throbbing, mild to moderately severe. She has missed work only once because of headaches when she felt nauseated, miserable and vomited several times. Otherwise, nausea is associated only occasionally. Headaches now average once or twice a week, usually are there when she wakes up and last all day. Little relief from aspirin. It helps to lie down, be quiet, use cold wet towel on head. No other related symptoms, no local weakness, no numbness or visual symptoms.

Mrs. N. first began to have headaches at age 15. "Sick headaches" recurred through her mid-20s, then diminished to one every 2 or 3 months and finally almost disappeared.

Has recently had increased pressure at work, is also worried about daughter (see psychosocial). Thinks headaches may be like those in the past, but wants to be sure since mother died of a stroke. Is concerned that they make her irritable with her family.

Past Medical History

  General Health: Good

  Childhood Illnesses: Only measles and chickenpox

  Immunizations. Smallpox vaccination as child; oral polio vaccine, year uncertain; tetanus shots X 2 three years ago followed by a booster a year later; others uncertain

Adult Illnesses: None serious

Psychiatric Illnesses: None

Operations: Tonsillectomy, age 6; appendectomy, age 13

Injuries: Stepped on glass at beach 3 years ago, laceration, sutured, healed

* *Hospitalizations:* St. Mary's, acute kidney infection, age 42

Current Medications: Aspirin for headaches, multivitamins. Has taken "water pill" for ankle swelling, but none in past several months.

* *Allergies:* Generalized skin rash with itching from *sulfa*, age 42

Habits:

Diet. Breakfast: Orange juice, two sweet rolls, black coffee
Mid-morning: Doughnut, coffee
Lunch: Hamburger and bun or fish sandwich, coffee
Dinner: Meat or fish, vegetable, potato, sometimes fruit, sometimes cookies
Snacks in evening: e.g., chips, cola
Has almost no milk or cheese

Exercise. Prolonged standing at work, little other exercise

Alcohol. Rare, doesn't like it

Tobacco. About one pack cigarettes per day from age 18 (36 pack years)

Sleep. Generally good, average 7 hours, sometimes has trouble falling asleep, is waked by alarm

Family History. (There are two methods of recording the family history. The diagrammatic format is more helpful in tracing genetic disorders. The negative family information follows either format.)
Diagrammatic:

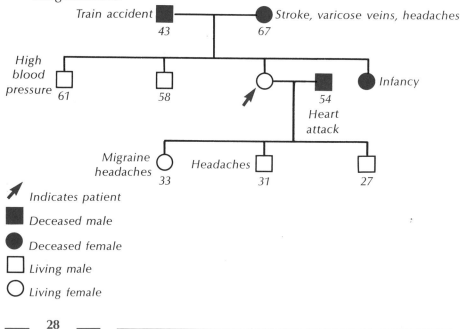

Indicates patient

Deceased male

Deceased female

Living male

Living female

Narrative Outline:
    Father died age 43, train accident
    Mother died age 67, stroke, had had varicose veins, headaches
    One brother, age 61, has high blood pressure, otherwise well
    One brother, age 58, apparently well, but for mild arthritis
    One sister, died in infancy, ?cause
    Husband died age 54, heart attack
    One daughter, age 33, "migraine headaches," otherwise well
    One son, age 31, headaches
    One son, age 27, well

    No family history of diabetes, tuberculosis, heart or kidney disease, cancer, anemia or mental illness

* *Psychosocial.* Born and raised in Lake City, finished high school, married at age 19. Worked in store for 2 years, then moved with husband to Capital City, had three children. Mr. N. had steady factory job but to help with income Mrs. N. went back to work 10 years ago. Children have all married. Four years ago Mr. N. died suddenly of a heart attack. Finances now tight. Has moved to small apartment to be near daughter, Dorothy. Dorothy's husband has a drinking problem and Mrs. N.'s apartment serves as a haven for Dorothy and her two young children. Mrs. N. feels responsible for helping the family, is tense and nervous, but denies depression.

Typically up at 7:00 a.m., works 9:00 to 5:30, eats dinner alone. Dorothy or children visit most evenings and weekends. Moderate number of squabbles and considerable strain.

Review of Systems

* *General:* Has *gained* about *10 pounds* in the past 4 years

Skin: No rashes or other changes

Head: No head injury (See present illness.)

Eyes: Reading glasses for 5 years, last checked a year ago; no other symptoms

Ears: Hearing good; no tinnitus, vertigo, infections

Nose, Sinuses: Occasional mild cold; no hay fever or sinus trouble

* *Mouth and Throat:* Some *bleeding of gums* recently; last to dentist 2 years ago; occasional canker sore, has had one for 4 days

Neck: No lumps, goiter or pain

Breasts: No lumps, pain, discharge; does breast self exams sporadically

Respiratory: No cough, wheezing, pneumonia, tuberculosis; last chest X-ray 12 years ago, St. Mary's Hospital, normal

Cardiac: No known heart disease or high blood pressure; last blood pressure taken 3 years ago; no dyspnea, orthopnea, chest pain, palpitations; no EKG

* *GI:* Appetite good; no nausea, vomiting, indigestion; bowel movement about once daily though sometimes has *hard stools, q 2–3 days, when especially tense;* no diarrhea or bleeding; no pain, jaundice, gallbladder or liver trouble

* *Urinary: Acute kidney infection,* age 42, with fever and right flank pain; treated with pills, including sulfa; no recurrence; no frequency, dysuria or hematuria; nocturia X 1, large volume; *occasionally loses some urine when coughs hard*

Genito-reproductive: Menarche at 13, regular periods, tapered off in late 40's and stopped at 49; no bleeding since; mild hot flashes and sweats then, none now
Gravida 3, para 3, living children 3; prolonged labor during first pregnancy, otherwise normal; little sexual interest now

* *Musculoskeletal:* Mild *aching low back* often after a long day's work; no radiation down legs; used to do back exercises, but not now; no other joint pain

* *Peripheral Vascular:* Varicose veins appeared in both legs during first pregnancy; has had swollen ankles after prolonged standing for 10 years; wears light elastic pantyhose; tried "water pill" several months ago but it didn't help much; no history of phlebitis or leg pain

Neurologic: No faints, seizures, motor or sensory loss; memory good

Psychiatric: (See present illness and psychosocial.)

Endocrine: No known thyroid trouble, temperature intolerance; sweating average; no symptoms or history of diabetes

Hematologic: Except for bleeding gums, no easy bleeding, no anemia

the physical examination of the adult—an overview

This chapter is designed to give you an overview of the physical examination. In subsequent chapters you will learn in detail the approach to specific regions or systems of the body. As you learn the new steps, fit them into this more general context.

The sequence suggested here describes a quite comprehensive examination of an adult. Insofar as possible it minimizes patient effort, avoiding repetitious sitting up and lying back down. By learning a basic routine, you will improve your efficiency without forgetting important steps. It is not the only possible sequence, however, and you may alter it as the patient's needs or your own preferences dictate. Variations useful in examining infants and small children are described in Chapter 20.

* * *

General Survey: Observe the apparent state of health; signs of distress; skin color; stature and habitus; weight; posture, motor activity and gait; dress, grooming and personal hygiene; odors; facial expression; manner, mood and relationship to surroundings; speech; state of awareness.

Vital Signs: Measure the pulse, respiratory rate, blood pressure and, if indicated, temperature.

Skin: Note the color of the skin, its vascularity, any lesions, edema, moisture, temperature, texture, thickness, mobility and turgor; the condition of the nails.

Begin your assessment of the skin with the hands, forearms and face. Continue it throughout the remainder of the examination. Include in your inspection of the hands and arms observations relevant to the peripheral vascular, musculoskeletal and neurological systems.

The patient is sitting, unless his condition contraindicates this position.

Head: Examine the hair, scalp, skull, face.

Eyes: Check visual acuity and fields, the position and alignment of the eyes, the eyebrows, eyelids, lacrimal apparatus, conjunctivas and scleras, corneas, irises, pupils, extraocular movements, ocular fundi.

Ears: Inspect the auricles, canals and drums; check auditory acuity. If acuity is diminished, check lateralization and compare air and bone conduction.

Nose and Sinuses: Examine the external nose, mucosa, septum, turbinates; frontal and maxillary sinuses.

Mouth and Pharynx: Inspect the lips, buccal mucosa, gums and teeth, roof of the mouth, tongue, and pharynx.

Further Cranial Nerve Assessment: (Optional) If indicated, you may wish to complete your cranial nerve assessment here by checking facial and jaw movement, facial sensation and sternomastoid and trapezius function.

Neck: Inspect and palpate the cervical nodes, trachea and thyroid.

Back: Inspect and palpate the spine and muscles of the upper back; check for costovertebral angle tenderness.

Posterior Thorax and Lungs: Inspect, palpate, percuss and auscultate.

Breasts and Axillae: In a woman, inspect the breasts with her arms relaxed, then elevated, then with hands pressed on hips; examine the epitrochlear nodes and axillae.

NOTE: by this point you will have examined the hands, surveyed the back, and at least in women, made a fair estimate of the range of motion of the shoulders. Examination of the anterior thorax will include additional musculoskeletal structures. Use these observations, together with noting how the patient moves throughout the examination, in deciding whether or not to continue later with a full musculoskeletal examination.

Breasts: Inspect and palpate.

Anterior Thorax and Lungs: Inspect, palpate, percuss and auscultate.

Heart: Inspect, palpate and auscultate. Correlate your findings with the jugular venous pulse and the carotid artery pulse. Elevation of the patient's upper body somewhat may be helpful here. You may also wish him to lie on his left side or sit up and lean forward.

The patient is sitting, unless his condition contraindicates this position.

The patient is supine.

Abdomen: Inspect, auscultate, percuss, palpate lightly and deeply.

The patient is supine.

Inguinal Area: Identify the inguinal nodes and the femoral artery pulsations.

Genitalia and Rectal Examination in Men: Examine the penis, scrotal contents, anus, rectum and prostate.

If the examiner prefers the left lateral decubitus position for the rectal examination, it is conveniently done here. If the standing position is used, defer the examination until later.

Legs: Inspect the legs, noting evidence of peripheral vascular, musculoskeletal or neurological abnormalities. Palpate for edema. Check the dorsalis pedis and posterior tibial pulses.

Musculoskeletal System: Examine the range of motion of the spine, the alignment of the legs, and the feet.

The patient is standing, if this is feasible.

Peripheral Vascular System: Inspect for varicose veins.

Hernia and Rectal Examination: In men, check for hernias, and if the standing position is preferred, perform a rectal examination.

Screening Neurological Examination: Check the gait, Romberg's sign, and the ability to do a knee bend, to hop, walk on toes and heels, maintain the arms held forward, and grip the examiner's fingers. These maneuvers also serve to screen the *musculoskeletal* system.

Completion of a Screening Neurological Examination
   Screening the Sensory System: Pain and vibration in hands and feet, light touch on the limbs, and stereognosis in the hands.

The patient is sitting or supine.

   Reflexes: Deep tendon and superficial.

Full Neurological Examination: If indicated, go on to a more thorough examination, including:

   Motor: More detailed inspection; testing of muscle tone, strength, coordination.

   Sensory: Pain, temperature, light touch, position, vibration, discrimination.

Completion of Musculoskeletal Examination: If indicated, inspect and palpate each joint and check its range of motion. Use special maneuvers as indicated.

Mental Status: Evaluate mood, thought processes and perceptions, cognitive functions.

Genitalia and Rectal Examination in Women: Examine the external genitalia, vagina, cervix, uterus and adnexa; do a rectovaginal and rectal examination.

The patient is supine.

Alternatively, this may follow the abdominal and inguinal examination.

a method of recording the physical examination

The order in which you record your findings is similar although not identical to the sequence of your examination. As in the history, a routine format improves your efficiency, helps to avoid omissions and makes your record easier to use.

Strive for completeness without verbosity, be organized yet flexible, work for objectivity, accuracy and clarity.

A suggested format for recording a physical examination is outlined on the following pages along with cross references to the techniques and tables in the *GUIDE*. Words appearing in parentheses indicate sections frequently omitted when the examination is entirely negative. Such judgments, of course, are bound to be controversial.

Descriptive Paragraph.   Write a succinct paragraph describing the patient's appearance, including the characteristics noted in your general survey. Avoid trite phrases such as "well-developed, well-nourished." Develop your prose skills here and try to portray the patient so that another could pick him out in the waiting room. | 40–42*

   Pulse   Resp   BP   (Temp)   Ht   Wt | 185, 133

Skin and Nails | 45, 46–51

Head: Hair, scalp, skull (face) | 65, 86

Eyes: Acuity, (fields), (position and alignment), (eyebrows), (eyelids), (lacrimal apparatus); conjunctivas; scleras; (corneas); (irises); pupils, including their size, shape, equality and reaction to light and accommodation; extraocular movements; ophthalmoscopic examination | 66–75, 87–99

Ears: (Auricles), canals, drums, auditory acuity. If indicated, lateralization, air and bone conduction | 76–78, 100–102

* Page numbers in black refer to techniques; those in red to tables of abnormalities.

Nose and Sinuses: (External nose), mucosa, septum, (turbinates), sinus tenderness	78–80, 103
Mouth and Pharynx: (Lips), buccal mucosa, gums, teeth, (roof of mouth), tongue, pharynx	81–82, 104–110
Neck: Trachea, thyroid	82–85, 111
Nodes: Cervical, axillary, epitrochlear, inguinal	82–83, 194, 263, 264
Thorax: Inspection; (palpation, including fremitus); percussion including diaphragmatic movement; breath sounds, (voice sounds), and adventitious sounds	120–131, 132–138
Heart: Location and quality of the apical impulse, other impulses; heart sounds; murmurs and thrills	139–155, 156–172
Jugular venous pressure and pulse	181–184
Carotid artery pulse	177, 185
Breasts: Inspection, including (size), (symmetry), (contour), (nipples); palpation, including tenderness and nodules	189–193, 196–199
Abdomen: Contours, scars, (umbilicus); bowel sounds and bruits; tenderness, masses, palpable organs	203–212, 213–220
Genitalia and Rectum	
Female: External genitalia, (urethral meatus), vagina, cervix, uterus, adnexa, rectovaginal exam, anus and rectum	232–238, 252–253, 239–248, 254–255
Male: Penis, scrotal contents, hernias, anus, rectum, and prostate	223–224, 251–252, 225–229, 254–256
Peripheral Vascular: Color, temperature, pulses, edema, veins	262–267, 268–272
Musculoskeletal: Joints and range of motion; deformities	284–296, 297–310
Nervous System	
Cranial Nerves: These may be recorded here or under the appropriate sections of the head and neck.	321–324, 346–349
Motor: Gait, appearance, muscle tone, strength and coordination	325–332, 350–355
Sensory: Pain, temperature, light touch, position, vibration, discrimination	333–335, 356–358

* Page numbers in black refer to techniques; those in red to tables of abnormalities.

Reflexes: Deep tendon and superficial

336–344, 354–355

Mental Status: Appearance, mood, thought processes and content, cognitive functions

359–364, 345, 365–366

*   *   *

A sample physical examination follows. The patient is Mrs. N., whose history was detailed in Chapter 2.

Mrs. N. is a short, moderately obese, middle-aged woman who walks and moves easily and responds quickly to questions. She wears no makeup but her hair is neatly fixed and her clothes immaculate. Although her ankles are swollen, her color is good and she lies flat without discomfort. She talks freely but is somewhat tense, with moist, cold hands.

P 94, regular   R 18   BP 164/98 right arm, lying
                             160/95 left arm, lying
                             152/88 right arm, lying (wide cuff)
                         Ht (without shoes) 157 cm (5'2")
Temp 37.1°C (oral)   Wt (dressed) 65kg (143 lbs.)

Skin: Palms cold and moist, but color good. Scattered cherry angiomas over the upper trunk.

Head: Hair of average texture. Scalp and skull normal.

Eyes: Vision 20/30 in both eyes. Fields not done. Conjunctivas show good color. Scleras clear. Pupils are round, regular, equal, react to light and accommodation. Extraocular movements intact. Discs well-delineated. No arteriolar narrowing, A-V nicking, hemorrhages or exudates.

Ears: Wax partially obscures the right drum. Left canal clear and drum negative. Acuity good (to whispered voice).

Nose: Mucosa pink, septum midline. No sinus tenderness.

* *Mouth:*   Mucosa pink. Gums healthy. Teeth in good repair. Tongue midline, negative but for a small (3 × 4 mm) shallow white <u>ulcer</u> on an erythematous base, located on the under surface near the tip. It is slightly tender but not indurated. Tonsils absent. Pharynx negative.

Neck: Trachea midline. Thyroid isthmus barely palpable, lobes not felt.

Nodes: Small (less than 1 cm), soft, non-tender and mobile tonsillar and posterior cervical nodes bilaterally. No axillary or epitrochlear nodes. Several small inguinal nodes bilaterally—soft and non-tender.

Thorax and Lungs: Thorax symmetrical. Good excursion. Lungs resonant. Diaphragm descends 4 cm on inspiration. Breath sounds vesicular without rales or wheezes.

---

* Page numbers in black refer to techniques; those in red to tables of abnormalities.

Heart: Apical impulse barely palpable in the 5th left interspace 8 cm from the midsternal line. Physiologic splitting of S_2. No S_3 or S_4. A grade 2/6 medium pitched midsystolic <u>murmur</u> heard at the aortic area; does not radiate to the neck.

Jugular venous pressure at the level of the sternal angle, while the patient elevated at 30 degrees. Carotid pulses normal and symmetrical.

Breasts: Large, pendulous, symmetrical. No masses. Nipples erect and without discharge.

Abdomen: Obese, but symmetrical. Well-healed right lower quadrant scar. Bowel sounds normal. But for a slightly tender sigmoid colon, no masses or tenderness. Liver, spleen and kidneys not felt. Liver span 7 cm in the right midclavicular line.

Genitalia: Vulva normal. On straining, a mild <u>cystocele</u> appears. Vagina negative. Parous cervix without redness or tenderness. Uterus anterior, midline, smooth, not enlarged. Adnexa are difficult to delineate because of obesity and poor relaxation, but there is no tenderness. Pap smears taken. Rectovaginal examination confirms above.

Rectal: Negative. Brown stool, negative for occult blood.

Peripheral Vascular
  Pulses (4+ = normal)

	Radial	*Femoral*	*Popliteal*	*Dorsalis Pedis*	*Posterior Tibial*
Rt	4+	4+	4+	4+	4+
Lt	4+	4+	4+	4+	4+

2+ <u>edema</u> of feet and ankles with 1+ edema extending up to just below the knees. Moderate <u>varicosities</u> of the saphenous veins bilaterally from mid thigh to the ankles, with venous stars on both lower legs. No stasis pigmentation or ulcers. No calf tenderness. Homans's sign negative bilaterally.

Musculoskeletal: No joint deformities. Range of motion, including hands, wrists, elbows, shoulders, spine, hips, knees, ankles is normal.

Neurological
  Cranial nerves: See head and neck. Also—
      N5 —Sensation intact, strength good.
      N7 —Facial movement good.
      N11—Sternomastoids and trapezii strong.

Motor: No atrophy, fasciculations, tremors. Gait, heel-to-toe, heel and toe walking, knee bends, hops well done. Romberg negative. Grip and arms strong.

Sensory: Screening for pain, vibration, light touch, stereognosis intact.

Reflexes: (Two methods of recording may be used, depending upon personal preference: a tabular form or a stick figure diagram, as shown below.)

	Biceps	*Triceps*	*Sup*	*Abd*	*Knee*	*Ankle*	*Pl*
Rt	2+	2+	2+	2+/2+	2+	1+	↓
Lt	2+	2+	2+	2+/2+	2+	1+	↓

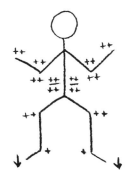

Mental Status: Tense but alert and cooperative. Thought coherent. Oriented. Cognitive testing not done in detail.

the general survey

TECHNIQUES OF EXAMINATION

Begin the examination of the patient by observing him from the first moment you see him and shake hands with him. Continue your observations, systematically yet unobtrusively, throughout the interview. After the interview it is useful to initiate physical contact by taking the patient's vital signs and examining his hands—maneuvers which are relatively non-threatening. Throughout the process make note of the following:

EXAMPLES OF ABNORMALITIES

Apparent State of Health

Frail, acutely or chronically ill

Signs of Distress, for example:

    Cardiorespiratory distress

Labored breathing, wheezing, cough

    Pain

Facial expression, sweating, protectiveness of a painful part

    Anxiety

Anxious face, fidgety movements, cold moist palms

Skin Color: See Chapter 6 for further details.

Pallor, cyanosis, jaundice, changes in pigmentation

Stature and Habitus: If possible, measure the patient's height in stocking feet. Note his body build, his general bodily proportions and any gross deformities.

Long limbs in proportion to the trunk in hypogonadism and Marfan's syndrome

Weight: Note if the patient is obese or thin for his body build. Observe the distribution of fat over the body.

Generalized fat in simple obesity; truncal fat with relatively thin limbs in Cushing's syndrome

Weigh him and compare the results with the desirable weights prepared by the Metropolitan Life Insurance Company (see overleaf). These figures apply to persons who are weighed while dressed, with shoes on. If you measure height and weight under different conditions, make the appropriate corrections.

DESIRABLE WEIGHTS

FOR MEN 25 YEARS OF AGE OR OLDER				FOR WOMEN 25 YEARS OF AGE OR OLDER				
HEIGHT a		SMALL FRAME	MEDIUM FRAME	LARGE FRAME	HEIGHT b		SMALL FRAME	MEDIUM FRAME	LARGE FRAME
Feet	Inches				Feet	Inches			
5	2	112-120	118-129	126-141	4	10	92- 98	96-107	104-119
5	3	115-123	121-133	129-144	4	11	94-101	98-110	106-122
5	4	118-126	124-136	132-148	5	0	96-104	101-113	109-125
5	5	121-129	127-139	135-152	5	1	99-107	104-116	112-128
5	6	124-133	130-143	138-156	5	2	102-110	107-119	115-131
5	7	128-137	134-147	142-161	5	3	105-113	110-122	118-134
5	8	132-141	138-152	147-166	5	4	108-116	113-126	121-138
5	9	136-145	142-156	151-170	5	5	111-119	116-130	125-142
5	10	140-150	146-160	155-174	5	6	114-123	120-135	129-146
5	11	144-154	150-165	159-179	5	7	118-127	124-139	133-150
6	0	148-158	154-170	164-184	5	8	122-131	128-143	137-154
6	1	152-162	158-175	168-189	5	9	126-135	132-147	141-158
6	2	156-167	162-180	173-194	5	10	130-140	136-151	145-163
6	3	160-171	167-185	178-199	5	11	134-144	140-155	149-168
6	4	164-175	172-190	182-204	6	·0	138-148	144-159	153-173

a. with shoes on, 1-inch heels   b. with shoes on, 2-inch heels

SOURCE: Metropolitan Life Insurance Company, Statistical Bureau. Derived primarily from data of the Build and Blood Pressure Study, 1959, Society of Actuaries.

Posture, Motor Activity and, if possible, Gait

Slumped posture and slowed activity of depression; tremor, paralysis, ataxia

Dress, Grooming and Personal Hygiene

Unkempt appearance in depression and chronic organic brain disease

Odors: of body or breath.
   CAUTION: Never assume that alcohol on the breath indicates alcohol as the sole cause of mental or neurological symptoms.

Breath odor of alcohol, acetone (diabetes), oral or pulmonary infections, uremia or liver failure

Facial Expression: at rest and in interaction with others.

Anxiety, depression, pain, apathy

Manner, Mood and Relationship to Persons and Things Around Him

Uncooperativeness, hostility, anger, resentment, depression, tearfulness, distrustfulness, elation

Speech: including the pace of speech, its pitch and clarity.

Fast speech of hyperthyroidism; slow, thick, hoarse voice of myxedema; dysphasia, dysarthria

State of Awareness, Consciousness: including the speed of response to questions and apparent comprehension.

Inattentiveness, drowsiness, stupor, coma

Vital Signs: including the pulse, respiratory rate and blood pressure, as described in detail in Chapters 8, 9 and 10. Although measurement of the patient's temperature may be omitted in many ambulatory visits, take it if symptoms or signs suggest a possible abnormality.

Fever, hypothermia

The average oral temperature, usually quoted at 37°C (98.6°F), fluctuates considerably and must be interpreted accordingly. In the early morning hours, it may be as low as 35.8°C (96.4°F), in the late afternoon or evening as high as 37.3°C (99.1°F). Rectal temperatures average 0.4 to 0.5°C (0.7 to 0.9°F) higher than oral readings, but this difference varies considerably.

For accurate measurements with a glass thermometer, take a rectal temperature over a 3-minute period; an oral reading often requires 8 minutes—considerably longer than our usual routines.

the skin

ANATOMY AND PHYSIOLOGY

The skin is composed of three layers: the epidermis, the dermis, and the subcutaneous tissues.

The most superficial layer, the *epidermis,* is thin, devoid of blood vessels and itself divided into two layers: an outer horny layer of dead keratinized cells; and an inner cellular layer where both melanin and keratin are formed.

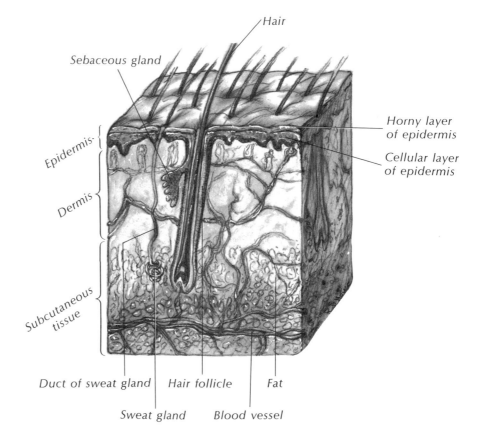

The epidermis depends on the underlying *dermis* for its nutrition. The dermis is well supplied with blood. It contains connective tissue, the sebaceous glands and some of the hair follicles. It merges below with the *subcutaneous tissues* which contain fat, the sweat glands and the remainder of the hair follicles.

Hair, nails, sebaceous and sweat glands are considered appendages of the skin. The sebaceous glands secrete a protective fatty substance which gains access to the skin surface through the hair follicles. These glands are present on all skin surfaces except for the palms and soles. Sweat glands are of two types: eccrine and apocrine. The eccrine glands are widely distributed, open directly onto the skin surface and by their sweat production help to control body temperature. In contrast, the apocrine glands are found chiefly in the axillary and genital regions, usually open into hair follicles and are stimulated by emotional stress. Bacterial decomposition of apocrine sweat is responsible for body odor.

Begin your observation of the skin with your general survey and continue it throughout the rest of your examination.
Inspect and palpate the skin, noting its:

Color: e.g., brownness, cyanosis, redness, yellowness or pallor

See Table 6-1, Variations in Skin Color (pp. 46–47).

Vascularity and evidence of *bleeding* or *bruising*

See Table 6-2, Vascular and Purpuric Lesions of the Skin (p. 48).

Lesions: If present, identify their:
1. *Color*
2. *Type:* e.g., macule, papule, vesicle, ulcer, scale
3. *Grouping or Configuration:* e.g., clustered, linear, annular
4. *Distribution Over the Body:* e.g., localized, generalized, involving the exposed surfaces, or involving the intertriginous (skin fold) areas

See Table 6-3, Basic Types of Skin Lesions (pp. 49–50).

Edema

Moisture: e.g., dryness, sweating, oiliness

Dryness in hypothyroidism, oiliness in acne

Temperature: Feel the skin with the backs of your fingers to assess temperature.

Texture: e.g., roughness, smoothness

Thickness

Roughness in hypothyroidism

Mobility and Turgor: Lift a fold of skin and note the ease with which it is moved (mobility) and the speed with which it returns into place (turgor).

Decreased mobility in edema, scleroderma; decreased turgor in dehydration

Inspect and palpate the fingernails and toenails, noting their color, shape and any lesions.

See Table 6-4, Abnormalities and Variations of the Nails (p. 51).

Inspect and palpate the hair, noting its quantity, distribution and texture.

The differential diagnosis of skin abnormalities is beyond the scope of this book. After describing an abnormality in the terms listed above, however, the practitioner should be well equipped to consult textbooks of dermatology. The diagnosis of skin diseases is basically accomplished by careful observation of the individual single lesion together with the distribution of the lesions.

TABLE 6-1

TABLE 6-1. VARIATIONS IN SKIN COLOR

COLOR	PROCESS	SELECTED CAUSES	TYPICAL LOCALIZATION
Brown	Deposition of melanin	Genetic	Generalized
		Sunlight	Exposed area
		Pregnancy	Face, nipples, and areolae, linea nigra, vulva
		Addison's disease and some pituitary tumors	Exposed areas, points of pressure and friction, nipples, genitalia, palmar creases, recent scars, often generalized
Grayish-tan or bronze	Deposition of melanin and hemosiderin	Hemochromatosis	Exposed areas, genitalia and scars, often generalized
Blue (cyanosis)	Increased amount of reduced hemoglobin secondary to hypoxia. This may be either:		
	Peripheral, or	Anxiety or cold environment	The nails, sometimes lips
	Central (arterial)	Heart or lung disease	Lips, mouth and nails
	Abnormal hemoglobin	Congenital or acquired methemoglobinemia; sulfhemoglobinemia	Lips, mouth and nails
Reddish blue	Combination of increase in total amount of hemoglobin, increase in reduced hemoglobin and capillary stasis	Polycythemia	Face, conjunctivas, mouth, hands and feet
Red	Increased visibility of normal oxyhemoglobin because of—		
	Dilatation or increased numbers of superficial blood vessels or increased blood flow	Fever, blushing, alcohol intake, local inflammation	Face and upper chest or local area of inflammation
	Decreased oxygen utilization in the skin	Cold exposure	The cold area, e.g., ears

TABLE 6-1. (CONT'D)

COLOR	PROCESS	SELECTED CAUSES	TYPICAL LOCALIZATION
Yellow			
Jaundice	Increased bilirubin levels	Liver disease, red blood cell hemolysis	First in scleras, then mucous membranes and generalized
Carotenemia	Increased levels of carotenoid pigments	Increased intake of carotene containing vegetables and fruits; myxedema, hypopituitarism, diabetes	Palms, soles, face; does not involve scleras or mucous membranes
Chronic uremia	Retention of urinary chromogens, superimposed on the pallor of anemia	Chronic renal disease	Most evident in exposed areas, may be generalized; does not involve scleras or mucous membranes
Decreased color	Decreased melanin		
	Congenital inability to form melanin	Albinism	Generalized lack of pigment in skin, hair, eyes
	Acquired loss of melanin	Vitiligo	Patchy, symmetrical, often involving the exposed areas
		Tinea versicolor (a common fungus infection)	Chest, upper back and neck
	Decreased visibility of oxyhemoglobin		
	Decreased blood flow in superficial vessels	Syncope, shock, some normal variations	Most evident in face, conjunctivas, mouth, nails
	Decreased amount of oxyhemoglobin	Anemia	Most evident in face, conjunctivas, mouth, nails
	Edema (Edema of the skin masks the colors of melanin and hemoglobin and prevents the appearance of jaundice.)	Nephrotic syndrome	The edematous areas

TABLE 6-2

TABLE 6-2. VASCULAR AND PURPURIC LESIONS OF THE SKIN

	VASCULAR			PURPURIC	
	CHERRY ANGIOMA	SPIDER ANGIOMA	VENOUS STAR	PETECHIA	ECCHYMOSIS
Color	Bright or ruby red; may become brownish with age	Fiery red	Bluish	Deep red or reddish purple	Purple or purplish-blue, fading to green, yellow and brown with time
Size	1–3 mm	Very small up to 2 cm	Variable, from very small to several inches	Usually 1–3mm	Variable, larger than petechiae
Shape	Round, sometimes raised, may be surrounded by a pale halo	Central body, sometimes raised, surrounded by erythema and radiating legs	Variable. May resemble a spider or be linear, irregular, cascading	Round, flat	Round, oval or irregular; may have a central subcutaneous flat nodule
Pulsatility	Absent	Often demonstrable in the body of the spider, when pressure with a glass slide is applied	Absent	Absent	Absent
Effect of pressure	May show partial blanching, especially if pressure is applied with a pinpoint's edge.	Pressure over the body causes blanching of the spider	Pressure over center does not cause blanching	None	None
Distribution	Trunk, also extremities	Face, neck, arms and upper trunk, almost never below the waist	Most often on the legs, near veins; also anterior chest	Variable	Variable
Significance	None; increase in size and numbers with aging	Liver disease, pregnancy, vitamin B deficiency, occurs in some normal people	Often accompanies increased pressure in the superficial veins, as in varicose veins	Blood extravasated outside the vessels; may suggest increased bleeding tendency or emboli to skin	Blood extravasated outside the vessels; often secondary to trauma; also seen in bleeding disorders

TABLE 6-3

TABLE 6-3. BASIC TYPES OF SKIN LESIONS

PRIMARY LESIONS (May arise from previously normal skin)

CIRCUMSCRIBED, FLAT, NON-PALPABLE CHANGES IN SKIN COLOR

Macule—Small, up to 1 cm.* Example: freckle, petechia

Patch—Larger than 1 cm. Example: vitiligo

PALPABLE ELEVATED SOLID MASSES

Papule—Up to 0.5 cm. Example: an elevated nevus

Plaque—A flat, elevated surface larger than 0.5 cm, often formed by the coalescence of papules

Nodule—0.5 to 1–2 cm; often deeper and firmer than a papule

Tumor—Larger than 1–2 cm.

Wheal—A slightly irregular, relatively transient, superficial area of localized skin edema. Example: mosquito bite, hive

CIRCUMSCRIBED SUPERFICIAL ELEVATIONS OF THE SKIN FORMED BY FREE FLUID IN A CAVITY WITHIN THE SKIN LAYERS

Vesicle—Up to 0.5 cm; filled with serous fluid. Example: Herpes simplex

Bulla—Greater than 0.5 cm; filled with serous fluid. Example: 2nd degree burn

Pustule—filled with pus. Examples: acne, impetigo

SECONDARY LESIONS (Result from changes in primary lesions)

LOSS OF SKIN SURFACE

Erosion—Loss of the superficial epidermis; surface is moist but does not bleed. Example: moist area after the rupture of a vesicle, as in chickenpox

Ulcer—A deeper loss of skin surface; may bleed and scar. Examples: stasis ulcer of venous insufficiency, syphilitic chancre

Fissure—A linear crack in the skin. Example: athlete's foot

MATERIAL ON THE SKIN SURFACE

Crust—The dried residue of serum, pus or blood. Example: impetigo

Scale—A thin flake of exfoliated epidermis. Examples: dandruff, dry skin, psoriasis

*Authorities vary somewhat in their definitions of skin lesions by size. Dimensions given in this table should be considered approximate, not rigid.

TABLE 6-3

TABLE 6-3. (CONT'D)

SECONDARY LESIONS (Result from changes in primary lesions)

MISCELLANEOUS

Lichenification—Thickening and roughening of the skin with increased visibility of the normal skin furrows. Example: atopic dermatitis

Scar—Replacement of destroyed tissue by fibrous tissue

Atrophy—Thinning of the skin with loss of the normal skin furrows; the skin looks shinier and more translucent than normal. Example: arterial insufficiency

Keloid—A hypertrophied scar

Excoriation—A scratch mark

TABLE 6-4

TABLE 6-4. ABNORMALITIES AND VARIATIONS OF THE NAILS

CLUBBING OF THE NAILS

NORMAL

Normal angle 160°

The angle between the normal finger nail and nail base is about 160 degrees. When palpated the nail base feels firm.

EARLY CLUBBING

Springy, floating / *Straightened angle (180°)*

In early clubbing, the angle between nail and nail base straightens out. The nail base gives a springy or floating sensation when palpated. You can simulate this by squeezing your middle finger from each side between your thumb and ring finger of the same hand, just behind the nail. Then palpate the nail base with the index finger of the opposite hand.

LATE CLUBBING

Swollen, springy, floating / *Angle greater than 180°*

In late clubbing the base of the nail becomes visibly swollen and the angle between nail and nail base exceeds 180 degrees.

Clubbing has many causes, including hypoxia and lung cancer.

CURVED NAILS

Normal angle / *Curved nail*

Clubbing should not be confused with curved nails, a variant of normal. Here, although the nails show a convex curve, as they may in clubbing, the normal angle between nail and nail base is preserved.

SPOON NAILS (KOILONYCHIA)

Spoon nails are characterized by concave curves. Spoon nails are sometimes seen in iron deficiency anemia although they are not specific for this disorder.

BEAU'S LINES

Beau's lines are transverse depressions in the nails associated with acute severe illness. Appearing some weeks later, they grow out with the nail gradually over several months.

PARONYCHIA

The term paronychia refers to inflammation of the skin around the nail. It is characterized by swelling and sometimes redness and tenderness.

SPLINTER HEMORRHAGES

Splinter hemorrhages are red or brown linear streaks in the nail bed, parallel to the long axis of the fingers. Although traditionally associated with subacute bacterial endocarditis and trichinosis, they are nonspecific, often occurring with minor trauma or without apparent cause. They have been described in from 10–20 percent of hospitalized adults.

the head and neck

ANATOMY AND PHYSIOLOGY

The Head

Regions of the head take their names from the underlying bones, e.g., frontal area, occipital area. Familiarity with the anatomy of the skull is helpful, therefore, in localizing and describing physical findings. Shown also in this diagram are the two salivary glands that can be examined clinically: the parotid gland, which when enlarged is sometimes visible and palpable superficial to and behind the mandible, and the submaxillary gland which is located deep to the mandible. The openings of the parotid and submaxillary glands are visible within the oral cavity.

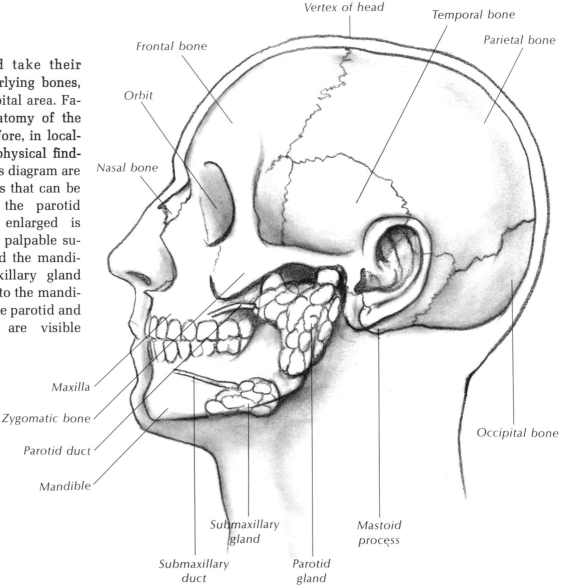

Frontal bone

Vertex of head

Temporal bone

Parietal bone

Orbit

Nasal bone

Maxilla

Zygomatic bone

Parotid duct

Mandible

Submaxillary gland

Submaxillary duct

Parotid gland

Mastoid process

Occipital bone

The Eye

Gross Anatomy. Review the external anatomy of the eye, identifying the diagrammed structures.

Note that the upper eyelid normally covers a portion of the iris. The white sclera may be somewhat buff-colored peripherally.

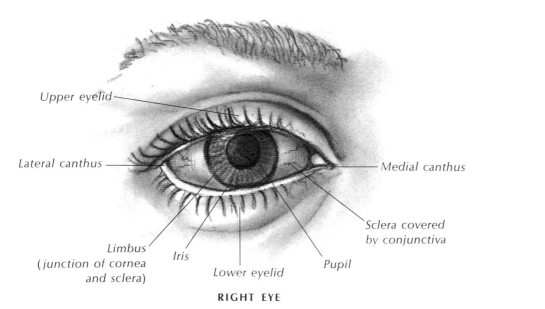

RIGHT EYE

Except for the cornea, the parts of the eyeball visible anteriorly are covered by the conjunctiva. At the margin of the cornea (limbus), the conjunctiva merges with the corneal epithelium. A portion of the conjunctiva with its vessels lies loosely on the surface of the sclera and is called the bulbar conjunctiva. Above and below, it forms a deep recess and then folds forward to join the tissues of the eyelids (palpebral conjunctiva). The eyelids themselves are given form and consistency by thin strips of connective tissue known as the tarsal plates. These relationships are best shown in the cross-section at the right.

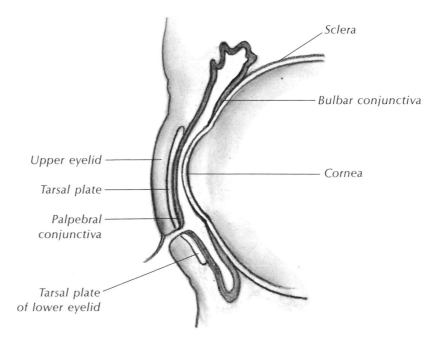

The conjunctiva and cornea are lubricated by secretions from the lacrimal gland and conjunctiva. Tears are drained out through the puncta at the lid margins, into the lacrimal ducts and sac, and on into the nose through the nasolacrimal duct. The puncta are the only portions of the lacrimal apparatus normally visible without special maneuvers.

The eyeball itself is a spherical structure designed to focus a controlled amount of light on the neurosensory elements within the retina. Muscles within the iris control pupillary size. Muscles of the ciliary body control the thickness of the lens, enabling the normal eye to focus in turn on objects both near and far away. At the posterior pole of the eye the retinal surface shows a slight depression—the fovea centralis—which marks the point of central vision. The retina immediately around it is called the macula. The optic nerve with its retinal vessels joins the eye somewhat medial to this point. It is visible ophthalmoscopically as the optic disc. That portion of the eye posterior to the lens is termed the fundus of the eye. It includes all the structures normally inspected with the ophthalmoscope: retina, choroid, fovea, macula, optic disc and retinal vessels. The most anterior parts of the retina and the ciliary body are visible with the ophthalmoscope only by use of special techniques.

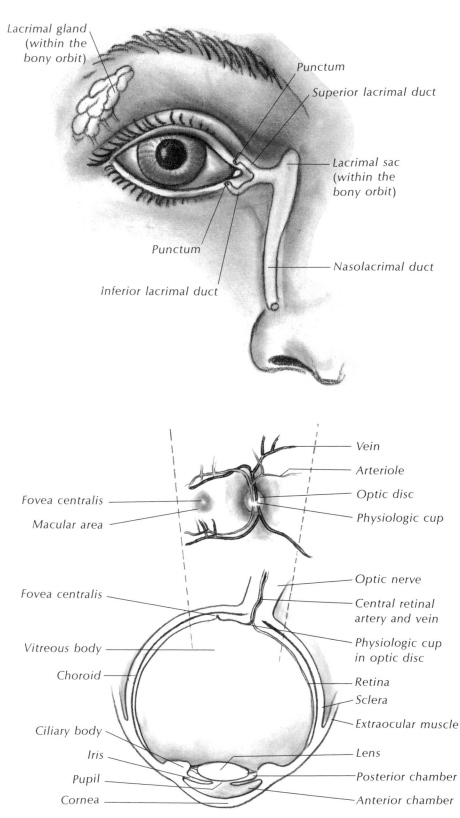

Cross Section of the Right Eye from above Showing a Portion of the Fundus Commonly Seen With the Ophthalmoscope

Visual Pathways. For a clear visual image, reflected light from an object must pass through cornea and lens and be focused on the retina. Images so formed are upside down and reversed right to left. An object in the upper temporal visual field, therefore, strikes the lower nasal quadrant of the retina.

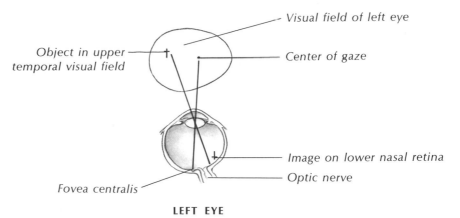

LEFT EYE

In response to this light stimulus, nerve impulses are conducted through the retina, the optic nerve, the optic tract and thence to the visual cortex of the occipital lobes. The spatial arrangements of nerve fibers in the retina are preserved in the optic nerves: temporal fibers run laterally in the nerve; nasal fibers run medially. At the optic chiasm, however, the nasal or medial fibers cross over so that the left optic tract contains fibers only from the left half of each retina; the right optic tract contains fibers from only the right.

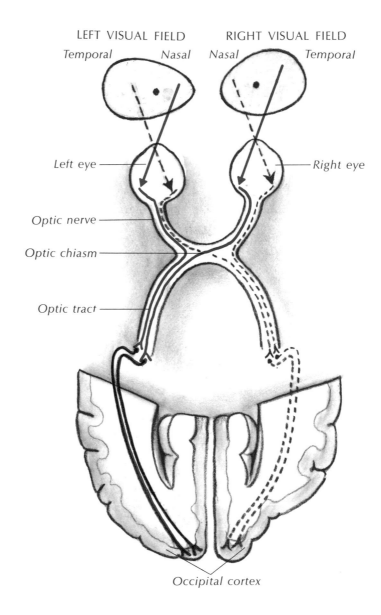

Visual Reflexes. By the sequence of events just described, light rays produce conscious vision. Light also stimulates reflex action of two kinds.

The Light Reflex. A light beam shining onto the retina causes reflex pupillary constriction of that eye *(direct light reflex)* and also of the opposite eye *(consensual light reflex).* The initial sensory pathways are similar to those described above: retina, optic nerve and optic tract. The pathways diverge, however, in the midbrain, and through a series of synapses impulses are transmitted through the oculomotor nerve (3rd cranial nerve) and thence to the constrictor muscles of the iris on each side.

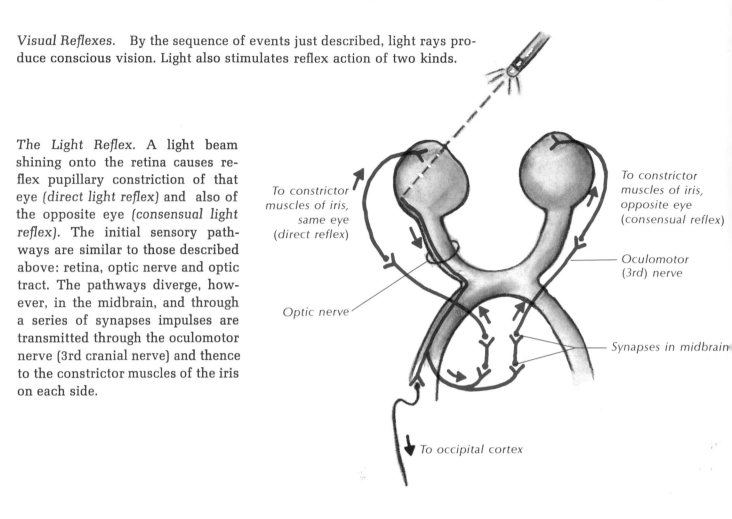

To constrictor muscles of iris, same eye (direct reflex)

To constrictor muscles of iris, opposite eye (consensual reflex)

Oculomotor (3rd) nerve

Optic nerve

Synapses in midbrain

To occipital cortex

Accommodation. Accommodation is the process by which a clear visual image is maintained as the gaze is shifted from a distant to a near point. There are three components of the accommodation reaction: convergence of the eyes, pupillary constriction, and thickening of the lens through contraction of the ciliary muscles. Only the first two are visible to the examiner.

Sensory pathways for accommodation are similar to those involving conscious vision. Nerve impulses then pass from the occipital cortex to the frontal cortex, thence to the midbrain and the oculomotor nerve.

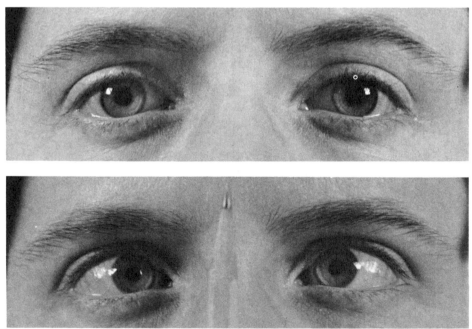

Autonomic Nerve Supply to the Eyes. Fibers traveling in the oculomotor nerve and producing pupillary constriction as described above are part of the parasympathetic nervous system. The iris is also supplied by sympathetic fibers. When these are stimulated, pupillary dilatation and also some elevation of the eyelid result. The sympathetic fibers travel through the sympathetic trunk and ganglia in the neck, then follow a nerve plexus around the carotid artery and its branches into the orbit.

Extraocular Movements. The movement of each eye is controlled by the coordinated action of six muscles, the four rectus and two oblique muscles. The function of each muscle, together with that of the nerve that supplies it, may be tested by asking the patient to move his eye in the direction predominantly controlled by that muscle. There are six such directions, known as the cardinal fields of gaze. These are shown in the next diagram. When the patient looks down and to the right, for example, the right inferior rectus (third cranial nerve) is principally responsible for moving the right eye while the left superior oblique (fourth cranial nerve) is principally responsible for moving the left. If one of these muscles is paralyzed, deviation of the eyes from their normal conjugate, or parallel, positions will be most obvious in this direction of gaze.

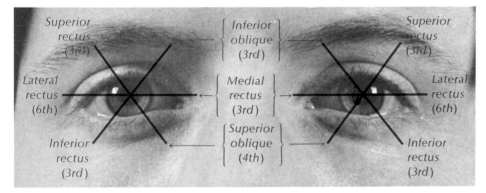

These muscles are correctly diagrammed for the intact human being but differ from the individual muscle functions described in most anatomy textbooks.*

*For further explanation, see:

Newell, F.W., Ernest, J.T. *Ophthalmology. Principles and Concepts.* St. Louis: The C.V. Mosby Company, 1974, pp. 35–36; and Duke-Elder Sir S., Wybar, K. *System of Ophthalmology, Vol. VI. Ocular Motility and Strabismus.* St. Louis: The C.V. Mosby Company, 1973, pp. 110–127.

The Ear

Anatomy. The ear has three compartments: the external ear, the middle ear and the inner ear.

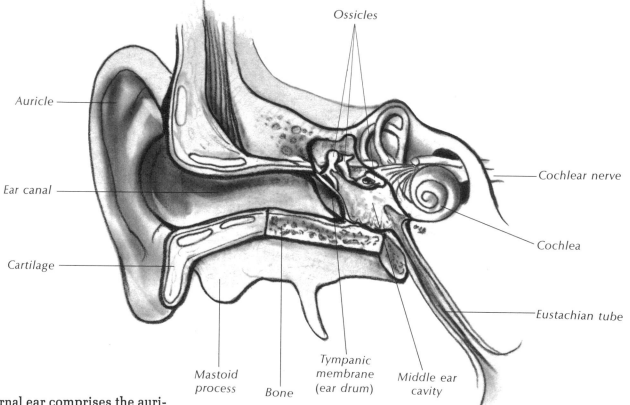

The external ear comprises the auricle and ear canal. The auricle consists chiefly of cartilage covered by skin and has a firm elastic consistency. The mastoid process, a bony prominence which is not part of the external ear, can be located just posterior to the lobule. It is the point of insertion for the sternomastoid muscle.

Behind the tragus of the ear opens the somewhat curving ear canal. Its outer portion is surrounded by cartilage, its inner portion by bone. The skin lining the bony portion is exquisitely sensitive, a point always to remember while examining the patient.

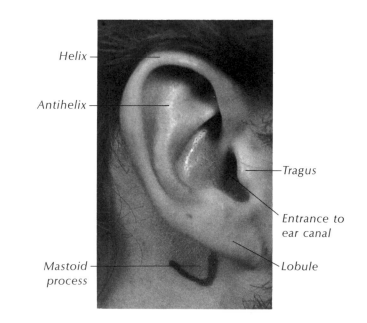

At the end of the ear canal lies the tympanic membrane or eardrum, marking the lateral limits of the middle ear. The middle ear is an air-filled cavity across which sound is transmitted by way of three tiny bones, the ossicles. It is connected by the Eustachian tube to the nasopharynx and is also contiguous with some air-filled cells in the adjacent mastoid portion of the temporal bone.

Inspection of the eardrum gives significant information about the condition of the middle ear; hence knowledge of its landmarks is important. The eardrum may be visualized as an oblique membrane pulled inward at its center by one of the ossicles, the malleus. The short process of the malleus protrudes into the eardrum above the handle. Most of the eardrum is rather taut—the pars tensa—and gives a characteristic reflection known as the cone of light. Superiorly the pars flaccida is less tensely stretched.

Much of the middle ear and all of the inner ear are inaccessible to direct examination. Some inferences concerning its condition can be made, however, by testing auditory function.

Pathways of Hearing. Vibrations of sound pass through the air of the external ear and are transmitted through the eardrum and ossicles of the middle ear into the cochlea or inner ear.

Here nerve impulses are initiated and sent to the brain via the cochlear nerve (a portion of the eighth cranial nerve). This pathway is the usual one in normal hearing. An alternate pathway used for testing purposes bypasses the external and middle ear by setting the bone of the skull into vibration and thereby stimulating the inner ear directly.

Pars flaccida
Short process of malleus
Posterior fold
Anterior fold
Pars tensa
Umbo
Cone of light
Handle of malleus
Posterior
Anterior

RIGHT EAR DRUM

Middle ear
Inner ear
Cochlear nerve
External ear
Air conduction pathway
Bone conduction pathway

Hearing over the usual pathways, including the air-filled external and middle ear, is called air conduction. Hearing dependent upon sound transmitted through bone to the inner ear is called bone conduction. In the normal individual, the usual pathway, i.e., air conduction, is the more sensitive.

Equilibrium. The inner ear has an additional important function in controlling balance. A discussion of this, however, is beyond the scope of this book.

The Nose and Paranasal Sinuses

Review the terms used to describe the external anatomy of the nose.

Approximately the upper third of the nose is supported by bone, the lower two-thirds by cartilage. Air enters the nasal cavity by way of the anterior naris on either side, then passes into a widened area known as the vestibule and on through the slit-like nasal passage to the nasopharynx. The medial wall of each nasal cavity is formed by the nasal septum, which like the external nose is supported by both bone and cartilage. It is covered by a mucous membrane well supplied with blood.

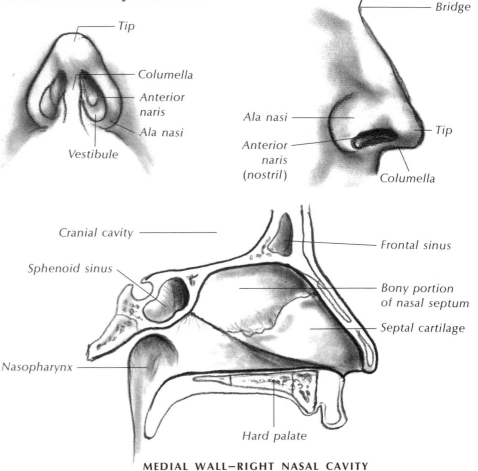

MEDIAL WALL—RIGHT NASAL CAVITY
(Mucous membrane removed to show the structure of the nasal septum)

Laterally the anatomy is more complex. Curving bony structures, the turbinates, covered by a highly vascular mucous membrane, protrude into the nasal cavity. Below each turbinate is a groove, or meatus, each named according to the turbinate above it. Into the inferior meatus drains the nasolacrimal duct; into the middle meatus drain most of the paranasal sinuses. Their openings, however, are not usually visible.

The additional surface area provided by the turbinates and the mucosa covering them aid the nasal cavities in their principal functions: cleansing, humidification, and temperature control of inspired air.

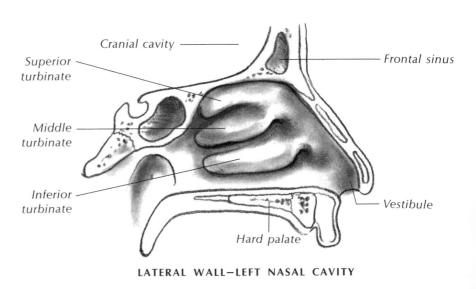

LATERAL WALL—LEFT NASAL CAVITY

Inspection of the nasal cavity through the anterior naris is usually limited to the vestibule, the anterior portion of the septum, and the lower and middle turbinates. Examination by means of a nasopharyngeal mirror is required for detection of posterior abnormalities. It is beyond the scope of this book.

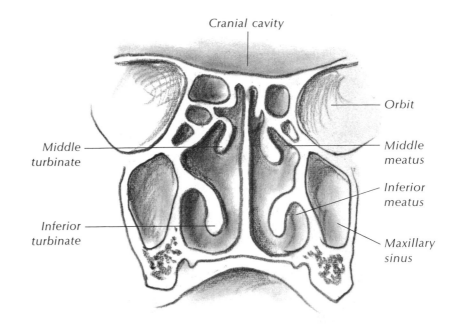

CROSS SECTION OF NASAL CAVITY—ANTERIOR VIEW

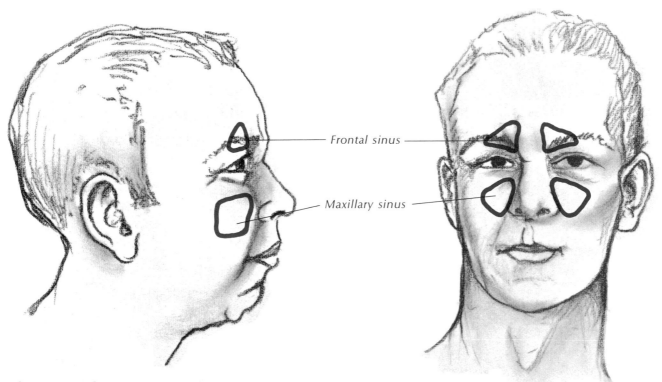

The paranasal sinuses are air-filled cavities within the bones of the skull. Like the nasal cavities into which they drain, they are lined by mucous membrane. Their locations are diagrammed above. Only the frontal and maxillary sinuses are readily accessible to clinical examination.

The Mouth and the Pharynx

Structures in the mouth and pharynx are illustrated below.

The dorsum of the tongue is covered by papillae, giving it a roughened surface. A thin white coating is frequent and normal. Often just visible toward the back of the tongue are the large vallate papillae. These should not be confused with tumor nodules.

Above and behind the tongue rises an arch formed by the anterior and posterior pillars, the soft palate and uvula. The tonsils can be seen in the fossae, or cavities, between the anterior and posterior pillars. The posterior pharynx may normally show small blood vessels and patches of lymphoid tissue on its surface.

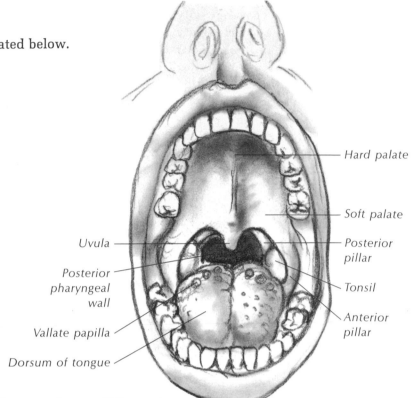

The under surface of the tongue is smooth. At its base can be seen Wharton's ducts—ducts of the submaxillary glands—and their openings. The parotid duct (Stensen's duct) opens onto the buccal mucosa near the upper second molar where its location is frequently marked by a small papilla.

A full complement of 32 teeth in the adult are identified below on the right.

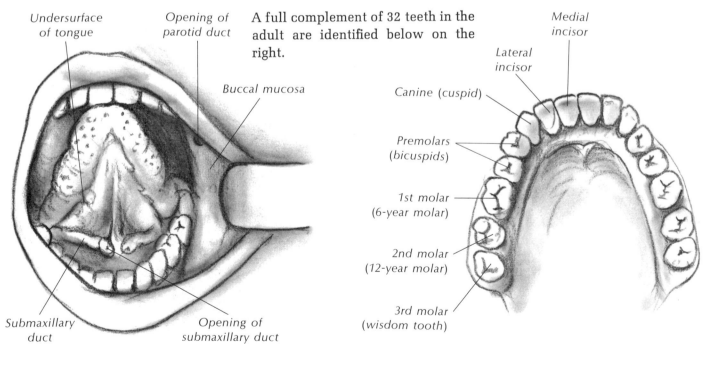

The Neck

For descriptive purposes each side of the neck is divided into two triangles by the sternomastoid muscle. The anterior triangle is bounded above by the mandible, laterally by the sternomastoid, and medially by the midline of the body. The posterior triangle extends from the sternomastoid to the trapezius and is bounded below by the clavicle. A portion of the omohyoid muscle crosses its lower portion and can be mistaken by the uninitiated for a lymph node or mass.

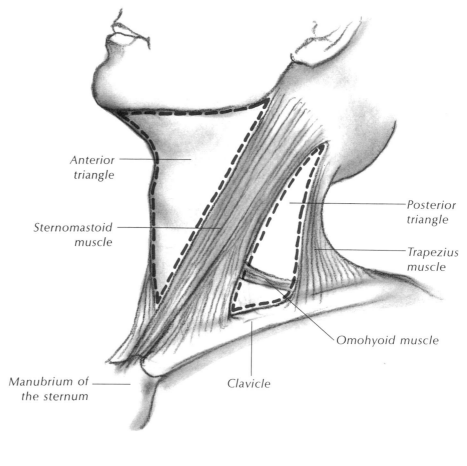

From above down identify the following midline structures: (1) the mobile hyoid bone just below the mandible, (2) the thyroid cartilage, readily identified by the notch on its superior edge, (3) the cricoid cartilage, (4) the tracheal rings and (5) the soft thyroid isthmus which lies across the trachea below the cricoid. The lateral lobes of the thyroid curve posteriorly around the sides of the trachea and the esophagus. They are partially covered by the sternomastoid muscles and are not usually palpable.

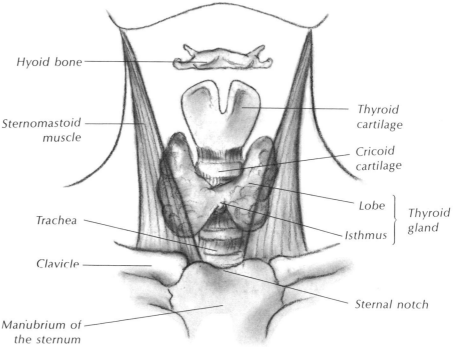

Deep to the sternomastoids run the great vessels of the neck: the carotid artery and internal jugular vein. The external jugular vein passes diagonally over the surface of the sternomastoid.

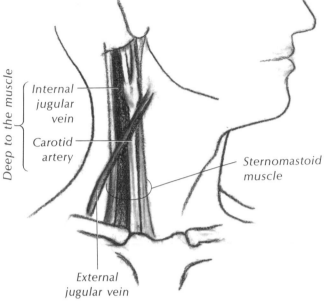

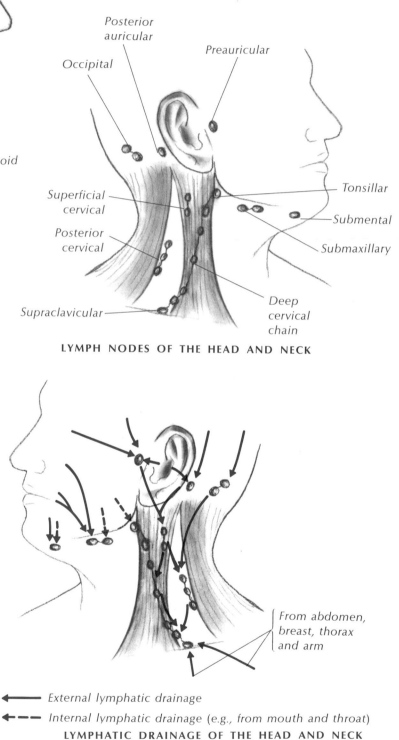

LYMPH NODES OF THE HEAD AND NECK

The lymph nodes of the head and neck have been classified in a variety of ways. One system of classification is shown here, together with the directions of lymphatic drainage. The deep cervical chain is largely obscured by the overlying sternomastoid muscle, but at its two extremes the tonsillar node and the supraclavicular nodes may be palpable. Note that the tonsillar, submaxillary and submental nodes drain portions of the mouth and throat as well as the more superficial tissues of the face. Knowledge of the lymphatic system is important to a sound clinical habit: whenever a malignant or inflammatory lesion is observed, look for involvement of the regional lymph nodes that drain it; whenever a node is enlarged or tender, look for a source in the area that it drains.

⬅——— *External lymphatic drainage*

⬅— — — *Internal lymphatic drainage (e.g., from mouth and throat)*

LYMPHATIC DRAINAGE OF THE HEAD AND NECK

The Head

Because abnormalities covered by the hair are so easily missed, ask the patient if he has noticed anything wrong with his scalp or hair.

Inspect and Palpate:

The Hair.   Note its quantity, distribution, pattern of loss if any, texture. Identify nits (the eggs of lice) if present, differentiating them from dandruff.

Fine hair in hyperthyroidism; coarse hair in hypothyroidism. Tiny white ovoid nits adherent to hairs; loose white flakes of dandruff

The Scalp.   Observe for scaliness, lumps or other lesions.

Redness and scaling in dandruff (seborrhea), psoriasis

The Skull.   Observe the general size and contour of the skull. Note any deformities, lumps or tenderness.

Enlarged skull in hydrocephalus, Paget's disease

The Face.   Note the patient's facial expression. Observe for symmetry, involuntary movements, edema, masses.

See Table 7-1, Selected Facies (p. 86).

The Skin.   Observe the skin, noting its color, pigmentation, texture, thickness, hair distribution, any lesions.

Acne, hirsutism

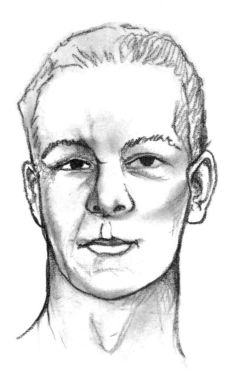

The Eyes

Visual Acuity.   For screening purposes, ask the patient to read any available print. He should use each eye separately, covering the other with an opaque card, not his fingers. With progressively worse acuity, ask him to count your upraised fingers and distinguish light from dark.

If more precise data are required, use a Snellen eye chart. The patient should wear glasses if he has them, but not if the glasses are intended only for reading. Position the patient 20 feet from the chart and ask him to read the smallest line of print possible. As before, test each eye separately. Determine the smallest line of print from which he is able to identify correctly more than half the figures. Record the visual acuity designated at the side of this line. Visual acuity is expressed as a fraction, e.g., 20/30, where the numerator indicates the distance of the patient from the chart, the denominator the distance at which a normal eye can read the chart.

The larger the denominator, the worse the vision

Visual Fields by the Confrontation Method.   This procedure is usually omitted in a routine examination but should be included whenever a neurological problem is suspected. Since it is a rather crude method, it should be supplemented, if indicated, by special techniques such as perimetry or a tangent screen.

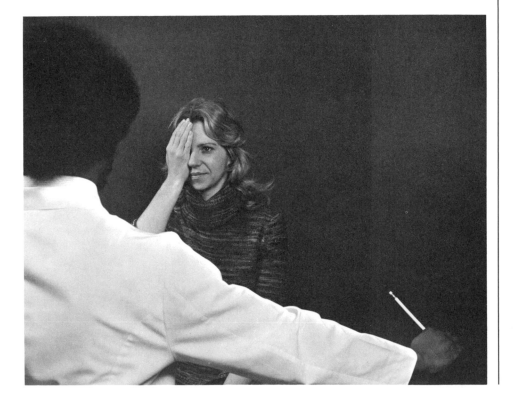

Ask the patient to cover one eye, without pressing on it, and to look at your eye directly opposite. Position yourself so that your face is directly in front and on the level with his, about 2 feet away. Close your other eye so that your own visual field is roughly superimposable on that of the patient. Bring a pencil or other small test object from the periphery into his field of vision from several directions as shown.

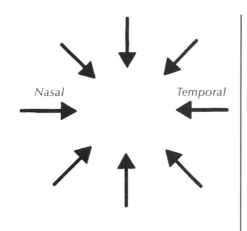

Nasal   Temporal

See Table 7-2, Visual Field Defects Produced by Selected Lesions in the Visual Pathways (p. 87).

The test object should be equidistant between you and the patient except in the temporal field. Because a normal person, even when looking straight ahead, can detect a moving object almost 90 degrees to the side, you must test his temporal field of vision by first placing the test object somewhat behind him, a location that is unavoidably well within your visual field. Moving slowly enough to give him time to respond, ask him to indicate when the object appears. Compare his field against your own.

Repeat with the other eye.

Position and Alignment of the Eyes.   Survey the eyes for their position and alignment with each other.

Exophthalmos, an abnormal protrusion of the eyeball

Eyebrows. Inspect the eyebrows, noting their quantity, distribution and any scaliness of the underlying skin.

Scaliness in seborrhea; loss of lateral 3rd in myxedema.

Eyelids. Note the position of the lids in relationship to the eyeballs. Inspect for:
   Edema
   Color, e.g., redness
   Lesions
   Condition and direction of the eyelashes

See Table 7-3, Abnormalities of the Eyelid (p. 88).

See Table 7-4, Lumps and Swellings in and Around the Eyes (p. 89).

Lacrimal Apparatus. Inspect the region of the lacrimal gland. If lacrimal gland enlargement is suspected, either because of the patient's history or your observation, elevate the temporal aspect of the upper lid and ask the patient to look down and to the opposite side. Observe for a swollen lacrimal gland protruding between the upper lid and eyeball. In many normal people a small portion of the lacrimal gland can be brought into view by this maneuver.

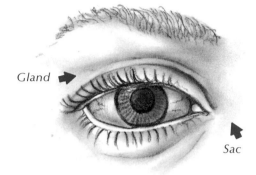

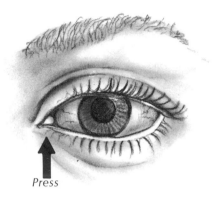

Inspect the area of the lacrimal sac for swelling. If tearing is excessive, check for nasolacrimal duct obstruction by pressing on the medial aspect of the lower eyelid just inside the orbital rim. Watch for regurgitation of fluid out of the lacrimal duct openings (puncta). Palpate the area for tenderness, but press only gently on an acutely inflamed lacrimal sac.

Regurgitation of fluid from the puncta suggests an obstructed nasolacrimal duct.

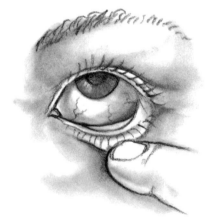

Conjunctiva and Sclera. Ask the patient to look up as you depress the lower lid of each eye with your thumb, exposing the sclera and conjunctiva.

Inspect both the sclera and the palpebral conjunctiva of the lower lid for color.

Note any nodules or swelling.

Yellow scleras of jaundice
Pale conjunctivas of anemia

See Table 7-5, Red Eyes (p. 90).

Special Technique for Inspection of the Upper Palpebral Conjunctiva. Adequate examination of the eye in search of a foreign body requires eversion of the upper eyelid. To do this:

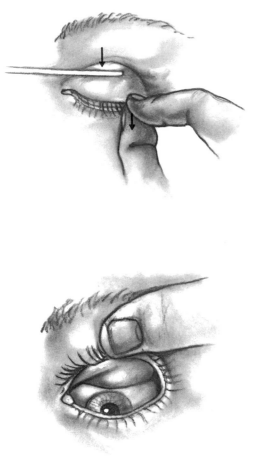

1. Instruct the patient to look down.
2. Get the patient to relax his eyes —by reassurance and by gentle, assured and deliberate movements.
3. Raise the upper eyelid slightly so that the eyelashes protrude, then grasp the upper eyelashes and pull them gently down and forward.
4. Place a small stick such as an applicator or tongue blade at least 1 cm above the lid margin (and thus at the upper border of the tarsal plate). Push down on the upper eyelid, thus everting it or turning it "inside out." Do not press on the eyeball itself.
5. Secure the upper lashes against the eyebrow with your fingers and inspect the palpebral conjunctiva.
6. After your inspection, grasp the upper eyelashes and pull them gently forward. Ask the patient to look up. The eyelid will return to its normal position.

Cornea and Lens. With oblique lighting inspect the cornea for opacities and note any opacities in the lens that may be visible through the pupil.

See Table 7-6, Opacities of the Cornea and Lens (p. 91).

Iris. Inspect the iris of each eye. Note its markings. Normally these are clearly defined.

Pupils. Inspect the size, shape and equality of the pupils.

See Table 7-7, Pupillary Abnormalities (pp. 92–93).

Test the *pupillary reaction to light.* Shine a bright light on each pupil in turn. Inspect for:

1. The direct reaction (pupillary constriction in the same eye)

2. The consensual reaction (pupillary constriction in the opposite eye)

Do not let the patient focus on the light during this maneuver lest pupillary constriction in response to near gaze confuse your observations. A darkened room and a bright light should always be used before deciding that a pupillary reaction is absent.

Test the *pupillary reaction to accommodation.* Ask the patient to look into the distance and then at your finger held 5 to 10 cm. from the bridge of his nose. Note:

1. The pupillary constriction
2. Convergence of the eyes   (Convergence is also part of the extra-ocular movement examination and if observed here need not be repeated.)

Extraocular Movements.   Test the range of extraocular movements through the six cardinal fields of gaze by asking the patient to follow your finger or pencil as you sweep through six motions: (1) to the patient's right; (2) upward, to the right of the midline; (3) then straight down; (4) to the left; (5) upward, to the left of the midline; (6) from there, straight down. Move your finger or pencil at a comfortable distance from the patient. Because middle aged or older people may have difficulty focusing on near objects (presbyopia), it is helpful to make this distance greater for them than for young people. Pause during upward and lateral gaze to detect nystagmus. In watching for nystagmus laterally, hold the patient's gaze within the field of binocular vision, avoiding extreme lateral fixation points.

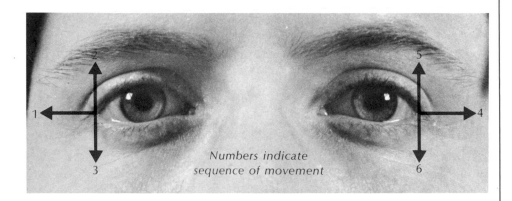

Numbers indicate
sequence of movement

Inspect for:
1. The normal conjugate, or parallel, movements of the eyes in each direction, or any deviation from normal.

   See Table 7-8, Deviations of the Eyes (p. 94).

2. Abnormal movements of the eyes, e.g., nystagmus, a rhythmic fine oscillation of the eyes. A few beats of nystagmus on extreme lateral gaze are within normal limits.

   Sustained nystagmus is seen in a variety of neurological conditions

3. The relation of the upper eyelid to the globe as he moves his eyes from above downward. Normally, the lid overlaps the iris slightly throughout this movement.

   Lid lag in hyperthyroidism: a rim of sclera is seen between the upper lid and iris; the lid appears to lag behind the globe.

Ask the patient to follow your finger or pencil as you move it in toward the bridge of his nose. Note convergence of the eyes. This is normally sustained to within 5 to 8 cm.

Poor convergence in hyperthyroidism

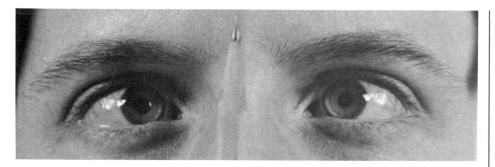

Ophthalmoscopic Examination. If possible, dilate the patient's pupils with an appropriate mydriatic drug such as tropicamide (Mydriacyl). Darken the room. Switch on the ophthalmoscope light and turn the lens disc to 0 diopters (a lens that neither converges nor diverges the light rays). Keep your index finger on the lens disc so that you can refocus the ophthalmoscope during the examination.

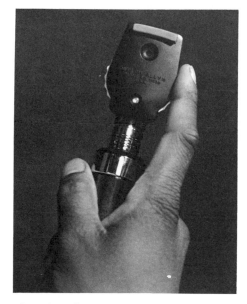

Use your *right hand* and *right eye* for the patient's *right eye;* your *left hand* and *left eye,* for the patient's *left eye.*

Place the thumb of your opposite hand on the patient's eyebrow. Ask the patient to look straight ahead or slightly toward the side you are examining. He should fix his gaze on a specific point on the wall. Hold the ophthalmoscope firmly braced against your face, with your eye directly behind its sight hole.

From a position about 15 inches away from the patient and about 15 degrees lateral to his line of vision, shine the light beam on his pupil.

Note the orange glow in the pupil—the red reflex. Also note any opacities interrupting the red reflex.

Absence of a red reflex suggests an opacity of the lens (cataract) or possibly of the vitreous. Less commonly, a detached retina may obscure this reflex. Do not be fooled by an artificial eye, which of course has no red reflex either.

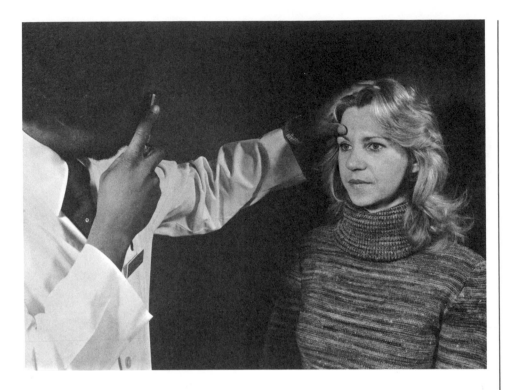

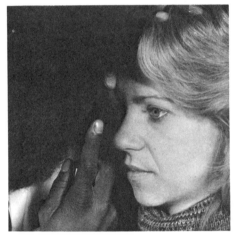

Keep your eyes relaxed, as if gazing into the distance. Try to keep both eyes open. Keeping the light beam focused on the red reflex, move in toward the pupil until your ophthalmoscope is very close to it. If you have approached on the 15 degree angle, you should now be seeing the retina in the vicinity of the optic disc, a yellowish round or oval structure. If not, follow a blood vessel centrally until you find it.

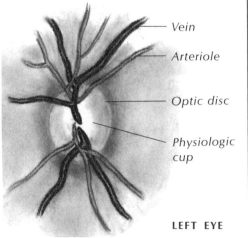

Vein

Arteriole

Optic disc

Physiologic cup

LEFT EYE

Bring it into sharp focus by adjusting the lens disc. When examining a near-sighted (myopic) patient, whose eyeball is somewhat longer than normal, you will need to use a lens with a longer focus. To do this, rotate the lens disc counterclockwise to the lenses identified by the red numbers, indicating minus diopters.* When examining a far-sighted patient or one whose own lens has been surgically removed, rotate the disc clockwise to the lenses of plus diopters, indicated by the black numbers.

A clear focus is obtained with a lens of 0 diopters (clear glass).

Normal eye

A lens with a longer focus (minus diopters) is needed to see the retina clearly.

Near-sighted eye

A lens with a shorter focus is needed (e.g., +1 or +2 diopters).

Far-sighted eye

NOTE:
1. The clarity of the disc outline. The nasal outline may normally be somewhat blurred.
2. The color of the disc, normally yellowish.
3. The possible presence of normal white or pigmented rings or crescents around the disc.
4. The size of the central physiologic cup, if present. This cup is normally yellowish-white.

See Table 7-9, Normal Variations of the Optic Disc (p. 95).

See Table 7-10, Abnormalities of the Optic Disc (p. 96).

*A diopter is a unit which measures the power of a lens to converge or diverge light.

Identify the arterioles and veins. They may be distinguished by the following features:

	ARTERIOLES	VEINS
Color	Light red	Dark red
Size	Smaller (2/3 to 4/5 the diameter of veins)	Larger
Light reflex (or reflection)	Bright	Inconspicuous or absent

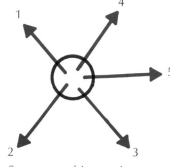

Sequence of inspection from disc to macula
LEFT EYE

Follow the vessels peripherally in each of four directions, noting their relative sizes and the character of the arteriovenous crossings. Move your head and instrument as a unit, using the patient's pupil as an imaginary fulcrum. Note any lesions of the surrounding retina.

Finally, by directing your light beam laterally or by asking the patient to look directly into the light, inspect the macular area. The tiny bright reflection from the fovea helps you to identify the relatively avascular macular region that surrounds it. Unfortunately, the patient frequently tears at this point, and the light reflection off his cornea may obscure your view.

See Table 7-11, Retinal Arterioles and Arteriovenous Crossings: Normal and Hypertensive (p. 97).

See Table 7-12, Red Spots in the Retina (p. 98).

See Table 7-13, Light Colored Spots in the Retina (p. 99).

— Macula

— Fovea

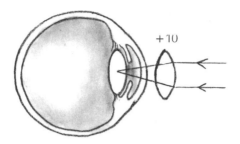

Anterior structures

If opacities in the vitreous or lens are suspected on clinical grounds or after initial inspection of the red reflex, inspect these normally transparent structures by rotating the lens disc progressively to diopters of around +10 or +12. This maneuver focuses on the anterior structures within the eyeball.

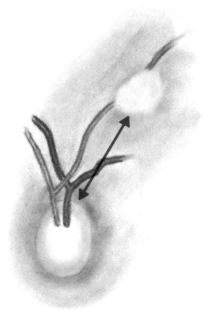

A Note on Measurement Within the Eye. Lesions of the retina can be located in relationship to the optic disc and are measured in terms of "disc diameters" and diopters. For example, "a lesion about 2/3 of a disc diameter in size located at 1 o'clock, almost 2 disc diameters from the disc" describes the abnormality shown on the left.

The elevated optic disc of papilledema can be measured by noting the differences in diopters of the two lenses used to focus clearly on the disc and on the uninvolved retina.

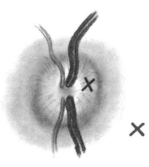

Clear focus here at +2 diopters

Clear focus here at −1 diopter

$+2 - (-1) = +3$, therefore a disc elevation of 3 diopters

For Interest. On ophthalmoscopic examination, the normal retina is magnified about 15 times, the normal iris about 4 times. The optic disc actually measures about 1.5 mm. At the retina, 3 diopters of elevation = 1 mm.

The Ears

The Auricle.   Inspect the auricle and surrounding tissues for deformities, lumps, skin lesions.

If ear pain, discharge or inflammation is present, check for tenderness by moving the auricle and by pressing on the tragus and mastoid process.

See Table 7-14, Nodules in and Around the Ears (p. 100).

Movement of the auricle and tragus is painful in acute otitis externa, but not in otitis media.

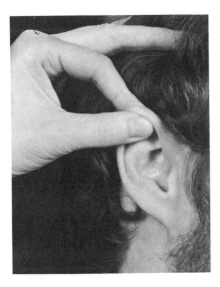

Ear Canal and Drum.   The patient's head should be tipped slightly to the opposite side. Grasp the auricle firmly but gently, pulling it upward, back and slightly out.

Using the largest speculum that the canal will accommodate, insert it slightly down and forward. Two possible grips are illustrated below. The first feels firm and natural. The second, because your hand is lightly braced against the patient's head, is especially helpful for active patients such as children.

Tenderness of the mastoid process suggests mastoiditis or posterior auricular lymphadenitis.

Non-tender nodular swellings covered by normal skin deep in the ear canals suggest osteomas. These are nonmalignant overgrowths that obscure the drum.

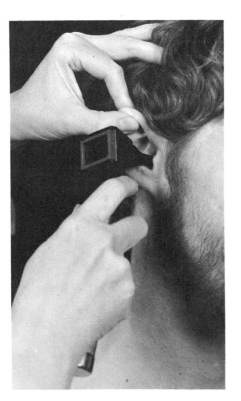

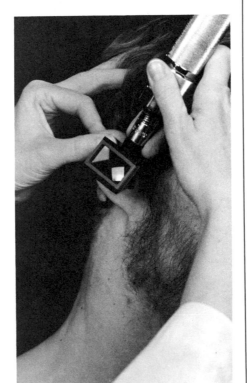

Identify wax, discharge or foreign bodies in the ear canal. Note any redness or swelling of the canal.

Redness, scaliness, narrowing, swelling and pain in acute otitis externa

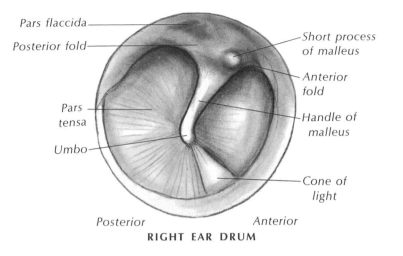

Pars flaccida

Posterior fold

Short process of malleus

Anterior fold

Pars tensa

Handle of malleus

Umbo

Cone of light

Posterior   Anterior

RIGHT EAR DRUM

Inspect the drum, identifying the landmarks: the pars tensa with its cone of light, the umbo, the handle and short process of the malleus, the anterior and posterior folds and the pars flaccida.

See Table 7-15, Abnormalities of the Eardrum (p. 101).

Gently move the speculum so that you can see the entire drum, including the periphery. Note the color, thickness and luster of the drum, the position of the light reflex and handle of the malleus or any perforations.

Fluid in the middle ear may be detected through the ear drum when a fluid level or air bubbles are identified. In most cases pneumatic otoscopy is required (see p. 399).

Auditory Acuity. To estimate hearing, test one ear at a time. Ask the patient to occlude one ear with his finger; or better still, occlude it for him. When auditory acuity on the two sides is quite different, simple occlusion of the better ear is inadequate. Under these circumstances move your finger rapidly, but gently, in the patient's ear canal. The noise so produced will help to prevent the occluded ear from doing the work of the ear you wish to test. Then standing 1 or 2 feet away, exhale fully (so as to minimize the intensity of your voice) and whisper numbers softly toward the unoccluded ear. Choose numbers that include two equally accented syllables, e.g., 14, 25. If necessary, increase the intensity of your voice to a medium whisper, a loud whisper, then a soft, medium and loud voice. To make sure the patient does not read your lips, cover your mouth or obstruct his vision.

Alternatively, a watch tick may be used. Since this sound is less relevant to functional hearing, it should not be used exclusively.

If hearing loss is present, distinguish between sensorineural deafness and conduction deafness by two maneuvers, both of which require tuning forks. Use a tuning fork of at least 512 or preferably 1024 cycles per second since it does not confuse sound with palpable vibrations and since it tests hearing within the frequency range of human speech (300–3000 cycles per second)—the functionally most important range. Set the fork into *light* vibration by stroking it between thumb and index finger or by tapping it on your knuckles.

1. *Test for lateralization (Weber Test).* Place the base of a lightly vibrating tuning fork firmly on the top of the patient's head or in the middle of his forehead. Ask where he hears it: on one or both sides. Normally the sound is perceived in the midline or equally in both ears. Sometimes the normal patient perceives the sound only vaguely. If he hears nothing, press the fork more firmly on his head.

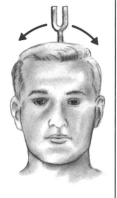

See Tables **7-16,** Patterns of Hearing Loss (p. 102).

2. *Compare air (AC) and bone con-duction (BC) (Rinne Test).* Place the base of a lightly vibrating tuning fork on the mastoid process until the patient can no longer hear the sound. Then quickly place the vibrating fork near the ear canal, with one side toward the ear as shown. Ascertain whether he can hear it. Normally the sound can be heard longer through air than through bone (AC > BC).

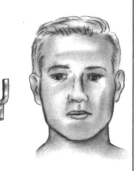

The Nose and Sinuses

Inspect the nose for deformity, asymmetry, inflammation.

Gently insert a nasal speculum through the nostril into the vestibule.

Two types of techniques may be used.

1. A nasal speculum, used with a head mirror or (by most who are not ENT specialists) a penlight. For this technique, grasp the speculum with your left hand, as shown, and insert the blades about 1 cm into the vestibule, stabilizing the instrument by placing your left finger on the patient's ala nasi. Open the blades widely in an anteroposterior direction, avoiding the sensitive septum. Do not switch examining hands for the opposite naris.

2. An otoscope, preferably equipped with a short, wide nasal speculum. This technique gives a narrower field of vision but has the advantages

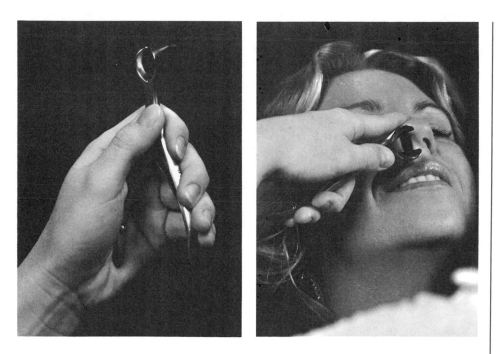

of good light and magnification. Again take care to avoid the nasal septum.

By either technique, inspect the lower portions of the nose, then tilt the patient's head backward with your other hand in order to visualize the upper portions.

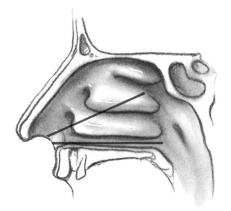

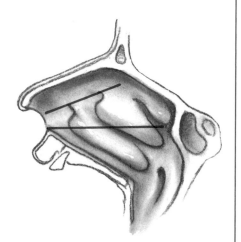

VIEW WITH HEAD ERECT   VIEW WITH HEAD TILTED BACK

Inspect:

1. The nasal mucosa, including its color (normally somewhat redder than the oral mucosa), swelling, exudate, bleeding.

2. The nasal septum, including evidence of bleeding, perforation, or deviation.

3. The inferior and middle turbinates and the middle meatus between them for color, swelling, exudate, polyps.

See Table 7-17, Common Abnormalities of the Nose (p. 103).

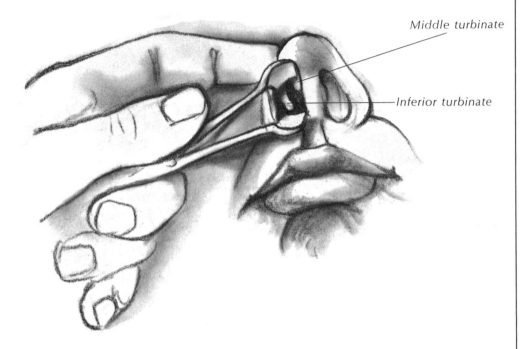

Middle turbinate

Inferior turbinate

Palpate for sinus tenderness by pressing up on the frontal and maxillary areas as shown. Avoid pressure on the eyes. (See p. 402 for the methods used to transilluminate the sinuses.)

Tenderness in acute sinusitis

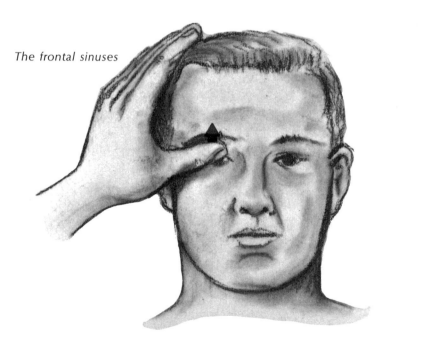

The frontal sinuses

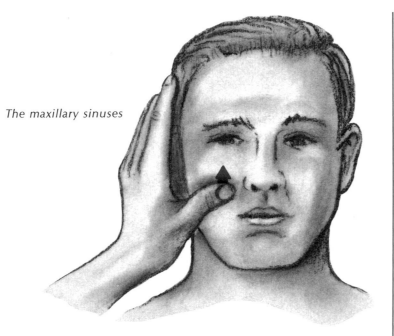

The maxillary sinuses

The Mouth and the Pharynx

If the patient wears dentures, offer him a paper towel and ask him to remove them. If suspicious ulcers or nodules are observed, put on a glove or finger cot and palpate the lesion, noting especially any thickening or infiltration of the tissues that might suggest malignancy.

Lips.   Inspect the lips for color, moisture, lumps, ulcers or cracking.

Cyanosis, pallor. **See Table 7-18,** Abnormalities of the Lips (pp. 104–105).

Buccal Mucosa.   Ask the patient to open his mouth. With a good light and the help of a tongue blade inspect the buccal mucosa for color, pigmentation, ulcers, nodules. Patchy pigmentation is normal in black people.

See Table 7-19, Abnormalities of the Buccal Mucosa and Hard Palate (p. 106).

Gums and Teeth.   Inspect for:

1. Inflammation, swelling, bleeding, retraction or discoloration of the gums.

2. Loose or carious teeth; abnormalities in the position or shape of the teeth.

See Table 7-20, Abnormalities of the Gums and Teeth (pp. 107–108).

Roof of the Mouth.   Inspect the color and architecture of the hard palate.

Tongue.   Inspect the dorsum of the tongue, its color and papillae. Note any abnormal smoothness.

See Table 7-21, Abnormalities of the Tongue (p. 109).

Ask the patient to put out his tongue and inspect it for symmetry—test of the 12th (hypoglossal) cranial nerve. Note its size.

Inspect the sides and the under surface of the tongue together with the floor of the mouth. These are the areas where malignancies are most likely to develop. Note any white or reddened areas, nodules or ulcerations. If any such abnormalities are present on or around the tongue, or indeed anywhere in the mouth, palpate the area, noting especially any induration.

Pharynx. Again ask the patient to open his mouth, this time without protruding his tongue. Grasp a tongue blade and press its free end firmly down upon the midpoint of the arched tongue—far enough back to get good visualization of the pharynx but not so far that you cause gagging. Simultaneously ask him to say "ah" or to yawn. Note the rise of the soft palate—test of the 10th cranial (vagus) nerve.

Inspect the soft palate, the anterior and posterior pillars, the uvula, tonsils and posterior pharynx. Note their color and symmetry, evidence of exudate, edema or ulceration, tonsillar enlargement. If possible, palpate any suspicious area for induration or tenderness.

Break or discard your tongue blade after use.

The Neck

Inspect the neck for symmetry, masses and scars.

Lymph Nodes. Palpate the lymph nodes. Using the pads of your index and middle fingers move the skin over the underlying tissues in each area, rather than moving your fingers over the skin. The patient should be relaxed, with his neck flexed slightly forward, and, if needed, slightly toward the side of the examination.

Feel in sequence for the following nodes:

1. Pre-auricular—in front of the ear
2. Posterior auricular—superficial to the mastoid process
3. Occipital—at the base of the skull posteriorly
4. Tonsillar—at the angle of the mandible

Tongue may enlarge in myxedema and amyloidosis.

Induration suggests malignancy.

See Table 7-22, Abnormalities of the Pharynx (p. 110).

5. Submaxillary—halfway between the angle and the tip of the mandible.

6. Submental—in the midline behind the tip of the mandible

7. Superficial cervical—superficial to the sternomastoid

8. Posterior cervical chain—along the anterior edge of the trapezius

9. Deep cervical chain—deep to the sternomastoid and often inaccessible to examination. Hook your thumb and fingers around either side of the sternomastoid muscle to find them.

10. Supraclavicular — deep in the angle formed by the clavicle and the sternomastoid

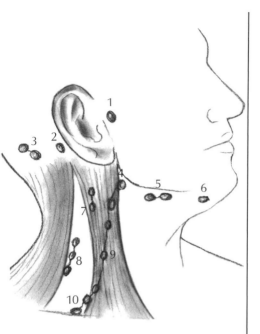

Note their size, shape, delimitation (discrete or matted together), mobility, consistency, tenderness. Small mobile discrete non-tender nodes are frequently found in normal persons. Detection of enlarged or tender nodes, if unexplained, calls for re-examination of the regions they drain.

Tender nodes suggest inflammation; hard or fixed nodes suggest malignancy.

Trachea and Thyroid.   Identify the hyoid bone, thyroid and cricoid cartilages, and the trachea.

Inspect the trachea for deviation.

Tracheal deviation from masses in the neck or mediastinum or from pleural and pulmonary abnormalities

Palpate the trachea for deviation. Place your finger on the trachea in the area of the sternal notch, slip it off the trachea to each side, noting any deviation from the midline.

Ask the patient to extend his neck slightly and to swallow. If he has difficulty swallowing give him some water, instructing him to hold it in his mouth and to swallow when asked. Inspect the neck for any visible thyroid tissue, noting its contour and symmetry.

Thyroid tissue rises with swallowing.

Palpate the thyroid, noting its size, shape, symmetry, tenderness, nodules. There are two approaches:

1. *Palpation from in Front.* With the pads of your index and middle fingers, feel below the cricoid cartilage for the thyroid isthmus. Ask the patient to swallow. Feel for the isthmus rising upward under your fingers.

The larynx, trachea and thyroid rise with swallowing; other structures such as lymph nodes do not.

Then move your fingers laterally and deep to the anterior border of the sternomastoid. Feel for each lateral lobe before and while the patient swallows.

Next, ask the patient to flex his neck slightly forward and to his right. Place your right thumb on the lower portion of his thyroid cartilage and displace it to the patient's right. Hook the tips of the index and middle fingers of your left hand behind the sternomastoid muscle while feeling in front of this muscle with your thumb. Your palpating fingers should be positioned below the level of the thyroid cartilage. Feel for the lateral lobe as the patient swallows. Reverse the procedure for the other side.

See Table 7-23, Thyroid Enlargement and Nodules (p. 111).

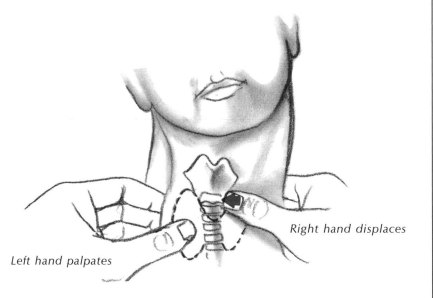

Left hand palpates

Right hand displaces

2. *Palpation from Behind.* Rest your thumbs on the nape of the patient's neck and with the index and middle fingers of both hands feel for the thyroid isthmus and for the anterior surfaces of the lateral lobes.

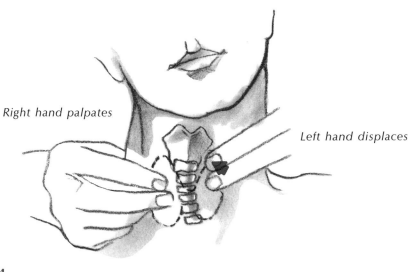

Right hand palpates

Left hand displaces

Then ask the patient to flex his neck slightly forward and to the right. Displace the thyroid cartilage to the right with the fingers of your left hand. Palpate with your right hand, placing your thumb deep to and behind the sternomastoid, and your index and middle fingers in front of it. Ask the patient to swallow. Reverse the procedure for the other side.

Occasionally palpation of the thyroid gland is more satisfactory with the patient's neck somewhat extended.

If the thyroid gland is enlarged, listen over the lateral lobes with the diaphragm of a stethoscope for a bruit (a sound similar to a cardiac murmur but of non-cardiac origin).

A localized systolic bruit may occur in hyperthyroidism and is to be distinguished from a carotid artery bruit or jugular venous hum.

NOTE: The ability to see or palpate a thyroid gland varies considerably not only with thyroid size but also with the patient's habitus. In a thin person, the isthmus is usually but not always palpable. It may be impossible to find in a stocky neck. Although normal lateral lobes are sometimes palpable, they more often are not.

The Carotid Arteries and Jugular Veins. You will probably wish to defer detailed examination of the great vessels of the neck until the patient lies down for the cardiovascular examination. Jugular venous distention, however, may be visible in the sitting position and should not be overlooked. Check the volume of each carotid arterial pulse by gently palpating the artery in the lower half of the neck. Examine one side at a time by gently placing your index and middle fingers just at or under the medial edge of the sternomastoid. Turning the patient's head slightly toward the side being examined may be helpful. (See Chapter 10 for further discussion.)

TABLE 7-1

TABLE 7-1. SELECTED FACIES

ACROMEGALY

The increased growth hormone of acromegaly produces enlargement of both bone and soft tissues. The head is elongated with bony prominence of the forehead, nose and lower jaw. Soft tissues of the nose, lips and ears also enlarge. The facial features appear generally coarsened.

Brow prominent

Soft tissues of nose, ears, lips enlarged

Jaw prominent

CUSHING'S SYNDROME

The increased adrenal hormone production of Cushing's syndrome produces a round or "moon" face with red cheeks. Excessive hair growth may be present in the mustache and sideburn areas and on the chin.

Red cheeks

Hirsutism

Moon face

MYXEDEMA

The patient with severe hypothyroidism, or myxedema, presents with a dull puffy facies. The edema, often especially pronounced around the eyes, does not pit with pressure. The hair and eyebrows are dry, coarse and thinned. The skin is dry.

Hair dry, coarse, sparse

Lateral eyebrows thin

Periorbital edema

Puffy dull face with dry skin

PAROTID GLAND ENLARGEMENT

Chronic bilateral asymptomatic parotid gland enlargement may be associated with obesity, diabetes, cirrhosis and other conditions. Note the swellings anterior to the ear lobes and above the angles of the jaw. Gradual unilateral enlargement suggests neoplasm. Acute enlargement is seen in mumps.

Local swelling obscures ear lobe

NEPHROTIC SYNDROME

The face is edematous and often pale. Swelling usually appears first around the eyes. The eyes may become slit-like when edema is severe.

Periorbital edema

Puffy pale face

Lips may be swollen

PARKINSON'S DISEASE

Decreased facial mobility blunts expression. A mask-like face may result, with decreased blinking and a characteristic stare. Since the neck and upper trunk tend to flex forward, the patient seems to peer upward toward the observer. Facial skin becomes oily, and drooling may occur.

Stare

Decreased Mobility

TABLE 7-2

TABLE 7-2 VISUAL FIELD DEFECTS PRODUCED BY SELECTED LESIONS IN THE VISUAL PATHWAYS

VISUAL PATHWAYS

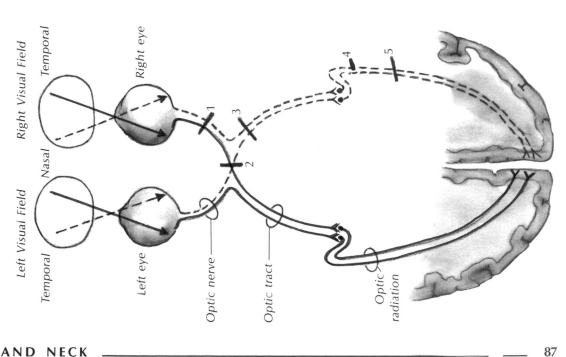

Left Visual Field   *Right Visual Field*

Temporal   *Nasal*   *Temporal*

Right eye

Left eye

Optic nerve

Optic tract

Optic radiation

VISUAL FIELDS

BLIND RIGHT EYE (Right optic nerve). A lesion of the optic nerve, and of course of the eye itself also, produces unilateral blindness.

BITEMPORAL HEMIANOPSIA (Optic chiasm). A lesion at the optic chiasm may involve only those fibers that are crossing over to the opposite side. Since these fibers originate in the nasal half of each retina, visual loss involves the temporal half of each field.

LEFT HOMONYMOUS HEMIANOPSIA (Right optic tract). A lesion of the optic tract interrupts fibers originating on the same side of both eyes. Visual loss in the eyes is therefore similar (homonymous) and involves half of each field (hemianopsia).

HOMONYMOUS LEFT UPPER QUADRANTIC DEFECT (Optic radiation, partial). A partial lesion of the optic radiation may involve only a portion of the nerve fibers, producing, e.g., a homonymous quadrantic defect.

LEFT HOMONYMOUS HEMIANOPSIA (Right optic radiation). A complete interruption of fibers in the optic radiation produces a visual defect similar to that produced by a lesion of the optic tract.

BLACKENED FIELD INDICATES AREA OF NO VISION

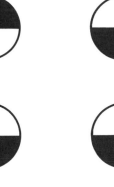
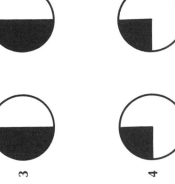
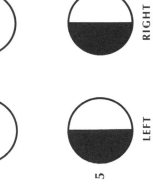

LEFT   RIGHT

1
2
3
4
5

TABLE 7-3

TABLE 7-3. ABNORMALITIES OF THE EYELIDS

ECTROPION

In ectropion, the margin of the lid is turned outward, exposing the palpebral conjunctiva. When the punctum of the lower lid turns outward, the eye no longer drains satisfactorily and tearing occurs.

RETRACTION OR SPASM OF THE UPPER EYELID AND EXOPHTHALMOS

A retracted upper lid is identified by noting a rim of sclera visible between the lid and iris. When this rim is visible as the eye moves from upward to downward gaze, it is called *lid lag.* A spastic lid and lid lag are signs of hyperthyroidism. They may simulate or accentuate the appearance of *exophthalmos* — an actual forward protrusion of the eyeball.

PERIORBITAL EDEMA

Caused by a variety of local and systemic conditions, periorbital edema exhibits a soft swelling of both lids.

PTOSIS

Ptosis refers to drooping of the upper eyelid. Causes include: (1) muscular weakness, (2) interference with the oculomotor nerve which controls voluntary elevation of the eyelid and (3) interference with the sympathetic nerves which maintain smooth muscle tone of the lid.

ENTROPION

An entropion is an inward turning of the lid margin. The lower eyelashes may produce irritation of the conjunctiva and cornea.

TABLE 7-4

TABLE 7-4. LUMPS AND SWELLINGS IN AND AROUND THE EYES

PINGUECULA

A yellowish triangular nodule in the bulbar conjunctiva on either side of the iris, a pinguecula is harmless. Pingueculae appear almost uniformly with aging, first on the nasal, then on the temporal side.

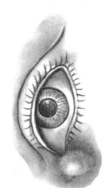

STY (ACUTE HORDEOLUM)

A painful, tender, red infection around a hair follicle of the eyelashes, a sty looks like a pimple or boil pointing on the lid margin.

CHALAZION

A beady nodule in an otherwise normal eyelid, a chalazion is usually painless. Occasionally a chalazion becomes acutely inflamed but, unlike a sty, usually points inside the lid rather than on the lid margin.

XANTHELASMA

Slightly raised, yellowish, well-circumscribed plaques in the skin, xanthelasmas appear along the nasal portions of one or both eyelids. They may accompany lipid disorders, e.g., hypercholesterolemia, but may also occur in normal individuals.

BASAL CELL CARCINOMA

A slowly progressive skin cancer, a basal cell carcinoma near the eye usually involves the lower lid. It appears as a papule with a pearly border and a depressed or ulcerated center.

INFLAMMATION OF THE LACRIMAL SAC (DACRYOCYSTITIS)

A swelling between the lower eyelid and nose indicates inflammation of the lacrimal sac. It may be acute or chronic. An *acute* inflammation is painful, red and tender and may have a surrounding cellulitis. *Chronic* inflammation is associated with obstruction of the nasolacrimal duct. Tearing is prominent and pressure on the sac produces regurgitation of material through the puncta of the eyelids.

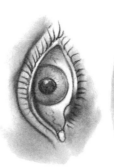

ENLARGEMENT OF THE LACRIMAL GLAND

An enlarged lacrimal gland may displace the eyeball downward, nasally and forward. A swelling is sometimes visible above the lateral third of the upper lid, giving the lid margin an S-shaped curve. Look for the enlarged gland between the elevated upper lid and the eyeball. Causes of lacrimal gland enlargement include inflammation and tumors.

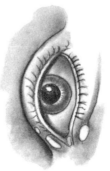

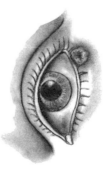

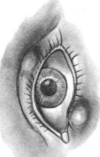

Tarsal plate and conjunctiva

Lacrimal gland

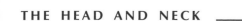

TABLE 7-5

TABLE 7-5. RED EYES

	CONJUNCTIVAL INJECTION	CILIARY INJECTION	ACUTE GLAUCOMA	SUBCONJUNCTIVAL HEMORRHAGE	BLEPHARITIS
Appearance					
Process	Dilatation of the conjunctival vessels	Dilatation of branches of the anterior ciliary artery which supply the iris and related structures	Dilatation of branches of the anterior ciliary artery; may also show some conjunctival vessel dilatation	Blood outside the vessels between the conjunctiva and sclera	Inflammation of the eyelids
Location of redness	Peripheral vessels of the conjunctivae, fading toward the iris	Central deeper vessels around the iris	Central deeper vessels around the iris; may also be peripheral	A homogeneous red patch, usually in an exposed part of the bulbar conjunctiva	Lid margins
Appearance of vessels	Irregularly branched	May radiate regularly or appear as a diffuse flush around the iris	Radiating regularly around the iris; peripherally may be irregularly branching	Vessels themselves not visible	Conjunctival and ciliary vessels normal unless there is associated disease
Color	Vessels bright red	Vessels more violet or rose colored	Vessels around iris violet or rose colored	Patch is bright red, fading with time to yellow.	Lid margins red, may have yellowish scales.
Movability	Conjunctival vessels can be moved against the globe by pressure on the lower lid.	Dilated vessels are deeper; cannot be moved by lid pressure.	Dilated vessels around the iris are deep; cannot be moved by lid pressure.	Not movable	Not relevant
Pupil size	Normal	Normal or small and irregular	Dilated, often oval, seen through a steamy cornea	Normal	Normal
Significance	Superficial conjunctival condition, as from irritation, infection, allergy, vasodilators	Disorder of cornea or inner eye. Requires prompt evaluation	Sudden increase in intraocular pressure because of blocked drainage from the anterior chamber. An ocular emergency	Often none. May result from trauma, sudden increase in venous pressure (e.g., cough), bleeding disorder	Often associated with seborrhea, staphylococcal infections

TABLE 7-6

TABLE 7-6. OPACITIES OF THE CORNEA AND LENS

ARCUS SENILIS

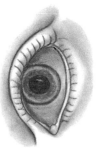

An arcus senilis is a thin grayish-white arc or circle not quite at the edge of the cornea. It accompanies normal aging. When present in young people it suggests the possibility of hypercholesterolemia.

CORNEAL SCAR

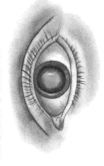

A corneal scar is a superficial grayish-white opacity in the cornea, secondary for example to an old injury or inflammation. Size and shape are variable. It should not be confused with the opaque lens of a cataract, visible on a deeper plane and only through the pupil.

PTERYGIUM

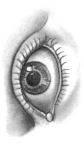

Not a true corneal opacity, a pterygium is a triangular thickening of the bulbar conjunctiva that grows slowly across the cornea usually from the nasal side. Reddening may occur intermittently. A pterygium may interfere with vision as it encroaches upon the pupil.

CATARACT

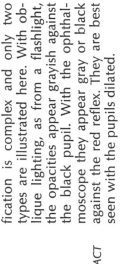

NUCLEAR CATARACT

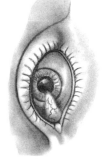

PERIPHERAL CORTICAL CATARACT

Cataracts are opacities of the lens and therefore can be viewed only through the pupil and on a deeper plane than corneal opacities. Classification is complex and only two types are illustrated here. With oblique lighting, as from a flashlight, the opacities appear grayish against the black pupil. With the ophthalmoscope they appear gray or black against the red reflex. They are best seen with the pupils dilated.

TABLE 7-7

TABLE 7-7. PUPILLARY ABNORMALITIES

BLIND EYE

Blind

Blind

When one eye is blind because of disease in the retina or optic nerve, the sensory limb of the light reflex arc is lost. A light shining into the blind eye produces no pupillary response in either eye. So long as the oculomotor nerve (the motor limb of the arc) is intact, however, a light directed into the sound eye produces normal responses in both eyes (normal direct and consensual reactions).

Sympathetic nerve lesion (Horner's syndrome)

Oculomotor nerve paralysis

Argyll-Robertson pupil

Retinal or optic nerve blindness

To occipital cortex

HORNER'S SYNDROME

This pupil is small, regular and unilateral. It is associated with ptosis of the eyelid and often with loss of sweating on the forehead of the involved side. Because of the ptosis, the eye may look small. Horner's syndrome is caused by interruption of the sympathetic nerve supply, most often in the neck. The pupil reacts to light and accommodation.

OCULOMOTOR NERVE PARALYSIS

A dilated pupil that reacts neither to light nor to accommodation results from injury to the oculomotor nerve. Ptosis and deviation of the eye laterally and downward may be associated.

TABLE 7-7

TABLE 7-7. (CONT'D)

ARGYLL-ROBERTSON PUPIL

Argyll-Robertson pupils are small, irregular and bilateral. They react to accommodation but not to light. They are often, but not necessarily, related to central nervous system syphilis (tabes dorsalis).

ANISOCORIA

Anisocoria is a descriptive, not a diagnostic, term and refers simply to inequality of the pupils. It is seen most often in dim light. Although slight pupillary inequality with normal pupillary reactions is a common normal variation, anisocoria should always be evaluated carefully.

DILATED FIXED PUPILS

Bilaterally dilated and fixed pupils result from anticholinergic agents (e.g., atropine, mushrooms) and from glutethimide (Doriden) poisoning. Additional causes that should be considered in the comatose patient are severe brain damage and profound hypoxia.

ADIE'S PUPIL (TONIC PUPIL)

This is a large, quite regular pupil usually confined to one side. The involved pupil reacts very slowly to light and accommodation. The disorder is benign and may be accompanied by diminished deep tendon reflexes.

IRIDECTOMY

COMPLETE   PERIPHERAL

A common cause of pupillary irregularity in the elderly is iridectomy, a surgical incision in the iris often made in the course of cataract extraction.

SMALL FIXED PUPILS

Bilaterally small fixed regular pupils result from morphine and related drugs, as well as from miotic drops given, for example, for glaucoma. In a comatose patient a pontine hemorrhage should also be considered.

TABLE 7-8

TABLE 7-8. DEVIATIONS OF THE EYES

Deviation of the eyes from their normally parallel position (often called strabismus or squint) may be classified into two general groups: (1) paralytic, in which either the extraocular muscles or one of the nerves that supplies them is paralyzed, or (2) non-paralytic.

PARALYTIC

Deviation during testing in the six cardinal fields of gaze

Present only in the field(s) of action of the involved muscles or nerves

Further observation

Note in which fields paralysis is present. For example, in a left 6th nerve paralysis:

Forward gaze—
Eyes parallel

Right lateral gaze—
Eyes parallel

Left lateral gaze—
Deviation apppears when the left eye does not move outward.

NON-PARALYTIC

Deviation during testing in the six cardinal fields of gaze

Constant in all fields

Further observation

Note whether the deviation is:

Convergent—

or Divergent

Check your findings with the cover test. Ask the patient to fix his gaze on a distant object.

Cover the right eye while you watch the left one.

Then cover the left eye while you watch the right.

If the uncovered eye swings into place as the opposite eye is covered, it must have been deviated. Repeat the test to be sure (see also pp. 392–394).

TABLE 7-9

TABLE 7-9. NORMAL VARIATIONS OF THE OPTIC DISC

PHYSIOLOGIC CUPPING

Central cup

Temporal cup

The physiologic cup is a small whitish depression in the optic disc from which the retinal vessels appear to emerge. Although sometimes absent, the cup is usually visible either centrally or toward the temporal side of the disc. Grayish spots are often seen at its base.

RINGS AND CRESCENTS

Choroidal crescent

Choroidal crescent

Scleral ring

Rings or crescents are often seen around the edges of the disc. They are of two types: (1) white scleral rings or crescents and (2) black pigmented choroidal rings or crescents.

MEDULLATED NERVE FIBERS

Medullated nerve fibers are a much less common but dramatic finding. Presenting as irregular white patches with feathered margins, they obscure the disc edge and retinal vessels.

TABLE 7-10

TABLE 7-10. ABNORMALITIES OF THE OPTIC DISC

	NORMAL	OPTIC ATROPHY	PAPILLEDEMA	GLAUCOMATOUS CUPPING
Process	Tiny disc vessels give normal color to disc.	Death of optic nerve fibers leads to loss of the tiny disc vessels.	Venous stasis leads to engorgement and swelling.	Increased pressure within the eye leads to increased cupping (backward depression of the disc) and atrophy.
Appearance	Color yellowish	Color white	Color pink, hyperemic	The base of the enlarged cup is pale.
	Disc vessels tiny	Disc vessels absent	Disc vessels more visible, more numerous, curve over the borders of the disc	—
	Disc margins sharp (except perhaps nasally)	—	Disc swollen with margins blurred	—
	The physiologic cup is located centrally or somewhat temporally. It may be conspicuous or absent, but its diameter from side to side is usually less than half that of the disc.	—	The physiologic cup is not visible.	The physiologic cup is enlarged, occupying more than half of the disc's diameter, at times extending to the edge of the disc. Retinal vessels sink in and under it, and may be displaced nasally.

TABLE 7-11

TABLE 7-11. RETINAL ARTERIOLES AND ARTERIOVENOUS CROSSINGS: NORMAL AND HYPERTENSIVE

NORMAL RETINAL ARTERIOLE AND ARTERIOVENOUS (A-V) CROSSING

Arteriolar wall (invisible)
Column of blood
Light reflex

The normal arteriolar wall is invisible. Only the column of blood within it can usually be seen. The normal light reflex is narrow—about ¼ the diameter of the blood column.

Vein
Arteriolar wall
Arteriole

Since the arteriolar wall is transparent, a vein crossing beneath the arteriole can be seen right up to the column of blood on either side.

THE RETINAL ARTERIOLE AND ARTERIOVENOUS CROSSING IN HYPERTENSION

FOCAL OR DIFFUSE SPASM

Narrowed column of blood
Narrowed light reflex
Focal narrowing

In hypertension the arterioles may exhibit areas of focal spasm causing an abrupt narrowing of the blood column. Or, the arteriole may be spastically narrowed along its entire course. The light reflex also is narrowed.

THICKENED ARTERIOLAR WALL WITH NARROWING AND INCREASED REFLEX

Thickened arteriolar wall
Narrowed column of blood
Widened light reflex

If the narrowing recurs or persists over many months or years, the arteriolar wall begins to thicken and becomes less transparent. These changes influence the color of the blood column within the vessel, giving it a yellow-red color, like a burnished copper wire. At this stage, the light reflex may be wider than normal.

Thickening of the arteriolar wall may also occur without hypertension, as a part of aging or as a result of other retinal diseases. It produces a variety of visible effects on arteriovenous crossings. These include:

CONCEALMENT OR A-V NICKING

TAPERING

SILVER WIRE ARTERIOLE

The vein appears to stop abruptly on either side of the arteriole.

The vein appears to taper down on either side of the arteriole.

Occasionally a portion of the arteriole has such an opaque wall that no blood is visible within it—a silver wire arteriole.

OTHER CHANGES IN HYPERTENSION

HEMORRHAGES AND EXUDATES
Soft exudate
A-V nicking
Hemorrhages

Hypertensive changes of a terminal arteriole may also stop the blood flow and result in a small infarct, visible as a "cotton wool" patch or "soft exudate." Small retinal hemorrhages may also be seen. (See **Tables 7-12** and **7-13**.)

TABLE 7-12

TABLE 7-12. RED SPOTS IN THE RETINA

1. *Flame-shaped hemorrhages* are small linear hemorrhages, often found in severe hypertension, but not specific to this condition.

2. *Deep hemorrhages* are small slightly irregular red spots often seen in diabetes. They may also be present in a number of other conditions.

3. *Microaneurysms* are tiny red spots commonly but not exclusively located in the macular area. They are characteristic of diabetic retinopathy.

4. *A preretinal hemorrhage*, located between retina and vitreous, is large and often characterized by a horizontal line separating red cells from plasma.

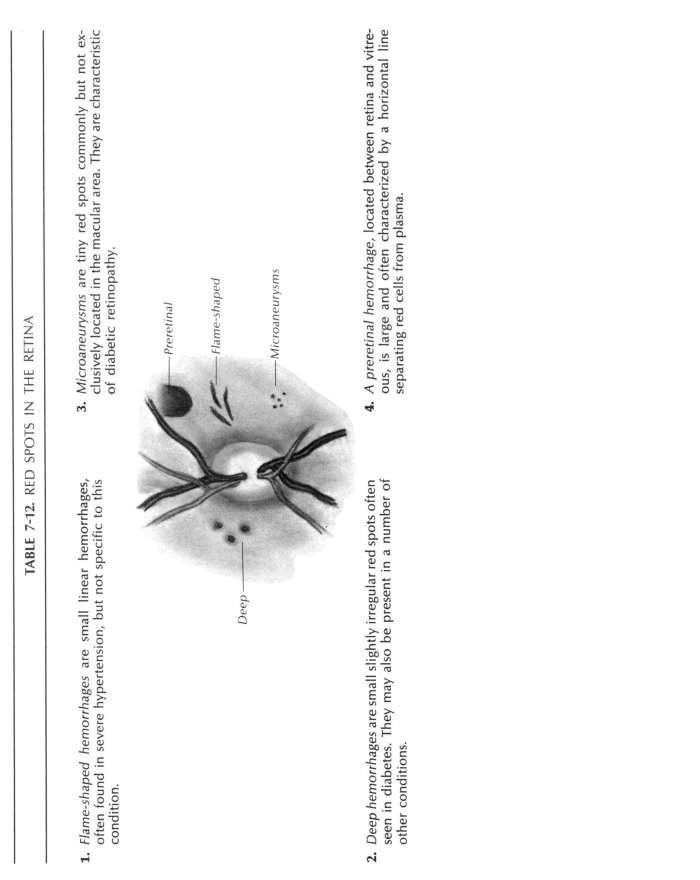

Preretinal

Flame-shaped

Microaneurysms

Deep

THE HEAD AND NECK

TABLE 7-13

TABLE 7-13. LIGHT COLORED SPOTS IN THE RETINA

	COTTON WOOL PATCHES (SOFT EXUDATES)	HARD EXUDATES	DRUSEN (COLLOID BODIES)	HEALED CHORIORETINITIS
Border	Ill-defined, fuzzy	Well-defined	Fairly well-defined	Well-defined, often outlined in pigment
Shape	Ovoid or polygonal; irregular	May be small and round or may coalesce into larger irregular spots	Round	Irregular
Size	Relatively large but smaller than optic disc	Small	Tiny to small	Variable: small to very large
Color	White or gray	Creamy or yellow, often bright	White to yellowish	White or gray with clumps of black pigment
Pattern	No definite pattern	Often in clusters, circular or linear patterns, or stars	Haphazardly and generally distributed, may concentrate at the posterior pole	Variable
Significance	Hypertension, other conditions	Diabetes, hypertension, other conditions	Concomitant of normal aging	Indicates old inflammation of many types

TABLE 7-14

TABLE 7-14. NODULES IN AND AROUND THE EARS

LYMPH NODES	SEBACEOUS CYSTS	TOPHUS	DARWIN'S TUBERCLE	CHONDRODERMATITIS HELICIS
Preauricular node / *Posterior auricular node* / *Mastoid process*	*Cyst* / *Punctum*	*Tophi*	*Typical location*	*Tender nodule*
Small lymph nodes just anterior to the tragus or overlying the mastoid process are quite common. Although sometimes visible, they are best detected by palpation.	Sebaceous cysts are common, especially behind the ear. They are characteristically *in* rather than beneath the skin and often show a central black dot or punctum which identifies the opening of the blocked sebaceous gland. Subcutaneous abscesses are also very common behind the ear.	Tophi are deposits of uric acid crystals characteristic of gout. They appear as hard nodules in the helix or antihelix. They occasionally discharge white chalky crystals.	A small elevation in the rim of the ear, a Darwin's tubercle is a harmless congenital variation from normal —the equivalent of the tip of a mammalian ear. It should not be mistaken for a tophus.	This entity is characterized by a small, chronic, painful, tender nodule in the helix of the ear. It usually affects men, involving the right ear more often than the left. It may be confused with a tophus or skin cancer. Biopsy is important.

TABLE 7-15

TABLE 7-15. ABNORMALITIES OF THE EARDRUM

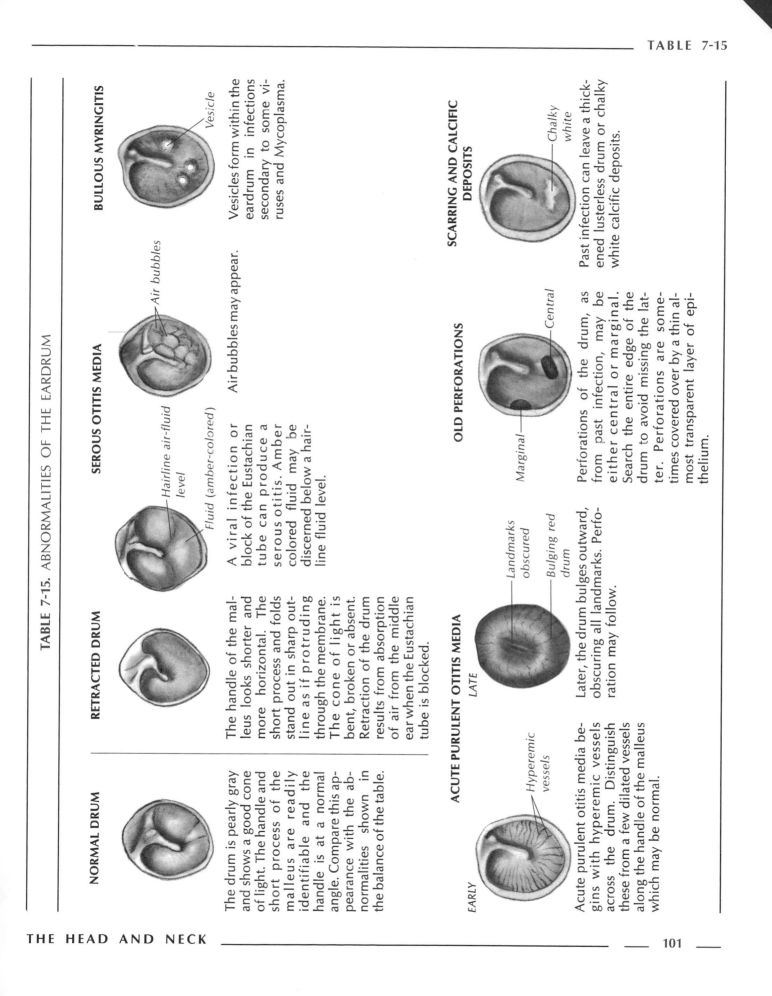

NORMAL DRUM

The drum is pearly gray and shows a good cone of light. The handle and short process of the malleus are readily identifiable and the handle is at a normal angle. Compare this appearance with the abnormalities shown in the balance of the table.

RETRACTED DRUM

The handle of the malleus looks shorter and more horizontal. The short process and folds stand out in sharp outline as if protruding through the membrane. The cone of light is bent, broken or absent. Retraction of the drum results from absorption of air from the middle ear when the Eustachian tube is blocked.

SEROUS OTITIS MEDIA

Air bubbles
Hairline air-fluid level
Fluid (amber-colored)

A viral infection or block of the Eustachian tube can produce a serous otitis. Amber colored fluid may be discerned below a hairline fluid level. Air bubbles may appear.

BULLOUS MYRINGITIS

Vesicle

Vesicles form within the eardrum in infections secondary to some viruses and Mycoplasma.

ACUTE PURULENT OTITIS MEDIA

EARLY
Hyperemic vessels

LATE
Landmarks obscured
Bulging red drum

Acute purulent otitis media begins with hyperemic vessels across the drum. Distinguish these from a few dilated vessels along the handle of the malleus which may be normal.

Later, the drum bulges outward, obscuring all landmarks. Perforation may follow.

OLD PERFORATIONS

Central
Marginal

Perforations of the drum, as from past infection, may be either central or marginal. Search the entire edge of the drum to avoid missing the latter. Perforations are sometimes covered over by a thin almost transparent layer of epithelium.

SCARRING AND CALCIFIC DEPOSITS

Chalky white

Past infection can leave a thickened lusterless drum or chalky white calcific deposits.

TABLE 7-16

TABLE 7-16. PATTERNS OF HEARING LOSS

Hearing loss is divided into two major types: (1) *conduction hearing loss* secondary to problems in the external or middle ear that impair the normal conduction of sound to the inner ear, and (2) *sensorineural (or perceptive) hearing loss,* produced by disease of the inner ear or 8th nerve. These two types may frequently be distinguished clinically. For example, consider a patient with a unilateral hearing loss.

CONDUCTION LOSS

PROCESS

Problem in the external or middle ear

WEBER TEST

Room noise blocked

Lateralizes to the poor ear. Because the poor ear is not distracted by room noise, it can detect bone vibrations better than normal. Test this on yourself by doing a Weber test while occluding one ear with your finger. This lateralization disappears in an absolutely quiet room.

RINNE TEST

Bone conduction lasts longer than air conduction (BC > AC). Pathways of normal conduction through the external or middle ear are blocked. Vibrations through bone bypass the obstruction.

SENSORINEURAL LOSS

PROCESS

Problem in the inner ear or nerve

WEBER TEST

Lateralizes to the good ear. The inner ear or nerve is less able to receive vibrations arriving by any route, including bone. The sound is therefore heard in the better ear.

RINNE TEST

Air conduction lasts longer than bone conduction (AC > BC). The inner ear or nerve is less able to perceive vibrations arriving by either route. The normal pattern prevails.

TABLE 7-17

TABLE 7-17. COMMON ABNORMALITIES OF THE NOSE

FURUNCLE OF THE NOSE

White center
Red margin

Furuncles are quite common in the nasal vestibule. The area is tender and may be red and swollen; then a typical pustule forms. Gentle examination is mandatory. Avoid manipulation since this may spread the infection.

ACUTE RHINITIS (THE COMMON COLD)

Red, swollen

The nasal mucosa is red and swollen. Nasal discharge, which is at first watery and copious, becomes thick and mucopurulent.

ALLERGIC RHINITIS

Pale, swollen

The nasal mucosa is swollen, pale, boggy, and usually gray. A dull red or bluish color may also be seen. Similar findings are seen in some patients with non-allergic vasomotor rhinitis.

NASAL POLYPS

Nasal polyps may develop in patients with allergic rhinitis. They are usually found in the middle meatus where they appear as gelatinous or soft, pale gray structures. Unlike the turbinates, for which they are sometimes mistaken, they are mobile.

SEPTAL DEVIATION

Displaced septum

Septal cartilage
Inferior turbinate
Displaced septal cartilage
Bone

CROSS SECTION VIEWED FROM THE FRONT

Some degree of septal deviation is common in most adults. Illustrated here is one of the most frequent types—displacement of the septal cartilage in the anterior portion of the nose. Septal deviation may produce nasal obstruction but the turbinates often accommodate to the asymmetry. Most septal deviations are asymptomatic.

TABLE 7-18

TABLE 7-18. ABNORMALITIES OF THE LIPS

HERPES SIMPLEX
(COLD SORE, FEVER BLISTER)

Blisters with crusting

The virus Herpes simplex may produce recurrent vesicular eruptions of the lips and surrounding tissues. A small cluster of blisters develops. As these break, a crust is formed and healing ensues within 10 to 14 days.

CHANCRE

Firm ulcer

The primary lesion of syphilis may appear on the lip instead of in its more common location on the genitalia. It is a firm button-like lesion which ulcerates and may become crusted. A chancre may resemble a carcinoma or a crusted cold sore. Use a glove for palpation. Dark field examination is necessary for diagnosis.

ANGULAR STOMATITIS
(CHEILOSIS)

Softening, fissuring

Softening of the skin at the angles of the mouth, followed by fissuring or cracking, is called angular stomatitis or cheilosis. Although rarely secondary to riboflavin deficiency, it more commonly is caused by over closure of the mouth, e.g., in patients without teeth or with dentures that are too short in their vertical dimension. Saliva then wets and macerates the infolded skin, often leading to secondary infection from Candida or bacteria. The mucous membrane remains uninvolved.

CHEILITIS

Fissures, scales and crusts

Painful fissuring with inflammation, scaling and crust formation characterizes cheilitis. Involving chiefly the lower lip, cheilitis is often chronic. Its causes are several and may be obscure.

TABLE 7-18

TABLE 7-18. (CONT'D)

MUCOUS RETENTION CYST (MUCOCELE)

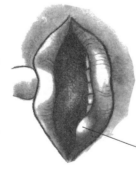

Round nodule

A round, regular, partially translucent or bluish nodule in the lip is probably a mucous retention cyst or mucocele. This is a benign lesion, having chiefly cosmetic importance. Size varies from tiny up to 1 to 2 cm in diameter. The cysts may also occur inside the lower lip in the buccal mucosa.

CARCINOMA OF THE LIP

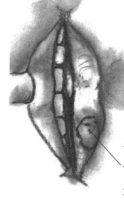

Non-healing

Carcinoma of the lip usually involves the lower lip and may appear as a thickened plaque, ulcer or warty growth. Any sore or crusting lesion on the lip that does not heal must be considered suspicious.

PEUTZ-JEGHERS SYNDROME

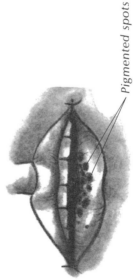

Pigmented spots

When pigmented spots on the lips are more prominent than freckling of the surrounding skin, suspect the Peutz-Jeghers syndrome. Look for abnormal pigment in the buccal mucosa to help confirm the diagnosis. Pigmented spots may also be found on the face, fingers and hands. These findings are important because they are often associated with multiple intestinal polyps.

ANGIONEUROTIC EDEMA

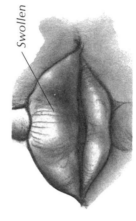

Swollen

Angioneurotic edema presents as a diffuse non-pitting, tense subcutaneous swelling that may involve a number of structures, including the lips. It appears rather rapidly, generally disappearing in a day or two. Although usually allergic in nature and sometimes associated with hives, it does not usually itch.

TABLE 7-19

TABLE 7-19. ABNORMALITIES OF THE BUCCAL MUCOSA AND HARD PALATE

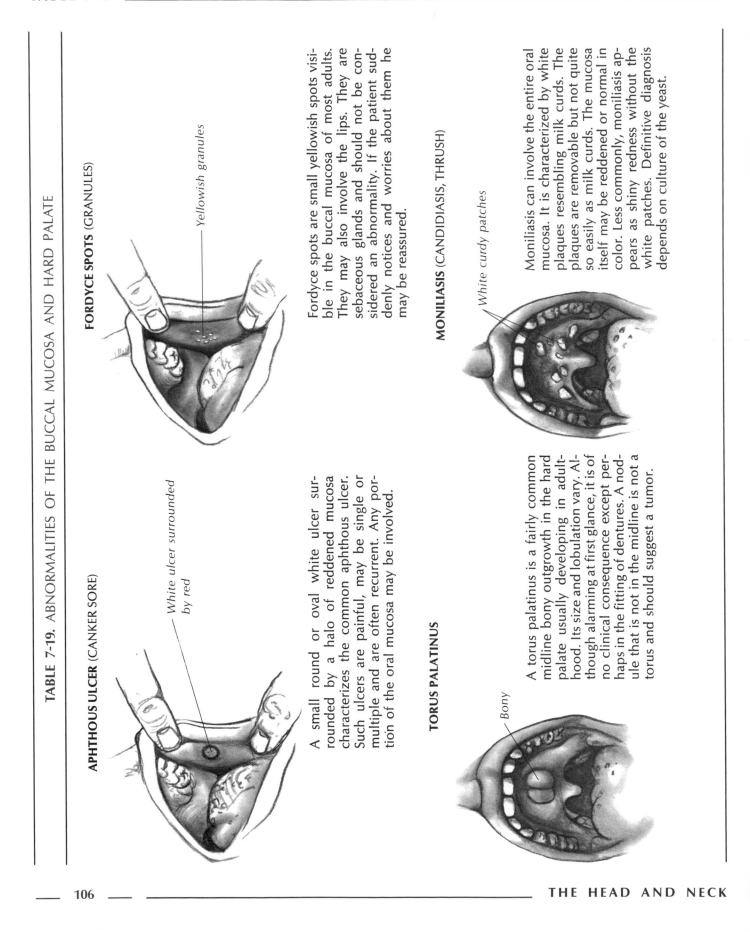

FORDYCE SPOTS (GRANULES)

Yellowish granules

Fordyce spots are small yellowish spots visible in the buccal mucosa of most adults. They may also involve the lips. They are sebaceous glands and should not be considered an abnormality. If the patient suddenly notices and worries about them he may be reassured.

APHTHOUS ULCER (CANKER SORE)

White ulcer surrounded by red

A small round or oval white ulcer surrounded by a halo of reddened mucosa characterizes the common aphthous ulcer. Such ulcers are painful, may be single or multiple and are often recurrent. Any portion of the oral mucosa may be involved.

MONILIASIS (CANDIDIASIS, THRUSH)

White curdy patches

Moniliasis can involve the entire oral mucosa. It is characterized by white plaques resembling milk curds. The plaques are removable but not quite so easily as milk curds. The mucosa itself may be reddened or normal in color. Less commonly, moniliasis appears as shiny redness without the white patches. Definitive diagnosis depends on culture of the yeast.

TORUS PALATINUS

Bony

A torus palatinus is a fairly common midline bony outgrowth in the hard palate usually developing in adulthood. Its size and lobulation vary. Although alarming at first glance, it is of no clinical consequence except perhaps in the fitting of dentures. A nodule that is not in the midline is not a torus and should suggest a tumor.

TABLE 7-20

TABLE 7-20. ABNORMALITIES OF THE GUMS AND TEETH

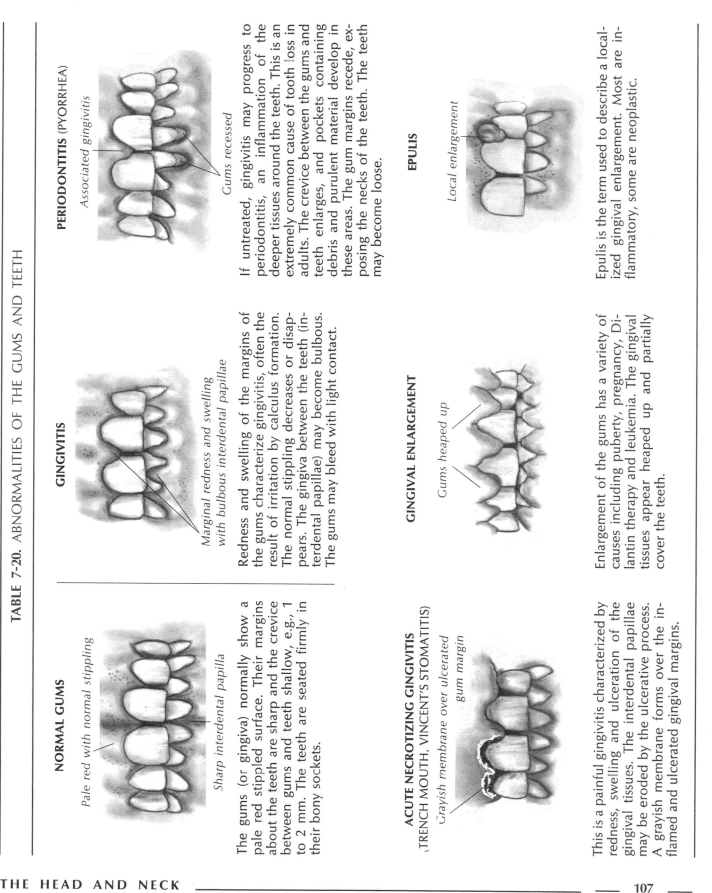

NORMAL GUMS

Pale red with normal stippling

Sharp interdental papilla

The gums (or gingiva) normally show a pale red stippled surface. Their margins about the teeth are sharp and the crevice between gums and teeth shallow, e.g., 1 to 2 mm. The teeth are seated firmly in their bony sockets.

GINGIVITIS

Marginal redness and swelling with bulbous interdental papillae

Redness and swelling of the margins of the gums characterize gingivitis, often the result of irritation by calculus formation. The normal stippling decreases or disappears. The gingiva between the teeth (interdental papillae) may become bulbous. The gums may bleed with light contact.

PERIODONTITIS (PYORRHEA)

Associated gingivitis

Gums recessed

If untreated, gingivitis may progress to periodontitis, an inflammation of the deeper tissues around the teeth. This is an extremely common cause of tooth loss in adults. The crevice between the gums and teeth enlarges, and pockets containing debris and purulent material develop in these areas. The gum margins recede, exposing the necks of the teeth. The teeth may become loose.

ACUTE NECROTIZING GINGIVITIS
(TRENCH MOUTH, VINCENT'S STOMATITIS)

Grayish membrane over ulcerated gum margin

This is a painful gingivitis characterized by redness, swelling and ulceration of the gingival tissues. The interdental papillae may be eroded by the ulcerative process. A grayish membrane forms over the inflamed and ulcerated gingival margins.

GINGIVAL ENLARGEMENT

Gums heaped up

Enlargement of the gums has a variety of causes including puberty, pregnancy, Dilantin therapy and leukemia. The gingival tissues appear heaped up and partially cover the teeth.

EPULIS

Local enlargement

Epulis is the term used to describe a localized gingival enlargement. Most are inflammatory, some are neoplastic.

TABLE 7-20

TABLE 7-20 (CONT'D)

LEAD OR BISMUTH LINE

Bluish black line

In chronic lead or bismuth poisoning a bluish-black line may appear on the gums about 1 mm from the gum margin. It does not appear where teeth are absent. Distinguish it from the much more common melanin pigmentation.

MELANIN PIGMENTATION

Patchy brown pigment

A brownish melanin pigmentation of the gums is frequently observed. It is normal in blacks and other dark-skinned individuals and may occasionally be seen even in light-skinned persons. A similar pigment pattern may be associated with Addison's disease.

DENTAL CARIES

Discolored, with cavitation

Chalky white

Dental caries is first visible as a chalky white deposit in the enamel surface of the tooth. This area may then discolor to brown or black, become soft and cavitate. Special dental techniques including X-rays are necessary for early detection.

HUTCHINSON'S TEETH

Smaller teeth, more widely spaced

Sides taper   Central notches

Hutchinson's teeth are notched on their biting surfaces, smaller than normal and more widely spaced. Their sides taper in. The upper central incisors are most often affected; the permanent, not the deciduous teeth, are involved. They are a sign of congenital syphilis.

ABRASION OF TEETH WITH NOTCHING

Notches

Sides normal, do not taper

The biting surface of the teeth may become abraded or notched by recurrent trauma, e.g., from opening bobby pins with one's teeth or holding nails between the teeth. Unlike Hutchinson's teeth, the sides of these teeth show their normal contours; size and spacing are unaffected.

ATTRITION OF TEETH

Exposed dentin

The teeth of many elderly people have been simply worn down by repetitive chewing. This flattening of the biting surfaces is called attrition. The enamel may be worn away, exposing the underlying dentin. The latter often takes on a yellow or brownish stain.

TABLE 7-21

TABLE 7-21. ABNORMALITIES OF THE TONGUE

SMOOTH TONGUE

In contrast to common lay ideas, a coated tongue is normal, a smooth red tongue is not. Loss of papillae gives the tongue a red slick appearance, often beginning at the edges. It suggests a deficiency of vitamin B₁₂, niacin or iron.

HAIRY TONGUE

The "hair" of hairy tongue consists of elongated papillae on the dorsum of the tongue and is yellowish to brown to black. Although alarming or annoying to the patient, it is clinically benign. The cause is unknown.

GEOGRAPHIC TONGUE

Geographic tongue is characterized by scattered red areas on the dorsum of the tongue that are denuded of their papillae and are smooth. The contrast of these areas with the normal roughened and coated surface gives a map-like pattern which changes over time. Of unknown cause, the condition is benign.

FISSURED TONGUE

Fissures may appear in the tongue with increasing age and at times become numerous, giving rise to the alternate term "scrotal tongue." Although food debris may accumulate in the crevices and become irritating, the fissured tongue has little significance.

12TH NERVE PARALYSIS

Paralysis of the 12th cranial (hypoglossal) nerve produces atrophy and fasciculations of the involved half of the tongue. Deviation toward the paralyzed side occurs when the tongue is protruded.

VARICOSE VEINS OF THE TONGUE

Small purplish or blue-black round swellings may appear under the tongue with age and have aptly been called "caviar lesions." They have no significance. As with several other tongue findings, familiarity with them pays dividends when the patient or the examiner first notices them. Reassurance is in order.

LEUKOPLAKIA

Leukoplakia is a term applied to a thickened white patch adherent to the mucous membrane. Its appearance has been likened to dried white paint. Although tongue involvement is illustrated here, leukoplakia may involve any part of the oral mucosa. Its primary significance lies in the fact that it may be pre-malignant.

CARCINOMA

Carcinoma of the tongue is uncommon on the dorsum of the tongue where it might be most readily noticed. Look for it at the base or edges of the tongue. Any ulcer or nodule which fails to heal in two or three weeks must be considered suspicious.

TABLE 7-22

TABLE 7-22. ABNORMALITIES OF THE PHARYNX

VIRAL PHARYNGITIS

Slight redness

Prominent lymphoid patches

Viral pharyngitis may present few if any signs. Mild redness, slight swelling of the pillars and prominence of the lymphoid patches on the posterior pharyngeal wall are frequently seen.

STREPTOCOCCAL PHARYNGITIS

Swollen uvula

Red

Enlarged tonsils with white patches

Classically streptococcal infection produces redness and swelling of the tonsils, pillars and uvula, with white or yellow patches of exudate on the tonsils. Accurate diagnosis on clinical grounds alone is frequently impossible, however, since streptococcal pharyngitis may occur without exudate and some viral illnesses and infectious mononucleosis may produce an exudative pharyngitis.

DIPHTHERIA

Swollen uvula   *Grayish membrane*

Swollen pillars   *Dull red*

Now rare, diphtheria is included here because without prompt diagnosis and treatment it may prove fatal. The throat is dull red and swollen. A thick exudate forms on the tonsils, and, unlike a streptococcal exudate, may spread over the soft palate and uvula. The throat is less painful than might be expected, the patient sick.

TONSILLAR HYPERTROPHY

Enlarged tonsils

The tonsils may be enlarged without being infected. They may protrude medially beyond the edges of the pillars even to the midline when the tongue is protruded. The size of the tonsils is not in itself an indicator of disease.

PARALYSIS OF THE 10TH CRANIAL (VAGUS) NERVE

Failure to rise   *Deviated to left*

When the patient says "ah" the soft palate on the paralyzed side fails to rise. The uvula deviates to the uninvolved side.

PERITONSILLAR ABSCESS (QUINSY SORE THROAT)

Uvula displaced

Red, tense, bulging

Peritonsillar abscess occasionally complicates acute tonsillitis. Usually caused by streptococci or staphylococci, the infection spreads from tonsil to adjacent soft tissue, producing a very painful, usually unilateral red bulge that may extend beyond the midline. Painful swallowing may cause drooling.

TABLE 7-23

TABLE 7-23. THYROID ENLARGEMENT AND NODULES

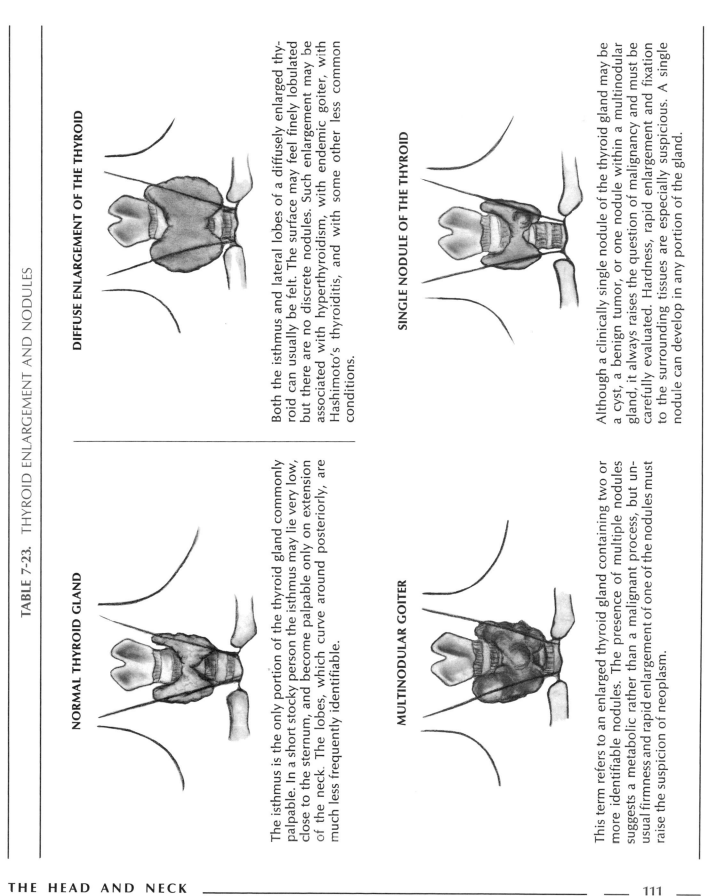

NORMAL THYROID GLAND

The isthmus is the only portion of the thyroid gland commonly palpable. In a short stocky person the isthmus may lie very low, close to the sternum, and become palpable only on extension of the neck. The lobes, which curve around posteriorly, are much less frequently identifiable.

DIFFUSE ENLARGEMENT OF THE THYROID

Both the isthmus and lateral lobes of a diffusely enlarged thyroid can usually be felt. The surface may feel finely lobulated but there are no discrete nodules. Such enlargement may be associated with hyperthyroidism, with endemic goiter, with Hashimoto's thyroiditis, and with some other less common conditions.

MULTINODULAR GOITER

This term refers to an enlarged thyroid gland containing two or more identifiable nodules. The presence of multiple nodules suggests a metabolic rather than a malignant process, but unusual firmness and rapid enlargement of one of the nodules must raise the suspicion of neoplasm.

SINGLE NODULE OF THE THYROID

Although a clinically single nodule of the thyroid gland may be a cyst, a benign tumor, or one nodule within a multinodular gland, it always raises the question of malignancy and must be carefully evaluated. Hardness, rapid enlargement and fixation to the surrounding tissues are especially suspicious. A single nodule can develop in any portion of the gland.

the thorax and lungs

ANATOMY AND PHYSIOLOGY

Review the anatomy of the chest wall, identifying the structures illustrated.

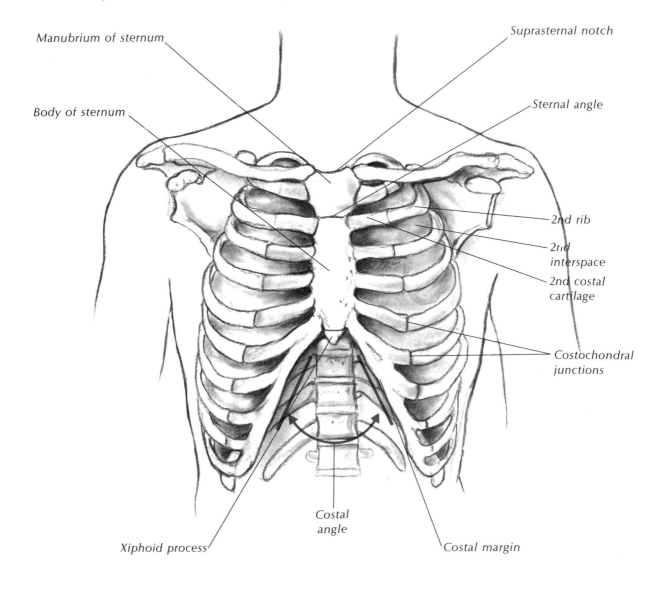

Manubrium of sternum

Suprasternal notch

Body of sternum

Sternal angle

2nd rib

2nd interspace

2nd costal cartilage

Costochondral junctions

Costal angle

Xiphoid process

Costal margin

Localization of a finding depends upon accurate numbering of ribs. The sternal angle (or angle of Louis) is the best guide. Identify it by finding the bony ridge joining the manubrium to the body of the sternum. A few centimeters below the suprasternal notch, this ridge lies adjacent to the second rib and its costal cartilage. The interspace immediately below is the second interspace. When locating ribs or interspaces lower in the anterior chest, start from the sternal angle and second rib, then count downward in an oblique line several centimeters lateral to the sternal edge or costal margin. Palpation more medially may be confused by the close approximation of the costal cartilages.

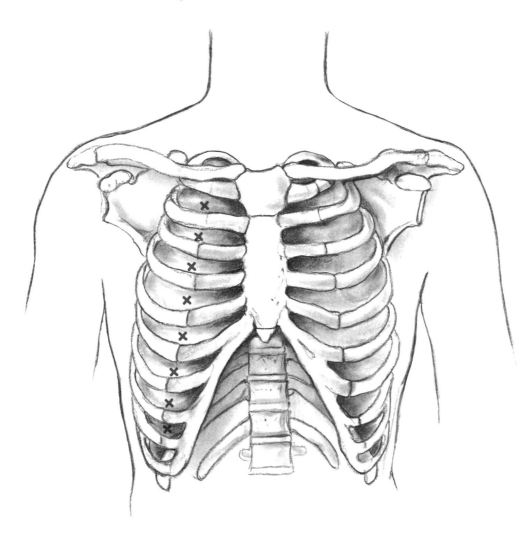

Note that the costal cartilages of only the first seven ribs articulate with the sternum. Those of the eighth, ninth and tenth ribs articulate with the costal cartilages just above. The eleventh and twelfth ribs, the so-called "floating ribs," have free anterior tips. The cartilaginous tip of the eleventh rib can usually be felt laterally, the twelfth may be felt posteriorly. Costal cartilages are not distinguishable from ribs by palpation.

Posteriorly the accurate numbering of ribs is more difficult. The inferior angle of the scapula is a helpful landmark, lying approximately at the level of the seventh rib or interspace. Findings may also be localized according to their relationship to the spinous processes. When the patient flexes his neck forward, the most prominent spinous process (the vertebra prominens) is usually that of the seventh cervical. It may, however, be the first thoracic. If two vertebrae appear equally prominent, they are the seventh cervical and first thoracic. The spinous processes below can usually be felt and counted, especially when the spine is flexed. Since the processes of T_4 through T_{12} angle obliquely downward, each overlies not its own vertebra but the body of the vertebra below. For example, the spinous process of T_6 overlies the seventh thoracic vertebra and is adjacent to the seventh rib.

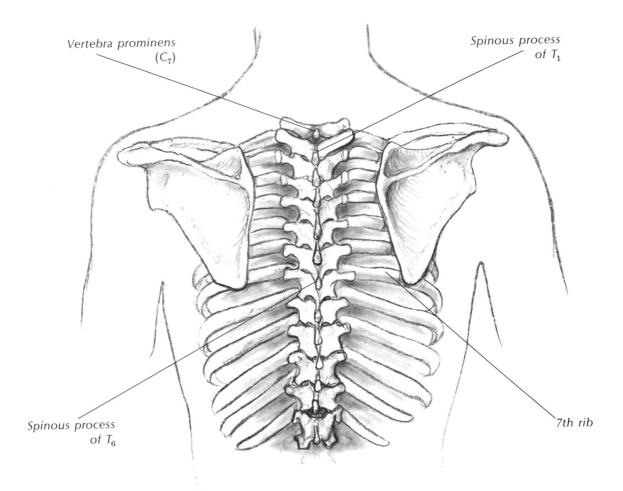

Vertebra prominens (C_7)

Spinous process of T_1

Spinous process of T_6

7th rib

Localization of findings depends upon their relationship not only to ribs and vertebrae but also to imaginary lines drawn on the chest. Become familiar with the following:

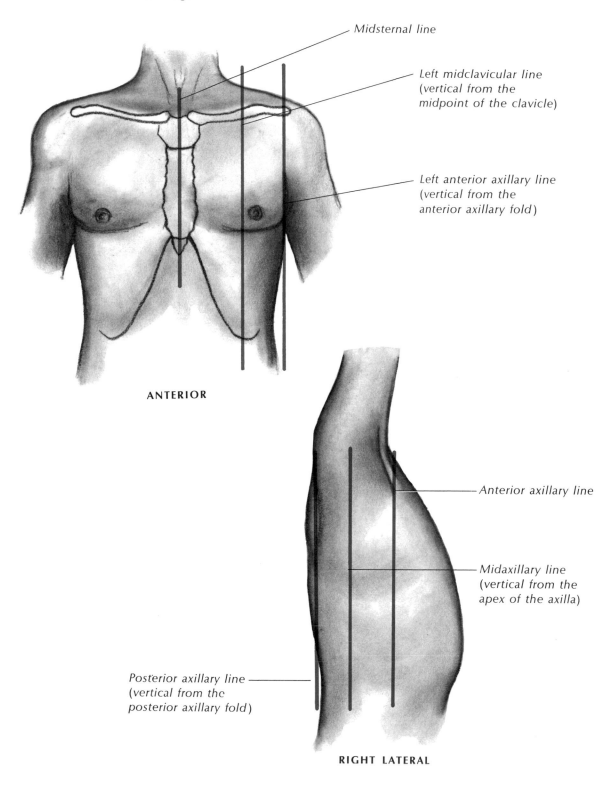

Midsternal line

Left midclavicular line (vertical from the midpoint of the clavicle)

Left anterior axillary line (vertical from the anterior axillary fold)

ANTERIOR

Anterior axillary line

Midaxillary line (vertical from the apex of the axilla)

Posterior axillary line (vertical from the posterior axillary fold)

RIGHT LATERAL

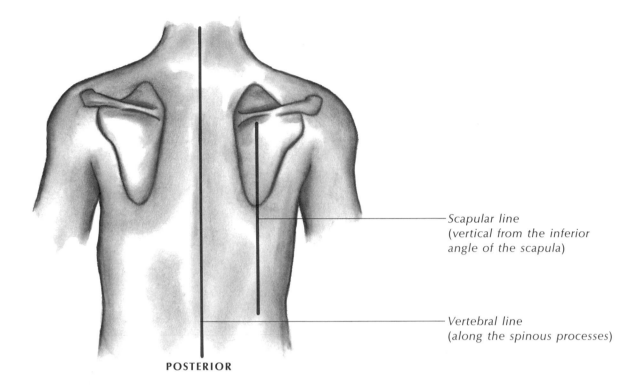

Scapular line
(vertical from the inferior
angle of the scapula)

Vertebral line
(along the spinous processes)

POSTERIOR

While examining the chest, keep in mind the probable location of the underlying lungs and their lobes. These locations can be mentally projected onto the chest wall. Key points in these surface projections include the following:

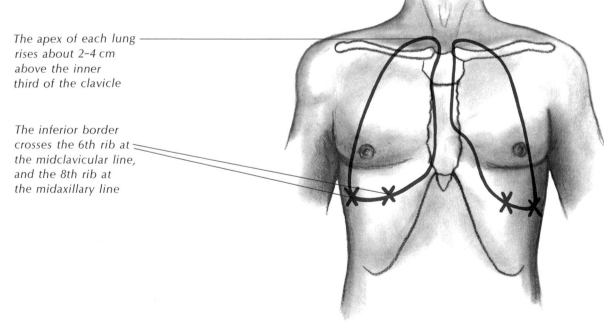

The apex of each lung
rises about 2–4 cm
above the inner
third of the clavicle

The inferior border
crosses the 6th rib at
the midclavicular line,
and the 8th rib at
the midaxillary line

ANTERIOR

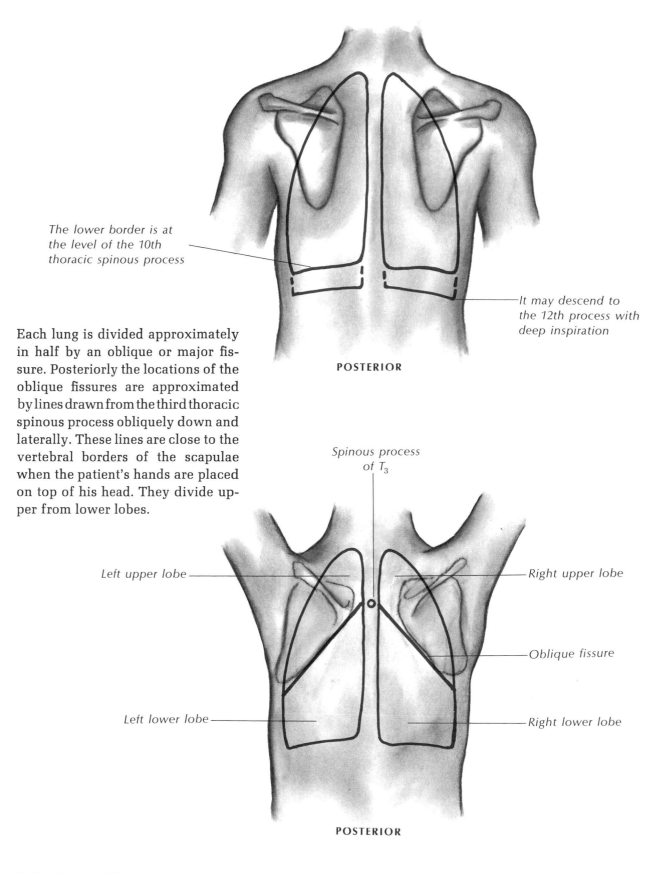

The lower border is at the level of the 10th thoracic spinous process

It may descend to the 12th process with deep inspiration

POSTERIOR

Each lung is divided approximately in half by an oblique or major fissure. Posteriorly the locations of the oblique fissures are approximated by lines drawn from the third thoracic spinous process obliquely down and laterally. These lines are close to the vertebral borders of the scapulae when the patient's hands are placed on top of his head. They divide upper from lower lobes.

Spinous process of T₃

Left upper lobe

Right upper lobe

Oblique fissure

Left lower lobe

Right lower lobe

POSTERIOR

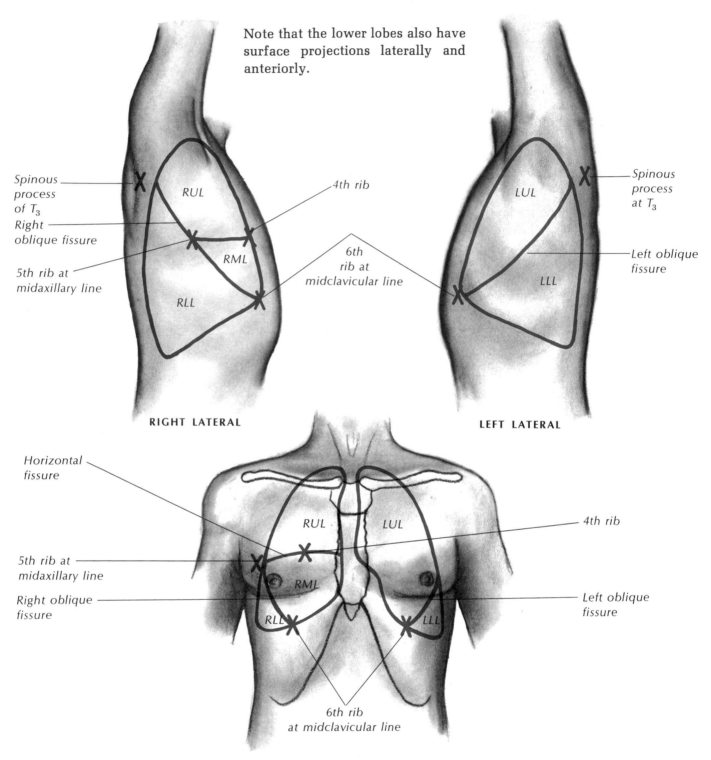

Note that the lower lobes also have surface projections laterally and anteriorly.

Spinous process of T_3

RUL

4th rib

Right oblique fissure

RML

6th rib at midclavicular line

5th rib at midaxillary line

RLL

RIGHT LATERAL

LUL

Spinous process at T_3

Left oblique fissure

LLL

LEFT LATERAL

Horizontal fissure

RUL

LUL

4th rib

5th rib at midaxillary line

RML

Right oblique fissure

Left oblique fissure

RLL

LLL

6th rib at midclavicular line

ANTERIOR

The right lung is further divided by the horizontal or minor fissure into the right upper and right middle lobes. This fissure runs from the right midaxillary line at the level of the fifth rib across anteriorly at the level of the fourth rib.

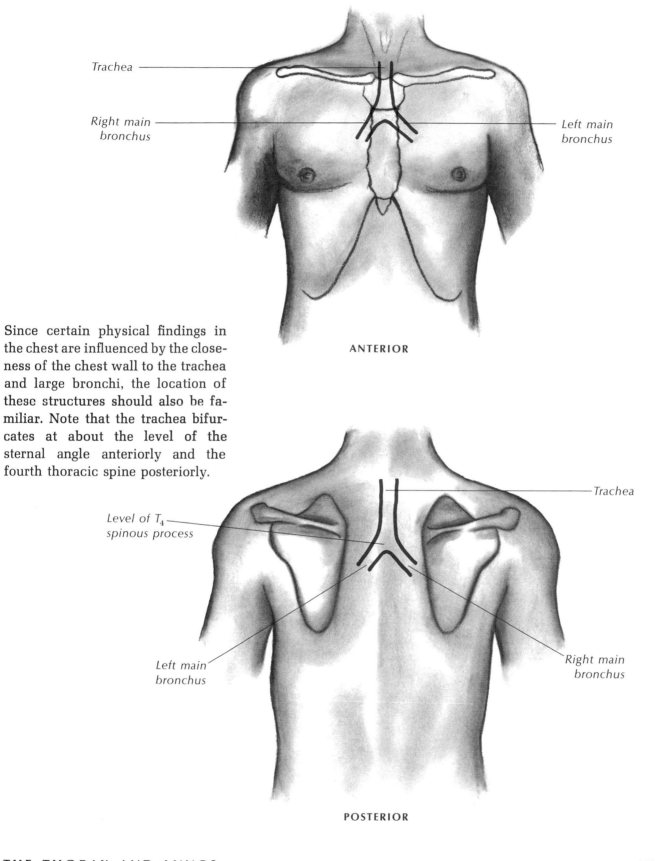

ANTERIOR

Since certain physical findings in the chest are influenced by the closeness of the chest wall to the trachea and large bronchi, the location of these structures should also be familiar. Note that the trachea bifurcates at about the level of the sternal angle anteriorly and the fourth thoracic spine posteriorly.

Trachea

Right main bronchus

Left main bronchus

Level of T₄ spinous process

Left main bronchus

Right main bronchus

POSTERIOR

General Approach

1. The patient should be undressed to the waist and examined with good lighting.
2. Proceed in an orderly fashion:
   a. Inspection, palpation, percussion, auscultation.
   b. Compare one side with the other. Variations between patients are great; and to some extent at least, comparison of one side with the other allows a patient to serve as his own control.
   c. Work from above down.
3. Throughout your examination, try to visualize the underlying tissues, including the lobes of the lungs.
4. Examine the posterior thorax and lungs while the patient is still in the sitting position. His arms should be folded across his chest so that his scapulae are partly out of the way. Then ask the patient to lie down while you examine his anterior thorax and lungs.

Examination of the Posterior Chest

INSPECTION

Note the shape of the patient's chest. Estimate its anteroposterior diameter in proportion to its lateral diameter (normally from 1:2 to about 5:7).

See Table 8-1, Deformities of the Thorax (p. 132).

From a midline position behind the patient, look for:

Deformities of the thorax

The slope of the ribs

More horizontal in emphysema

Abnormal retraction of the interspaces during inspiration

Severe asthma, emphysema, tracheal or laryngeal obstruction

Abnormal bulging of the interspaces during expiration

Asthma, emphysema

Local lag or impairment in respiratory movement

Underlying disease of lung or pleura

Rate and rhythm of breathing

See Table 8-2, Abnormalities in Rate and Rhythm of Breathing (p. 133).

PALPATION

Palpation of the chest has four uses:

1. *To identify areas of tenderness.* Carefully palpate any area where pain has been reported or where lesions are evident.
2. *To assess observed abnormalities* such as masses or sinus tracts (blind, inflammatory tube-like structures opening onto the skin).
3. *To assess further the respiratory excursion.* Place your thumbs about at the level of and parallel to the tenth ribs, your hands grasping the lateral rib cage. As you position your hands, slide them medially a bit in order to raise loose skin folds between thumbs and spine. Ask the patient to inhale deeply.

Although rare, sinus tracts usually indicate infection of the underlying pleura and lung, e.g., tuberculosis, actinomycosis.

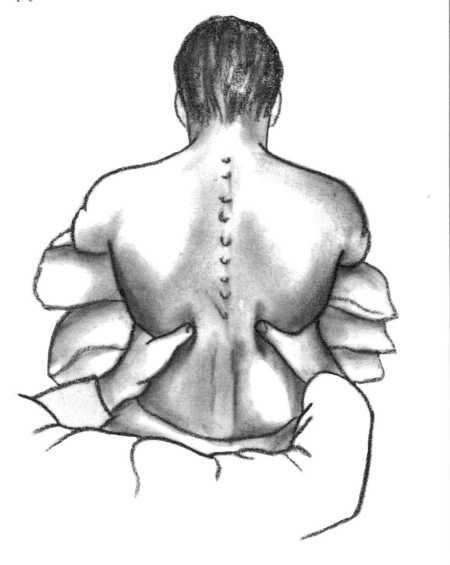

Lag or impairment of thoracic movement suggests underlying disease of the lung or pleura

Watch the excursion of your thumbs and feel for the range and symmetry of respiratory movement.

4. *To elicit vocal or tactile fremitus.* Fremitus refers to the palpable vibrations transmitted through the bronchopulmonary system to the chest wall when the patient speaks. Ask the patient to repeat the words "ninety-nine" or "one-one-one." If fremitus is faint, ask him to speak more loudly or lower his (and especially her) voice.

Fremitus is decreased or absent when the voice is decreased, the bronchus obstructed, or the pleural space occupied by fluid, air or solid tissue. Increased fremitus is noted near the large bronchi and over consolidated lung.

Palpate and compare symmetrical areas of the lungs, using the ball of the hand (the palm of the hand at the base of the fingers). Use one hand, not both, in order to maximize your accuracy.

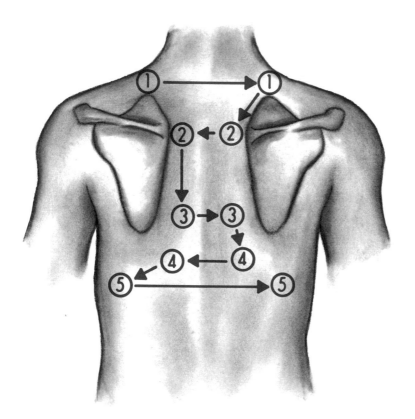

Numbers and arrows indicate sequence of examination

Identify, describe and localize any areas of increased or decreased fremitus.

Estimate the level of the diaphragm on each side using the ulnar side of the extended hand, held parallel to the expected diaphragmatic level. Move your hand downward in progressive steps until fremitus is no longer felt. This point gives an estimate of the diaphragmatic level. It is usually slightly higher on the right.

An abnormally high level suggests pleural effusion or a high diaphragm, as from paralysis or atelectasis.

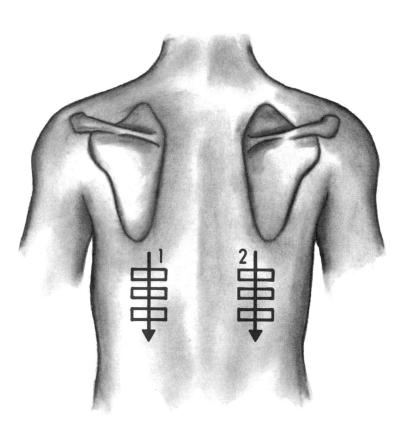

PERCUSSION

Percussion of the chest sets the chest wall and underlying tissues into motion, producing audible sounds and palpable vibrations. Percussion helps to determine whether the underlying tissues are air-filled, fluid-filled or solid. It penetrates only about 5 to 7 cm into the chest, however, and will therefore not detect deep-seated lesions.

The technique can be practiced on any surface. The key points are:

1. Hyperextend the middle finger of your left hand (the pleximeter finger). Press its distal phalanx and joint *firmly* on the surface to be percussed. Avoid contact by any other part of the hand, since this would damp the vibrations.

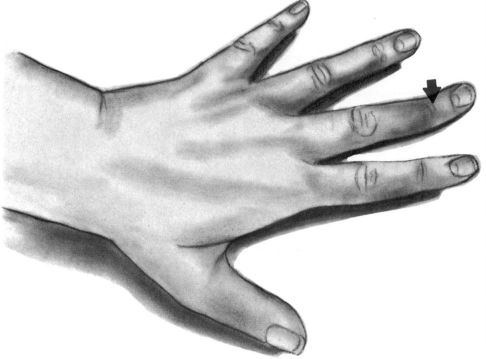

2. Position your right forearm quite close to the surface with the hand cocked upward. The right middle finger should be partially flexed, relaxed and poised to strike.

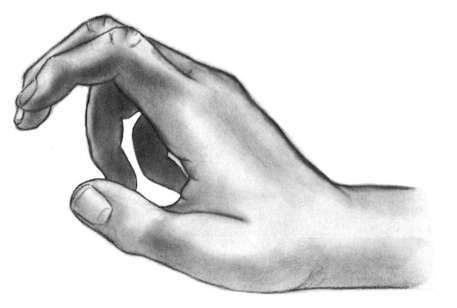

3. With a quick sharp but relaxed wrist motion, strike the pleximeter finger with the right middle finger (the plexor).

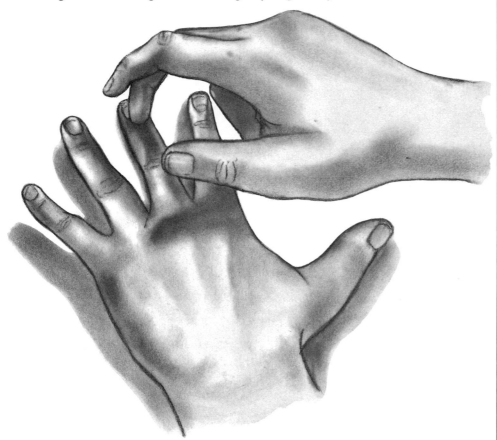

Aim at the base of the terminal phalanx or at the distal interphalangeal joint—the point overlying that portion of the pleximeter finger that is exerting maximum pressure on the surface.

Use the tip of the plexor finger, not the finger pad. The terminal phalanx should be almost at a right angle with the pleximeter. (A very short fingernail is required to avoid self-mutilation!) In percussing the lower posterior chest you can achieve the correct position more easily by standing somewhat to the side, not directly behind the patient.

4. Withdraw the plexor finger briskly to avoid damping the vibrations.

5. Strike one or two blows in one location and then move on. Keep your percussion technique uniform in comparing one part of the chest with another.

REMEMBER: The movement is at the wrist, not in the finger, elbow, or shoulder; it is a direct blow, not oblique or tangential. Use the lightest percussion that will produce a clear note.

The practitioner should learn to distinguish five percussion notes. Four of these are readily reproducible on himself. The notes can be distinguished by differences in their basic qualities as sounds, namely intensity, pitch and duration. Train your ear to detect these differences.

	Relative Intensity	Relative Pitch	Relative Duration	Example Location
Flatness	Soft	High	Short	Thigh
Dullness	Medium	Medium	Medium	Liver
Resonance	Loud	Low	Long	Normal lung
Hyperresonance	Very loud	Lower	Longer	Emphysematous lung
Tympany	Loud	*	*	Gastric air bubble or puffed out cheek

* Distinguished mainly by its musical timbre

Percuss across the top of each shoulder to identify the approximately 5-cm band of resonance overlying each lung apex. Then, while the patient continues to keep his arms folded across his chest, percuss symmetrical areas of the lungs at about 5-cm intervals down the chest wall. Below the scapulae, percuss symmetrical areas along the sides of the chest as well as medially.

Dullness replaces resonance when fluid or solid tissue replaces air-containing lung or occupies the pleural space.

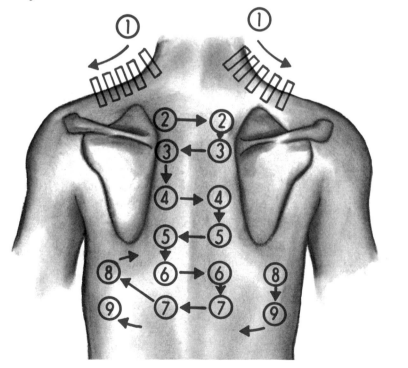

Omit the scapular areas since the thickness of musculoskeletal structures usually precludes worthwhile percussion there.

Identify, describe and localize any area of abnormal percussion note.

With the pleximeter finger held parallel to the expected border of diaphragmatic dullness, percuss in progressive steps downward. Identify the level of diaphragmatic dullness on each side during quiet respiration. This level is often slightly higher on the right. Check the level laterally as well as medially.

An abnormally high level suggests pleural effusion or a high diaphragm, as from paralysis or atelectasis.

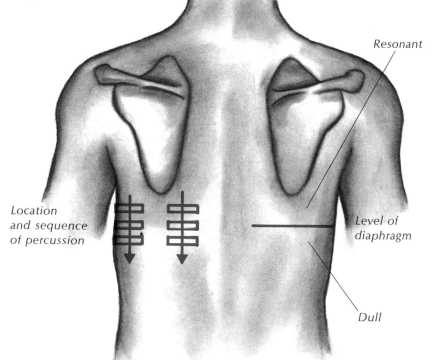

Resonant

Location and sequence of percussion

Level of diaphragm

Dull

Diaphragmatic excursion may be measured by noting the distance between the levels of dullness on full expiration and full inspiration, normally around 5 or 6 cm.

AUSCULTATION

Auscultation of the lungs is useful in assessing: (1) air flow through the tracheobronchial tree, (2) the presence of fluid, mucus or obstruction in the air passages and (3) the condition of the surrounding lungs and pleural space.

With a stethoscope, listen to the patient's lungs as he breathes through his mouth somewhat more deeply than normal. Using locations similar to those recommended for percussion, compare symmetrical areas of the lungs, from above down. Listen to at least one full breath in each location. Be alert for patient discomfort secondary to hyperventilation (e.g., light-headedness, faintness), and allow him to rest as needed. Listen for:

1. *The quality and intensity of breath sounds.* Breath sounds are produced by turbulent air flow in the pharynx and larger airways of the lungs. These can be heard most directly near the trachea. As the sounds are transmitted through the lungs, they are damped by surrounding tissues and their auscultatory characteristics are altered—from so-called bronchial breathing to vesicular breathing. Learn to distinguish three kinds of breath sounds by paying attention to their duration, pitch and intensity.

Breath sounds are decreased or absent when air flow is decreased (e.g., by bronchial obstruction, muscular weakness) or when fluid or tissue separates the air passages from the stethoscope (e.g., obesity, pleural disease).

Breath Sounds	Duration of Inspiration and Expiration	Pitch of Expiration	Intensity of Expiration	Sample Location
Vesicular	Insp. > Exp.	Low	Soft	Most of lungs
Broncho-vesicular	Insp. = Exp.	Medium	Medium	Near the main stem bronchi, i.e., below the clavicles and between the scapulae, especially on the right
Bronchial or tubular	Exp. > Insp.	High	Usually loud	Over the trachea

2. *Adventitious or abnormal sounds*, e.g., rales, rhonchi or friction rubs. Distinguish these from artifactual sounds produced, for example, by friction of the stethoscope on the chest and by muscular activity within the chest wall.

See Table 8-3, Adventitious Sounds in the Chest Examination (p. 134).

Identify, describe and locate any abnormality.

If breath sounds are diminished or if you suspect but cannot hear signs of obstructive breathing, ask the patient to breathe hard and fast with his mouth open. The diminished breath sounds associated with obesity may become readily audible; wheezes and rhonchi that were previously inaudible may appear.

Breath sounds remain decreased in emphysema. Wheezes or rhonchi may appear in asthma or bronchitis.

If you have discovered abnormalities in tactile fremitus, percussion or auscultation, continue on to check *spoken and whispered voice sounds.*

See Table 8-4, Alterations in Voice Sounds (p. 135).

Ask the patient to say "ninety-nine" or "eee." Listen in symmetrical areas of the lungs, noting the intensity and clarity of the sounds. Normally the sounds are muffled.

Ask the patient to whisper "ninety-nine." Normally the whispered voice is heard only faintly and indistinctly.

See Table 8-5, Physical Signs in Selected Abnormalities of Bronchi and Lungs (pp. 136–138).

Examination of the Anterior Chest

The patient should be supine and comfortable, with his arms slightly abducted away from his chest.

INSPECTION

Observe:

The shape of the chest, including any deformities

The width of the costal angle (usually less than 90 degrees except in patients with short heavy builds)

Abnormal retraction of the interspaces and supraclavicular fossae during inspiration

Abnormal bulging of the interspaces during expiration

Use of the normally quiet accessory muscles of breathing, especially the sternomastoids, scaleni and trapezii on inspiration and the abdominal muscles on expiration

Local lag or impairment in respiratory movement

Rate and rhythm of breathing

See Table 8-1, Deformities of the Thorax (p. 132).

Wider in emphysema

Severe asthma, emphysema, tracheal obstruction

Asthma, emphysema

Asthma, emphysema

Underlying disease of lung or pleura

PALPATION

Palpation has four uses:

1. *To identify areas of tenderness.*

2. *To assess any observed abnormality.*

3. *To assess further the respiratory excursion.* Place your thumbs along each costal margin, your hands along the lateral rib cage. As you position your hands, slide them medially a bit to raise a loose skin fold between the thumbs. Ask the patient to inhale deeply. Watch for divergence of your thumbs as the thorax expands and feel for the range and symmetry of respiratory movement.

Tender pectoral muscles or costal cartilages tend to corroborate, but do not prove, a musculoskeletal origin of chest pain.

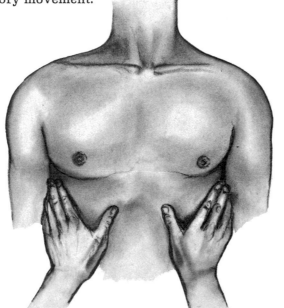

4. *To elicit vocal or tactile fremitus.* Compare symmetrical areas of the lungs, anteriorly and laterally, using the ball of your hand. When examining a woman, gently displace the breasts as necessary. Note that fremitus is usually decreased or absent over the precordium.

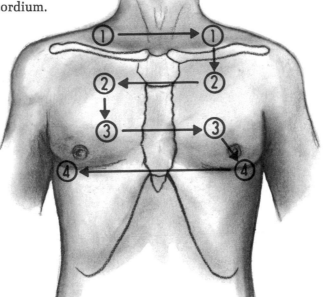

PERCUSSION

Percuss the anterior and lateral chest, again comparing symmetrical points, including the supraclavicular areas, the infraclavicular areas, and on down the chest wall at about 5-cm intervals. Displace the female breasts as necessary. The heart normally produces an area of dullness to the left of the sternum from the third to the fifth interspaces.

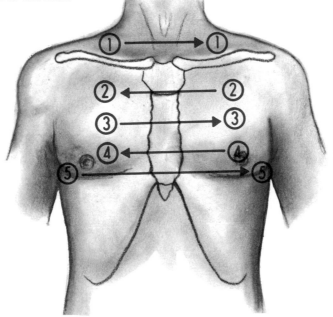

Identify, describe and localize any area of abnormal percussion note.

With your pleximeter finger parallel to the expected upper border of liver dullness, percuss in progressive steps downward in the right midclavicular line. Identify the upper border of liver dullness.

By a similar maneuver on the left, identify the usually tympanitic gastric air bubble.

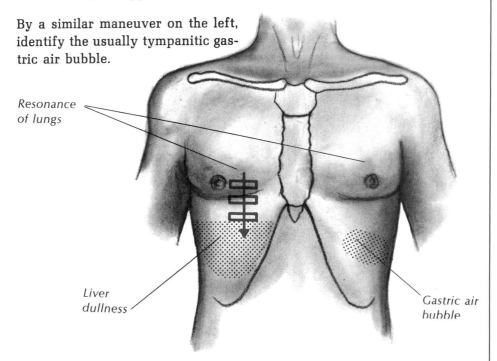

Resonance of lungs

Liver dullness

Gastric air bubble

AUSCULTATION

Listen to the patient's chest, anteriorly and laterally, as he breathes through his mouth somewhat more deeply than normal. Compare symmetrical areas of the lungs, from above downward. Listen for:

  1. *Quality and intensity of the breath sounds.*

  2. *Adventitious or abnormal sounds.*

Identify, describe and locate any abnormality.

If breath sounds are diminished or if you suspect but cannot hear signs of obstructive breathing, ask the patient to breathe hard and fast with his mouth open.

If indicated, proceed to *spoken and whispered voice sounds.*

A note on examining the patient who cannot sit up. Because physical signs in the chest are often masked or distorted in the supine patient, try to get help in sitting the patient up for an examination of his posterior lung fields. If this is not possible, position the patient alternately on each side and examine the upper lung.

TABLE 8-1

TABLE 8-1. DEFORMITIES OF THE THORAX

Normal Infant

CROSS SECTION OF THORAX CLINICAL APPEARANCE

Normal Adult

CROSS SECTION OF THORAX CLINICAL APPEARANCE

Barrel Chest

CROSS SECTION OF THORAX CLINICAL APPEARANCE

The chest of the normal infant is approximately round or barrel-shaped in cross section.

In the normal adult the ratio of anteroposterior to lateral diameter ranges from 1:2 to 5:7.

A barrel chest is associated with pulmonary emphysema or normal aging. The ratio of anteroposterior to lateral diameter approximates 1:1.

Funnel Chest (Pectus Excavatum)

CROSS SECTION OF THORAX CLINICAL APPEARANCE

Pigeon Chest (Pectus Carinatum)

CROSS SECTION OF THORAX CLINICAL APPEARANCE

Groove *Anteriorly displaced sternum*

Thoracic Kyphoscoliosis

CROSS SECTION OF THORAX CLINICAL APPEARANCE

High shoulder *High scapula* *Thoracic convexity to right* *Interspaces flared*

A funnel chest is characterized by a depression in the lower portion of the sternum. Compression of the heart and great vessels may cause murmurs.

In a pigeon chest the sternum is displaced anteriorly, increasing the anteroposterior diameter. Grooves in the chest wall accentuate the deformity.

In thoracic kyphoscoliosis the spine is curved and the thorax shows corresponding deformities. Distortion of the underlying lungs may make interpretation of lung findings very difficult.

TABLE 8-2

TABLE 8-2. ABNORMALITIES IN RATE AND RHYTHM OF BREATHING

When observing respiratory patterns, think in terms of rate, depth and regularity of the patient's breathing. Describe what you see in these terms. Traditional terms, such as tachypnea, are given below so that you will understand them, but simple descriptions are recommended for use.

NORMAL

Inspiration Expiration

Time

Volume of air

The respiratory rate is about 16 to 20 per minute in adults and up to 44 per minute in infants.

RAPID SHALLOW BREATHING (TACHYPNEA)

Rapid shallow breathing has a number of causes, including restrictive lung disease, pleuritic chest pain and an elevated diaphragm.

RAPID, DEEP BREATHING (HYPERPNEA, HYPERVENTILATION)

Rapid deep breathing also has a number of causes, including exercise, anxiety and metabolic acidosis. In the comatose patient, infarction, hypoxia or hypoglycemia affecting the midbrain or pons should be considered. *Kussmaul breathing* is deep breathing associated with metabolic acidosis. It may be fast, normal in rate or slow.

SLOW BREATHING (BRADYPNEA)

Slow breathing may be secondary to such causes as diabetic coma, drug-induced respiratory depression and increased intracranial pressure.

CHEYNE-STOKES BREATHING

Hyperpnea   Apnea

Respiration waxes and wanes cyclically so that periods of deep breathing alternate with periods of apnea (no breathing). Children and aging people may normally show this pattern in sleep. Other causes include heart failure, uremia, drug-induced respiratory depression and brain damage (typically on both sides of the cerebral hemispheres or diencephalon).

ATAXIC BREATHING (BIOT'S BREATHING)

Ataxic breathing is characterized by unpredictable irregularity. Breaths may be shallow or deep and stop for short periods. Causes include respiratory depression and brain damage, typically at the medullary level.

SIGHING RESPIRATION

Sighs

Breathing punctuated by frequent sighs should alert you to the possibility of hyperventilation syndrome—a common cause of dyspnea and dizziness.

Occasional sighs are normal.

OBSTRUCTIVE BREATHING

Prolonged expiration

Air trapping

In obstructive lung disease expiration is prolonged because of increased airway resistance. If the patient must increase his respiratory rate, he lacks sufficient time for full expiration. His chest overexpands (air trapping) and his breathing becomes more shallow.

TABLE 8-3

TABLE 8-3. ADVENTITIOUS SOUNDS IN THE CHEST EXAMINATION

RALES (CRACKLES)

Pitch

Inspiration   Expiration

Rales are discrete, noncontinuous crackling sounds that may be imagined as dots in time in contrast to dashes. They are represented here by open circles. They are usually inspiratory. Inspiratory rales are probably secondary to delayed reopening of previously deflated airways. Conditions in which they are heard include congestive heart failure, bronchitis, pneumonia and pulmonary fibrosis. Rales may or may not change with coughing.

RHONCHI OR WHEEZES

High, sibilant
Low, sonorous

Rhonchi or wheezes last longer than rales and are shown here as dashes. They may be inspiratory, expiratory or both. These sounds indicate partial obstruction to air flow in passages narrowed by secretions, mucosal swelling, tumors, and so on. They often change with coughing. Texts disagree in their definitions of wheezes versus rhonchi. The terms may be used interchangeably. Differences in pitch depend primarily on differences in velocity of air flow across the obstruction. Some sounds are high pitched, sibilant, and musical; others are lower and sonorous.

PLEURAL FRICTION RUB

A pleural friction rub is a crackling, grating sound produced when two roughened or inflamed pleural surfaces rub across each other during respiration. Friction rubs are usually heard in both inspiration and expiration but may be limited to inspiration. They are not affected by cough. Recordings have shown that rubs comprise a series of discrete crackles and may be difficult to differentiate from rales, especially when confined to inspiration. The crackles may be so frequent that they coalesce into a continuous sound.

---

*The mechanisms of rales and rhonchi are illustrated here and in Table 8-5 according to theories proposed by Forgacs.

TABLE 8-4

TABLE 8-4. ALTERATIONS IN VOICE SOUNDS

When a lung is consolidated by lobar pneumonia, or sometimes when it is compressed by a pleural effusion, voice sounds transmitted through it are often altered. The sounds are louder, clearer than usual and sometimes changed in quality. These changes may best be described simply, e.g., "increased intensity and clarity of spoken voice sounds." Three classical terms have been used in the past: bronchophony, egophony and whispered pectoriloquy. Since these terms are still used, become familiar with them.

BRONCHOPHONY

Bronchophony describes an increase in the intensity and clarity of spoken voice sounds as perceived through the stethoscope.

EGOPHONY

Egophony describes a nasal bleating quality of the voice sounds, often detected by the transformation of the patient's "ee" to what sounds like "ay."

WHISPERED PECTORILOQUY

Whispered pectoriloquy describes an unusually clear transmission of the whispered words through the stethoscope.

TABLE 8-5

TABLE 8-5. PHYSICAL SIGNS IN SELECTED ABNORMALITIES OF BRONCHI AND LUNGS

CONDITION	DESCRIPTION	PERCUSSION NOTE	TACTILE FREMITUS VOICE SOUNDS, WHISPERED VOICE SOUNDS	BREATH SOUNDS	ADVENTITIOUS SOUNDS
NORMAL	The tracheobronchial tree and alveoli are clear; the pleurae are thin and close together; the mobility of the chest wall is unimpaired.	Resonant	Normal	Vesicular, except perhaps for broncho-vesicular sounds near the large bronchi	None, except perhaps for a few transient, inspiratory rales at the bases after recumbency or sleep.
LEFT-SIDED HEART FAILURE	In left-sided heart failure, some airways in the dependent portions of the lungs are deflated abnormally during expiration. The bronchial mucosa may be swollen.	Resonant	Normal	Normal or sometimes prolonged expiration	Rales at lung bases; sometimes wheezes
PLEURAL FLUID OR THICKENING	Pleural fluid or fibrotic thickening muffles all sounds.	Dull to flat	Decreased to absent; however, when fluid compresses the underlying lung, bronchophony, egophony and whispered pectoriloquy may appear.	Decreased vesicular or absent; however, when fluid compresses the lung, a bronchial quality may appear.	None unless there is underlying disease

Bronchus

Pleura

Alveoli

Swollen mucosa (sometimes)

Deflated airway

Pleural fluid or thickening

THE THORAX AND LUNGS

TABLE 8-5

TABLE 8-5. (CONT'D)

CONDITION	DESCRIPTION	PERCUSSION NOTE	TACTILE FREMITUS VOICE SOUNDS, WHISPERED VOICE SOUNDS	BREATH SOUNDS	ADVENTITIOUS SOUNDS
PULMONARY CONSOLIDATION (e.g. LOBAR PNEUMONIA)	A consolidated lung is dull to percussion but so long as the large airways are clear, fremitus, breath and voice sounds are transmitted as if they came directly from the larynx and trachea. Abnormally deflated portions of the lungs produce rales.	Dull	Increased, with bronchophony, egophony, whispered pectoriloquy	Bronchial	Rales
BRONCHITIS	In bronchitis, there may be partial bronchial obstruction from secretions or constrictions. Abnormally deflated portions of lung may produce rales.	Resonant	Normal	Normal or prolonged expiration	Wheezes or rales
EMPHYSEMA	A hyperinflated lung of emphysema is hyperresonant. The overfilled air spaces muffle the voice and breath sounds.	Hyperresonant	Decreased	Decreased vesicular, often with prolonged expiration	None, or signs of bronchitis

Deflated airway

Alveoli filled with fluid, red and white cells

Bronchial constriction

Deflated airway

Overinflated alveoli with destruction of walls

TABLE 8-5

TABLE 8-5. (CONT'D)

CONDITION	DESCRIPTION	PERCUSSION NOTE	TACTILE FREMITUS VOICE SOUNDS, WHISPERED VOICE SOUNDS	BREATH SOUNDS	ADVENTITIOUS SOUNDS
PNEUMOTHORAX 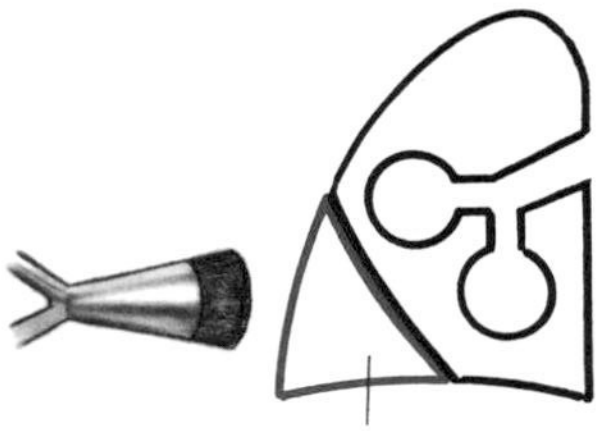 *Pleural air*	The free pleural air of pneumothorax may mimic obstructive lung disease but is usually unilateral and may shift the trachea to the opposite side. The air-filled pleural space gives a hyperresonant percussion note but muffles voice and breath sounds.	Hyperresonant	Decreased to absent	Decreased to absent	None
ATELECTASIS 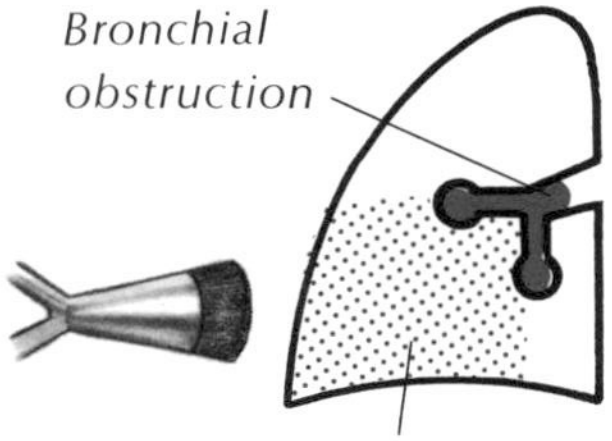 *Bronchial obstruction* *Collapsed portion of lung*	A collapsed or atelectatic lung is dull to percussion. Bronchial obstruction (shown here but not always present) prevents transmission of breath and voice sounds. The trachea may shift to the same side.	Dull	Decreased to absent	Decreased vesicular or absent	None

the heart

ANATOMY AND PHYSIOLOGY

Surface Projections of the Heart and Great Vessels

The heart is assessed chiefly by examination through the anterior chest wall. Most of the anterior cardiac surface is made up of right ventricle. This chamber and the pulmonary artery may be visualized roughly as a wedge lying behind and to the left of the sternum.

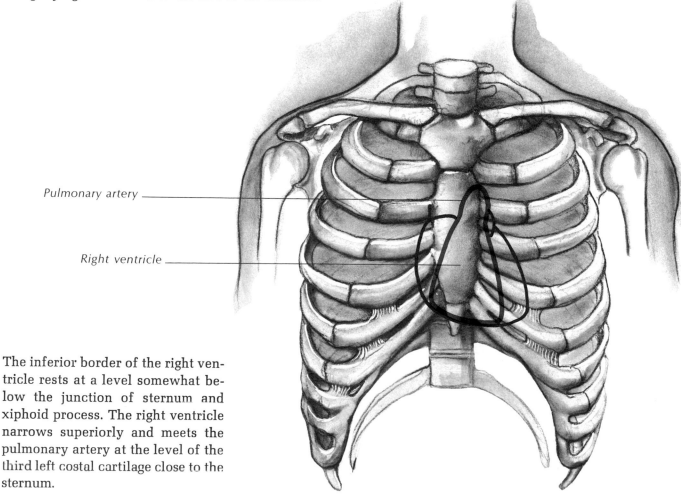

Pulmonary artery

Right ventricle

The inferior border of the right ventricle rests at a level somewhat below the junction of sternum and xiphoid process. The right ventricle narrows superiorly and meets the pulmonary artery at the level of the third left costal cartilage close to the sternum.

The left ventricle, lying to the left and behind the right ventricle, makes up only a small portion of the anterior cardiac surface. It is clinically important, however, forming the left border of the heart and producing the apical impulse.* This impulse is a brief systolic beat usually found in the fifth interspace, 7 to 9 cm from the midsternal line.

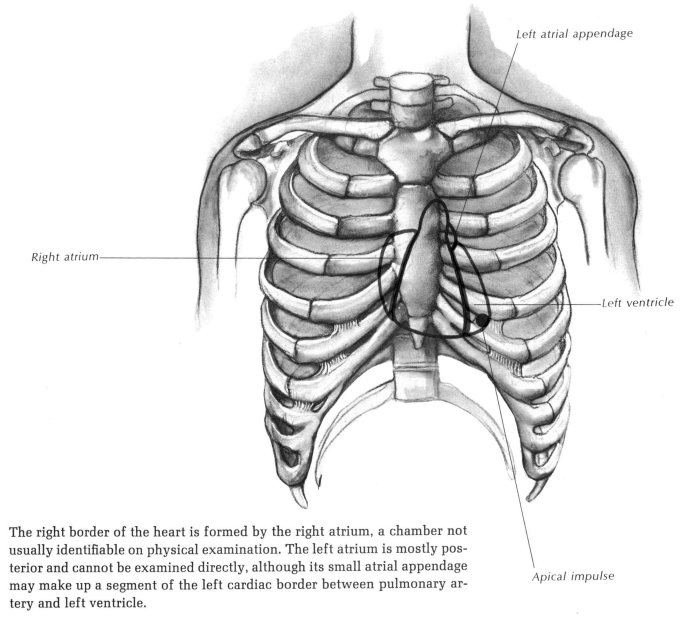

Left atrial appendage

Right atrium

Left ventricle

Apical impulse

The right border of the heart is formed by the right atrium, a chamber not usually identifiable on physical examination. The left atrium is mostly posterior and cannot be examined directly, although its small atrial appendage may make up a segment of the left cardiac border between pulmonary artery and left ventricle.

---

*The apical impulse is sometimes called the point of maximum impulse or P.M.I. Since in some conditions the most prominent cardiac impulse may not be apical, this term is not recommended.

Above the heart lie the great vessels. The pulmonary artery, already mentioned, bifurcates quickly into its left and right branches. The aorta curves upward from the left ventricle to the level of the sternal angle, where it arches backward and then down. On the right the superior vena cava empties into the right atrium.

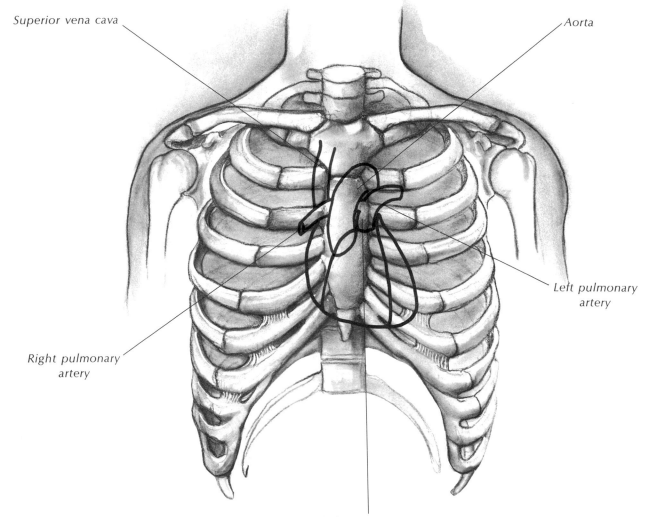

Superior vena cava

Aorta

Left pulmonary artery

Right pulmonary artery

Pulmonary artery

Although not illustrated above, the inferior vena cava also empties into the right atrium. The superior and inferior venae cavae carry venous blood from the upper and lower portions of the body respectively.

Cardiac Chambers, Valves and Circulation

Circulation through the heart is illustrated in the following diagram, which identifies the cardiac chambers, valves and direction of blood flow. Because of their positions, the tricuspid and mitral valves are often called atrioventricular valves. The aortic and pulmonic valves are called semilunar valves because their leaflets have a half-moon configuration.

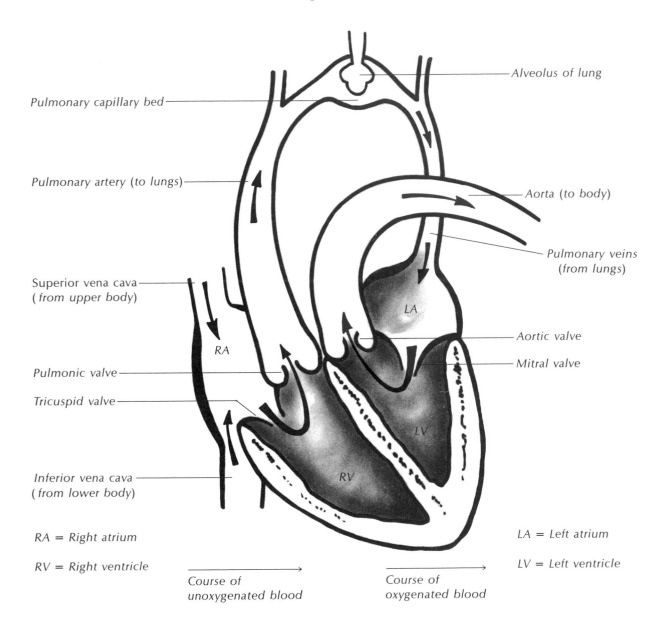

Pulmonary capillary bed

Pulmonary artery (to lungs)

Superior vena cava
(from upper body)

Pulmonic valve

Tricuspid valve

Inferior vena cava
(from lower body)

Alveolus of lung

Aorta (to body)

Pulmonary veins
(from lungs)

Aortic valve

Mitral valve

RA

LA

LV

RV

RA = Right atrium

RV = Right ventricle

LA = Left atrium

LV = Left ventricle

Course of
unoxygenated blood

Course of
oxygenated blood

Although this diagram shows all valves in an open position, they are not all open at the same time in the living heart. Closure of the valves is responsible for normal heart sounds. Their positions and movements must be understood in relation to events in the cardiac cycle.

Events in the Cardiac Cycle

If one were to measure the pressure in the left ventricle throughout the cardiac cycle, one would find a pressure curve like the following:

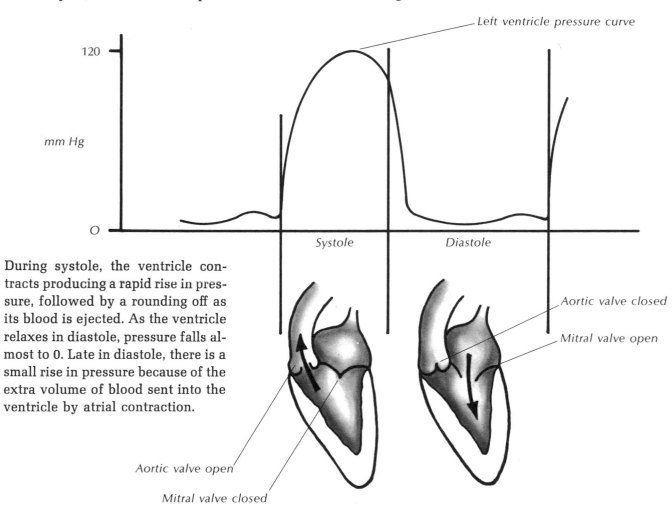

Left ventricle pressure curve

120

mm Hg

O

Systole   *Diastole*

During systole, the ventricle contracts producing a rapid rise in pressure, followed by a rounding off as its blood is ejected. As the ventricle relaxes in diastole, pressure falls almost to 0. Late in diastole, there is a small rise in pressure because of the extra volume of blood sent into the ventricle by atrial contraction.

Aortic valve closed

Mitral valve open

Aortic valve open

Mitral valve closed

Note that during systole, the aortic valve is open, allowing ejection of blood from the left ventricle into the aorta. The mitral valve is closed, preventing blood from regurgitating back into the left atrium. In contrast, during diastole the aortic valve is closed, preventing regurgitation of blood from the aorta back into the left ventricle. The mitral valve is open, allowing blood to flow from the left atrium into the relaxed left ventricle.

The interrelationships of the pressures in these three chambers—left atrium, left ventricle and aorta—together with the position and movement of the valves are fundamental to the understanding of heart sounds. Events on the right side of the heart also contribute, of course, but for the sake of clarity will be discussed later.

During diastole, pressure in the blood-filled left atrium slightly exceeds that in the relaxed left ventricle and blood flows from left atrium to left ventricle across the open mitral valve. Just before the onset of ventricular systole, atrial contraction produces a slight pressure rise in both chambers.

As the ventricle starts to contract, pressure within it rapidly exceeds left atrial pressure, thus shutting the mitral valve. Closure of the mitral valve produces the first heart sound (S_1).*

As the ventricular pressure continues to rise, it exceeds the diastolic pressure in the aorta and forces the aortic valve open. Opening of the aortic valve is not usually heard, but in some pathologic conditions is accompanied by an early systolic ejection click (Ej).

As the ventricle ejects most of its blood, its pressure begins to fall. When left ventricular pressure drops below the aortic pressure, the aortic valve shuts. Aortic valve closure causes the second heart sound.

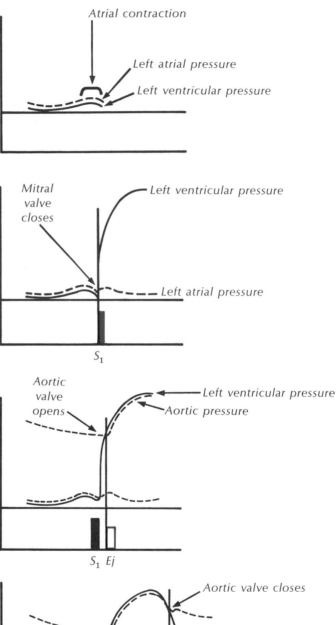

*An extensive literature deals with the exact causes of heart sounds, e.g., actual closure of valve leaflets, tensing of related structures, and the impact of columns of blood. The explanations given here are oversimplified but retain clinical usefulness.

As the left ventricular pressure continues to drop during ventricular relaxation, it falls below left atrial pressure. The mitral valve opens. This is usually a silent event but may be audible as an opening snap (O.S.) in mitral stenosis.

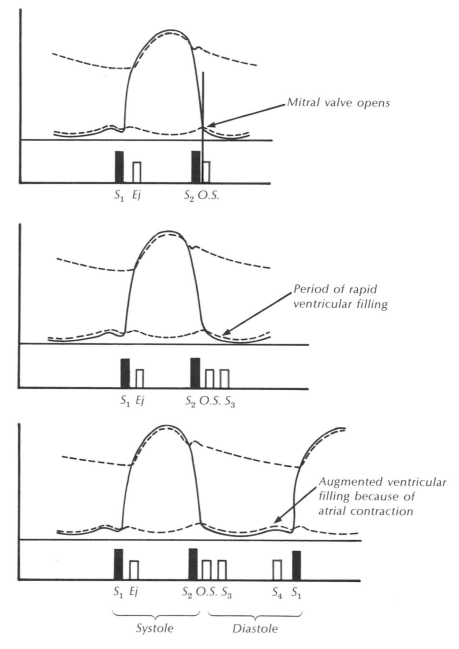

Mitral valve opens

S_1 Ej S_2 O.S.

Next occurs a period of rapid ventricular filling as blood flows early in diastole from left atrium to left ventricle. In children and young adults, this period may be marked by a third heart sound, S_3.

Period of rapid ventricular filling

S_1 Ej S_2 O.S. S_3

Finally, although not often heard in normal adults, a fourth heart sound or S_4 marks atrial contraction. It immediately precedes S_1 of the next beat.

Augmented ventricular filling because of atrial contraction

S_1 Ej S_2 O.S. S_3 S_4 S_1

Systole   Diastole

While these events are occurring on the left side of the heart, similar changes are occurring on the right, involving the right atrium, right ventricle, the tricuspid valve, the pulmonic valve and the pulmonary artery. Right ventricular and pulmonary arterial pressures are significantly lower than corresponding levels on the left side. Furthermore, right-sided events usually occur slightly later than those on the left. In auscultation, therefore, one often finds slight splitting of normal heart sounds, especially of S_2. Splitting of S_2 is normally more apparent during inspiration when flow into the right side of the heart is increased and right ventricular ejection is accordingly prolonged. During expiration when right-sided flow is decreased, the splitting diminishes or disappears.

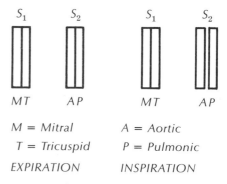

S_1 S_2 S_1 S_2

MT   AP   MT   AP

M = Mitral   A = Aortic

T = Tricuspid   P = Pulmonic

EXPIRATION   INSPIRATION

Relation of Heart Sounds to the Chest Wall

Events related to the movement of heart valves and to flow across them are best heard *not over their anatomic locations* but in the following *auscultatory areas* that bear their names. These names do not imply, however, that sounds heard there come only from those valves.

Aortic area—right 2nd interspace
close to the sternum

Pulmonic area—left 2nd interspace
close to the sternum

these two areas together are sometimes called the "base" of the heart

Aortic area

Pulmonic area

Tricuspid area—left 5th interspace
close to the sternum
Mitral (or apical) area—left 5th interspace just medial to the midclavicular line

Mitral area

Tricuspid area

When cardiovascular structures are altered by disease, the best areas for auscultation may change accordingly.

From a knowledge of pressure changes in the cardiac cycle, one can correctly predict the relative intensities of heart sounds in these areas. S_2 is produced by closure of the two semilunar valves, the aortic and pulmonic. Aortic valve closure under the relatively high aortic pressure produces the major component of S_2. This component (S_2A) is loudest in the aortic area and can be heard throughout the precordium. In the pulmonic area, one can additionally distinguish that component of S_2 produced by closure of the pulmonic valve (S_2P). S_2P is softer because of the lower pressure in the pulmonary artery. It can be heard normally only in the vicinity of the left second interspace. Physiologic splitting of S_2, therefore, is usually heard only at or near the pulmonic area.

The first sound, S_1, is produced by the closure of the atrioventricular valves, primarily the mitral, with probably an additional soft tricuspid component. Although usually audible throughout the precordium, S_1 is loudest, as expected, in the mitral area.

The Conduction System

Muscular contraction of the cardiac chambers should be distinguished from the electrical conduction system that stimulates and coordinates it.

Each normal impulse is initiated in a group of cardiac cells known as the sinus node. Located in the right atrium, the sinus node acts as cardiac pacemaker and automatically discharges an impulse about 60 to 100 times a minute. This impulse travels through both atria to the atrioventricular (or AV) node, a specialized group of cells located low in the atrial septum. Here the impulse is delayed somewhat before its passage down the bundle of His and its branches and thence to the ventricular myocardium. Muscular contraction follows, first the atria, then the ventricles. The normal conduction pathway is diagrammed in simplified form at the right.

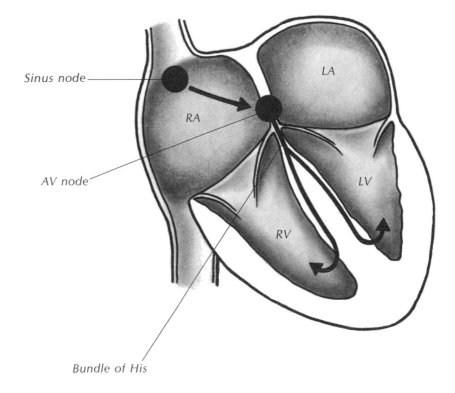

Sinus node

AV node

Bundle of His

LA

RA

RV

LV

The electrocardiogram records these events. Each normal impulse produces a series of waves:

A small P wave of atrial depolarization (electrical activation).

A larger QRS complex of ventricular depolarization, each consisting of one or more of the following:

A Q wave, formed whenever the initial deflection is downward.

An R wave, the upward deflection.

An S wave, a downward deflection following an R wave.

A T wave of ventricular repolarization (or recovery).

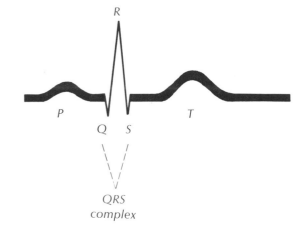

The electrical impulse slightly precedes the myocardial contraction that it stimulates. The relation of electrocardiographic waves to the cardiac cycle is shown below.

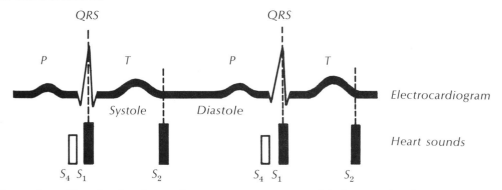

Disorders of cardiac rhythm have three common causes: (1) changes in the rate of the sinus pacemaker; (2) an abnormal or ectopic pacemaker which competes with the sinus node; and (3) delayed or abnormal conduction of the electrical impulse. When an impulse travels through the myocardium by an aberrant pathway, as it does for example when it originates in an ectopic pacemaker, it produces waves of altered configuration: altered P waves when atrial conduction is aberrant, altered QRS complexes and T waves when ventricular conduction is aberrant.

TECHNIQUES OF EXAMINATION

General Approach

The patient should be supine or lying with his upper body somewhat elevated. The latter position is especially helpful when the patient is orthopneic or when you are correlating cardiac signs with the jugular venous pulse. Stand at the patient's right side. When examining a woman with large breasts, you may need to displace the left breast upward or to the left. Alternatively, ask her to do this for you. The room must be quiet.

Abnormalities should be described in terms of:

1. Their timing in relation to the cardiac cycle.

2. Their location, i.e., the interspace and distance from the midsternal, the midclavicular or axillary lines. The midsternal line has the advantage of being the most reliable from one observer to another. When using it, hold the ruler tangential to the anterior chest, not curving around it.

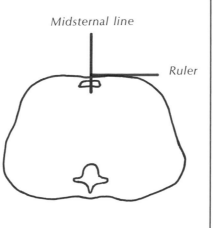

Midsternal line

Ruler

INSPECTION AND PALPATION

As you examine the patient's anterior chest, visualize the underlying cardiac chambers and great vessels: the right and left ventricles, the aorta and pulmonary artery. Try to detect any abnormal pulsations that they may produce. You may sometimes actually feel accentuated heart sounds, extra heart sounds and the vibrations of loud cardiac murmurs. These last vibrations, which feel like a cat's purr, are called thrills (a term that should be explained to the patient when it is used at the bedside!).

Since inspection and palpation reinforce each other, they will be described together. Note that:

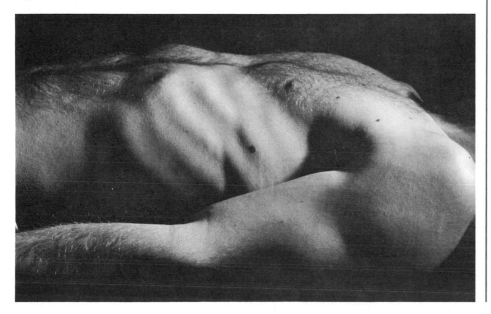

1. Tangential lighting helps you detect pulsations. Observing the chest surface tangentially is also useful, allowing you to see the pulsation "on edge."

2. The "ball of the hand" (the palmar surface of the hand at the base of the fingers) is most sensitive to vibrations. It may, therefore, be especially useful in detecting thrills. The finger pads are more helpful in detecting and analyzing pulsations.

3. In order to time puzzling pulsations or thrills in relation to systole and diastole, feel the carotid pulse or listen to the heart as you palpate (see pp. 152–153 for the relationships of these events).

Proceed in an orderly fashion to examine:

1. *The Aortic Area.* (Second interspace to the right of the sternum). Observe for any pulsation, thrill, the vibration of aortic valve closure.

Pulsation of aortic aneurysm; thrill of aortic stenosis; accentuated aortic valve closure sound of hypertension

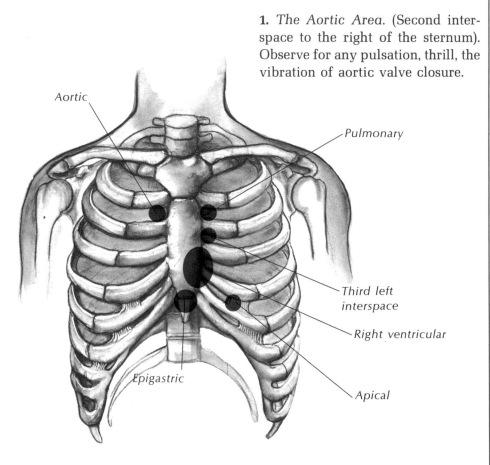

Aortic

Pulmonary

Third left interspace

Right ventricular

Epigastric

Apical

2. *The Pulmonary Area.* (Second left interspace; observe also the third left interspace for events of the pulmonic valve and artery). Observe for any pulsation, thrill, vibration of pulmonic valve closure.

Pulsation of increased pressure or flow in the pulmonary artery; thrill of pulmonic stenosis; accentuated pulmonic valve closure sound of pulmonary hypertension

3. *The Right Ventricular Area* (lower half of the sternum and the parasternal area, especially on the left). Observe for a diffuse lift or heave, thrills.

Note that in thin adults or in patients with anemia, anxiety, hyperthyroidism, fever or pregnancy (where cardiac output is increased) a brief right ventricular impulse is frequently felt here and does not necessarily indicate heart disease.

Sustained systolic lift of right ventricular hypertrophy; thrill of ventricular septal defect

4. *The Apical or Left Ventricular Area* (the fifth intercostal space at or just medial to the midclavicular line. Look for the apical impulse.

With the palm of your hand try to locate the apical impulse. If you

The apical impulse may be displaced upward and the left by pregnancy or a high left diaphragm.

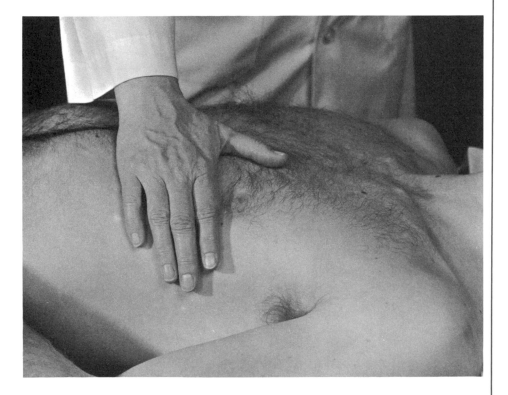

cannot find it, ask the patient to roll to his left side. This maneuver helps you find and assess the qualities of the apical impulse. Since it displaces the impulse, however, it should *not* be used in identifying its location. When the impulse is palpable, make finer observations with your fingertips. Assess its location, diameter, amplitude and duration. To estimate the duration of the impulse, listen to the heart sounds while you are palpating. Estimate the proportion of systole occupied by the palpable pulsation. Normally the apical impulse is a light tap, felt in an area about 1 to 2 cm in diameter, often smaller. It begins about at the time of the first heart sound and is sustained during the first $\frac{1}{3}$ to $\frac{1}{2}$ of systole.

See Table 9-1, Comparison of the Apical Impulse in Normal People and in Those with Left Ventricular Enlargement (p. 156).

Observe any thrills.

Thrills of mitral valve disease

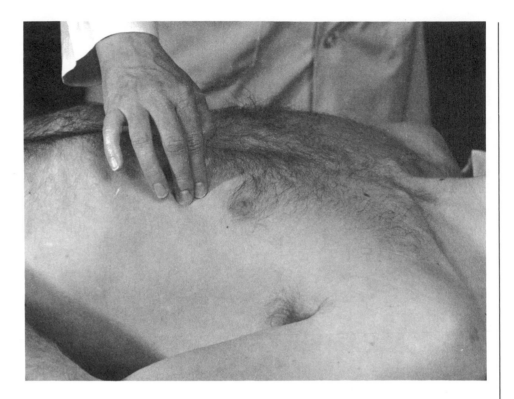

Observe any extra impulses, e.g., a palpable S_3 or S_4 (see heart sounds, p. 155).

A brief early diastolic impulse suggests a palpable S_3.

5. *The Epigastric Area.* Note any pulsations. The pulsation of the abdominal aorta may often be seen and felt here in the normal patient. In addition, the pulsation of an enlarged right ventricle can sometimes be felt. To distinguish these two, place the palm of your hand on the epigastric area and slide your fingers up under the rib cage. Note the aorta pulsating forward against the palmar surface of your fingers, the right ventricle beating downward against your fingertips.

Increased aortic pulse in aneurysm of the abdominal aorta, aortic regurgitation; right ventricular pulsation in right ventricular hypertrophy

AUSCULTATION

With your stethoscope identify the first and second heart sounds (S_1 and S_2), starting at the aortic or pulmonic area. The following clues are helpful:

1. At normal and slow rates S_1 is the first of the paired heart sounds, following the longer diastolic period and preceding the shorter systole.

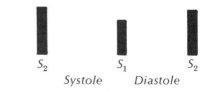

S_1 S_2 S_1 S_2
Systole   *Diastole*

2. At the base (aortic and pulmonic areas) S_2 is normally louder than S_1. This fact is especially helpful at rapid heart rates when systole and diastole may be approximately equal in length. Through a process of "inching," auscultation at the base may serve as a guide when listening in other areas of the heart. Having identified S_2 at the base, gradually

move or "inch" your stethoscope down toward the apex. Concentrate on S_2 and its rhythmic recurrence in the cardiac cycle, using it as a guide to time other sounds. If you get confused, inch back up to the base and down again.

3. S_1 is approximately synchronous with the onset of the apical impulse.

4. S_1 just precedes the carotid impulse

Identify the heart rate and rhythm.

Count the rate per minute. If the rhythm is perfectly regular, count for 15 seconds and multiply by 4. If there is any irregularity, however, or if the rate is slow, count for at least a minute.

Identify the rhythm. Is it regular or irregular? If irregular, try to identify a pattern: (1) Do early beats appear on a basically regular rhythm? (2) Does the irregularity vary consistently with respiration? (3) Or is the rhythm totally irregular?

See Tables 9-2 to 9-4, Differentiation of Selected Heart Rates and Rhythms (pp. 157–160).

Listen in order in the following locations:

1. Aortic area (second right interspace close to the sternum)
2. Pulmonic area (second left interspace close to the sternum)
3. Third left interspace close to the sternum (sometimes called Erb's point) where murmurs of both aortic and pulmonic origin may often be heard.
4. Tricuspid area (fifth left interspace close to the sternum)
5. Mitral (apical) area (fifth left interspace just medial to the midclavicular line).

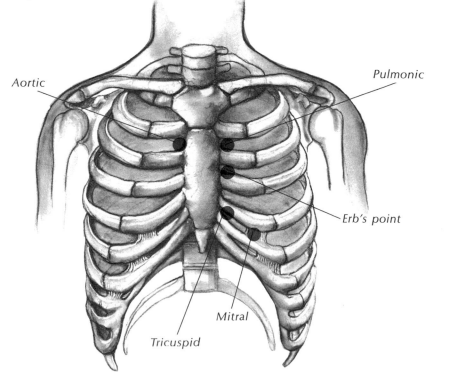

All heart sounds may be diminished in the presence of a thick chest wall or pulmonary emphysema.

At each auscultatory area:

1. Concentrate on the first heart sound. Note its intensity, splitting.

2. Concentrate on the second heart sound. Note its intensity, splitting. Pay special attention to splitting of S_2 in the left second and third interspaces. When listening for splitting, ask the patient to breathe quietly, then slightly more deeply than normal, but through his nose. (Mouth breathing makes louder breath sounds that obscure the heart sounds.)

3. Listen for extra sounds in systole. Note their timing, intensity, pitch.

4. Listen for extra sounds in diastole. Note their timing, intensity, pitch.

5. Listen for systolic murmurs. Murmurs are differentiated from heart sounds by their longer duration.

6. Listen for diastolic murmurs.

} If present, note the following characteristics:

Timing, for example:
    Systolic—early, mid or late systole
        —midsystolic ejection vs. pansystolic (holosystolic) regurgitant
    Diastolic—early, mid and late (or presystolic)

Location, described in terms of interspace and centimeters from the midsternal, midclavicular or one of the axillary lines

Radiation or transmission

Intensity
    Grade 1—very faint, heard only after the listener has "tuned in"; may not be heard in all positions
    Grade 2—quiet but heard immediately upon placing the stethoscope on the chest
    Grade 3—moderately loud, not associated with a thrill
    Grade 4—loud, may be associated with a thrill
    Grade 5—very loud, may be heard with stethoscope partly off the chest
    Grade 6—may be heard with stethoscope off the chest } thrills are associated

Pitch—high, medium or low

Quality—blowing, rumbling, harsh or musical

See Table 9-5, Variations in the First Heart Sound (p. 161).
See Table 9-6, Variations in the Second Heart Sound (p. 162).

See Table 9-7, Extra Heart Sounds in Systole (p. 163).
See Table 9-8, Extra Heart Sounds in Diastole (p. 164).
See Table 9-9, Three Causes of an Apparently Split First Heart Sound.

See Table 9-10, Mechanisms of Heart Murmurs (p. 166).

See Table 9-11, Midsystolic Ejection Murmurs (pp. 167–168).

See Table 9-12, Pansystolic Regurgitant Murmurs (p. 169).

See Table 9-13, Diastolic Murmurs (pp. 170–171).

7. Listen for murmurs or other cardiovascular sounds that have both systolic and diastolic components, such as pericardial friction rubs and venous hums.

Use first the diaphragm, which is best for picking up relatively high pitched sounds such as S₁, S₂, the murmurs of aortic and mitral regurgitation and pericardial friction rubs. Press the diaphragm firmly onto the chest. *Then use the bell* which is best for hearing low pitched sounds such as S₃, S₄ and the diastolic murmur of mitral stenosis. Apply the bell very lightly, with just enough pressure to produce an air seal with its full rim.

If an abnormality is heard, *explore the surrounding chest surface* to determine its distribution and radiation. For example, murmurs in the aortic area may radiate to the neck or down the left sternal border to the apex; those in the mitral area may radiate to the axilla.

See Table 9-14, Differentiation of Cardiovascular Sounds with Both Systolic and Diastolic Components (p. 172).

Use special positions or other maneuvers to elicit or accentuate abnormalities. For example, if you suspect an aortic murmur, especially the murmur of aortic regurgitation, ask the patient to sit up, lean forward, exhale completely and hold his breath in expiration. With the diaphragm of your stethoscope pressed on the chest, listen at the aortic area and down the left sternal border to the apex, pausing periodically so the patient may breathe.

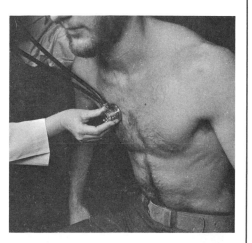

If you wish to bring out mitral murmurs or an S₃, ask the patient to roll onto his left side. Find the apical impulse. Then, using the bell of your stethoscope in light contact with the chest, listen carefully in and around the apical area.

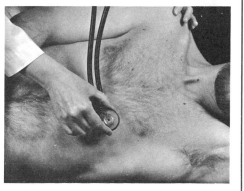

TABLE 9-1

TABLE 9-1. COMPARISON OF THE APICAL IMPULSE IN NORMAL PEOPLE AND IN THOSE WITH LEFT VENTRICULAR ENLARGEMENT

NORMAL HEART

Left ventricle

Apical impulse

AMPLITUDE	DURATION	LOCATION	DIAMETER
Small amplitude, light or even absent	Less than 2/3 and usually less than half of systole	5th or sometimes the 4th interspace, 7–9 cm from the midsternal line	1–2 cm; occupies only one interspace

LEFT VENTRICULAR ENLARGEMENT

Enlargement of left ventricle

Apical impulse

AMPLITUDE	DURATION	LOCATION	DIAMETER
Larger amplitude, feels more forceful and thrusting. When the left ventricle is hypertrophied but not dilated, increased amplitude and duration of the impulse are the principal signs.	Usually lasts throughout systole, up to S₂.	May be displaced to the left and down.	3 cm or more; occupies 2 or more interspaces. When the left ventricle is dilated as well as hypertrophied, the apical impulse is also both displaced and enlarged.

TABLE 9-2

TABLE 9-2. APPROACH TO THE DIFFERENTIATION OF SELECTED HEART RATES AND RHYTHMS

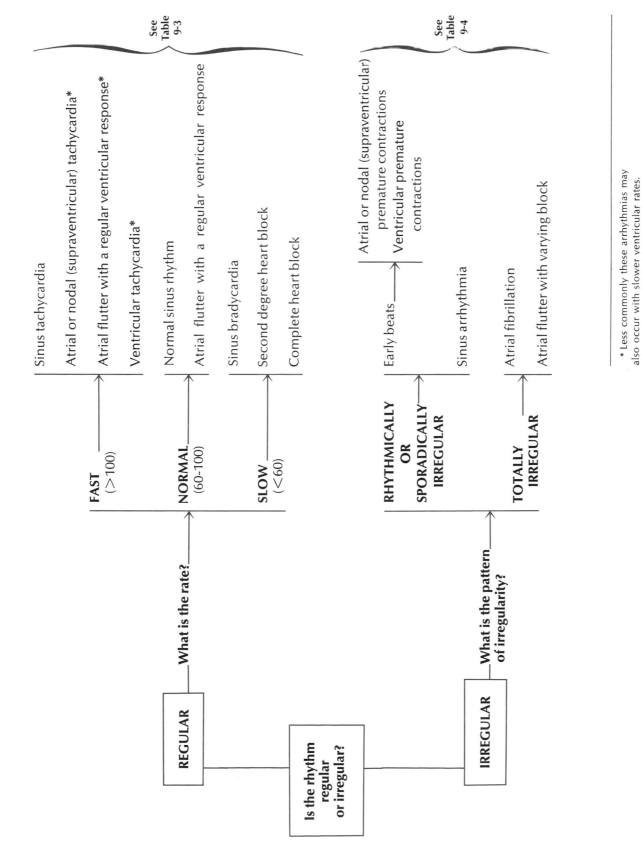

Is the rhythm regular or irregular?

REGULAR — What is the rate?

FAST (>100)
- Sinus tachycardia
- Atrial or nodal (supraventricular) tachycardia*
- Atrial flutter with a regular ventricular response*
- Ventricular tachycardia*

See Table 9-3

NORMAL (60–100)
- Normal sinus rhythm
- Atrial flutter with a regular ventricular response

SLOW (<60)
- Sinus bradycardia
- Second degree heart block
- Complete heart block

IRREGULAR — What is the pattern of irregularity?

RHYTHMICALLY OR SPORADICALLY IRREGULAR
- Early beats
  - Atrial or nodal (supraventricular) premature contractions
  - Ventricular premature contractions
- Sinus arrhythmia

See Table 9-4

TOTALLY IRREGULAR
- Atrial fibrillation
- Atrial flutter with varying block

* Less commonly these arrhythmias may also occur with slower ventricular rates.

TABLE 9-3

TABLE 9-3. DIFFERENTIATION OF SELECTED REGULAR RHYTHMS

| RHYTHMS WITH FAST VENTRICULAR RATES | PATHOPHYSIOLOGY | | | CLINICAL MANIFESTATIONS | | | | |
| | CONDUCTION PATHWAY | ORIGIN OF BEAT | CONDUCTION THROUGH AV NODE | VENTRICULAR RATE | | | | 1ST & 2ND HEART SOUNDS |
				USUAL RESTING RATE	RESPONSE TO EXERCISE	RESPONSE TO VAGAL STIMULATION *		
Sinus Tachycardia		Sinus node	Normal	100–150	–	Smooth slowing		Normal
Atrial or Nodal (Supraventricular) Tachycardia		Ectopic atrial	Normal	160–200	–	Abrupt slowing or no change		Normal
Atrial Flutter with a Regular Ventricular Response		Ectopic atrial, very rapid	Partial block at AV node, usually 2:1, i.e., 2 atrial beats to 1 ventricular	150–160	–	Abrupt slowing or no change		Normal
Ventricular Tachycardia		Ectopic ventricular	Ventricular rate too fast to permit AV conduction	150–200	–	No change		Split S_1, S_2; varying intensity of S_1

* Vagal stimulation may be produced by holding a deep breath, by the induction of gagging or retching and by carotid sinus massage. Careful monitoring is required.

TABLE 9-3

TABLE 9-3. (CONT'D)

RHYTHMS WITH NORMAL VENTRICULAR RATES	CONDUCTION PATHWAY	ORIGIN OF BEAT	CONDUCTION THROUGH AV NODE	USUAL RESTING RATE	RESPONSE TO EXERCISE	RESPONSE TO VAGAL STIMULATION *	1ST & 2ND HEART SOUNDS
Normal Sinus Rhythm		Sinus node	Normal	60–100	Smooth increase	Smooth slowing	Normal
Atrial Flutter with a Regular Ventricular Response		Ectopic atrial	Partial block at AV node, usually 3:1 or 4:1, i.e., 3 or 4 atrial beats to 1 ventricular	60–100	Abrupt increase or no change	Abrupt slowing or no change	Normal
RHYTHMS WITH SLOW VENTRICULAR RATES	CONDUCTION PATHWAY	ORIGIN OF BEAT	CONDUCTION THROUGH AV NODE	USUAL RESTING RATE	RESPONSE TO EXERCISE	RESPONSE TO VAGAL STIMULATION *	1ST & 2ND HEART SOUNDS
Sinus Bradycardia		Sinus node	Normal	50–60 may be down to 40	Smooth increase	–	Normal
Second Degree Heart Block		Sinus node	Partial block at AV node	35–60	Smooth increase	–	Normal S_1, S_2; atrial sounds may also be heard
Complete Heart Block		Sinus node and ventricle	Complete block at AV node	25–45, may be up to 60	No change	–	Varying S_1

* Vagal stimulation may be produced by holding a deep breath, by the induction of gagging or retching and by carotid sinus massage. Careful monitoring is required.

TABLE 9-4

TABLE 9-4. DIFFERENTIATION OF SELECTED IRREGULAR RHYTHMS

Type of Rhythm	Diagrammatic Representation	Rhythm	Heart Sounds
Atrial or Nodal (Supraventricular) Premature Contractions	QRS, Aberrant P wave, Normal QRS and T; P, T; S_1 S_2; Early beat, Pause	A beat of atrial or nodal origin comes earlier than the expected normal beat. A pause follows and the rhythm resumes.	S_1 may differ in intensity from normal beats, S_2 may be decreased, but both sounds are otherwise similar to normal beats.
Ventricular Premature Contractions	No P wave, Aberrant QRS and T; S_1 S_2; Early beat with split sounds, Pause	A beat of ventricular origin comes earlier than the expected normal beat. A pause follows and the rhythm resumes.	S_1 may differ in intensity from the normal beats, S_2 may be decreased but both sounds are likely to be split.
Sinus Arrhythmia	S_1 S_2; INSPIRATION, EXPIRATION	The heart varies cyclically, usually speeding up with inspiration and slowing down with expiration.	Normal although S_1 may vary with the heart rate.
Atrial Fibrillation and Atrial Flutter with Varying A-V Block	No P waves, Fibrillation waves; S_1 S_2	The ventricular rhythm is totally irregular, although short runs may seem regular.	S_1 varies in intensity.

TABLE 9-5

TABLE 9-5. VARIATIONS IN THE FIRST HEART SOUND

	Diagram	Description
NORMAL VARIATIONS	S_1 — S_2	S_1 is softer than S_2 at the *base* (aortic and pulmonic areas).
	S_1 — S_2	S_1 is often but not always louder than S_2 at the *apex*.
ACCENTUATED S_1	S_1 — S_2	S_1 is accentuated (1) during rapid heart action (e.g., exercise, anemia, hyperthyroidism), (2) in mitral stenosis. In both situations the mitral valve is still open wide at the onset of ventricular systole. The valve then slams shut.
DIMINISHED S_1	S_1 — S_2	S_1 is diminished in first degree heart block (delayed conduction from atria to ventricles). Here the mitral valve has had time after atrial contraction to float back into an almost closed position before ventricular contraction shuts it. It closes less loudly. S_1 is also diminished when the mitral valve is calcified and relatively immobile, as in mitral regurgitation.
VARYING S_1	S_1 — S_2 (varying)	S_1 varies in intensity (1) in complete heart block, where atria and ventricles are beating independently of each other, and (2) in any totally irregular rhythm, e.g., atrial fibrillation. In these situations the mitral valve is in varying positions before being shut by ventricular contraction. Its closure sound, therefore, varies in loudness.
SPLIT S_1	S_1 (split) — S_2	S_1 may normally be split in the tricuspid area where the tricuspid component, usually too faint to be heard, becomes audible. An apparently split S_1 that is heard easily at the apex is usually due instead to an S_4 or to an early systolic ejection click (see Table 9-9, p. 165).

TABLE 9-6

TABLE 9-6. VARIATIONS IN THE SECOND HEART SOUND

	EXPIRATION	INSPIRATION	

PHYSIOLOGICAL SPLITTING

Physiological splitting of the second heart sound can usually be detected in the pulmonic area. The pulmonic component of S_2 is usually too faint to be heard at the apex or aortic area where S_2 is single and derived from aortic valve closure alone. Normal splitting is accentuated by inspiration and usually disappears on expiration. In some patients, however, especially younger ones, S_2 may not become completely single on expiration.

PATHOLOGICAL SPLITTING

(All of these suggest heart disease.)

Wide splitting refers to an increase in the usual splitting and can be heard throughout the respiratory cycle. Wide splitting can be caused by delayed closure of the pulmonic valve, e.g., by pulmonic stenosis or right bundle branch block. As illustrated here, right bundle branch block also causes splitting of S_1 into its mitral and tricuspid components. Wide splitting can also be caused by early closure of the aortic valve, as in mitral regurgitation.

Fixed splitting refers to wide splitting that does not vary with respiration. It occurs in atrial septal defect and right ventricular failure.

Paradoxical splitting refers to splitting that appears on expiration, disappears on inspiration. Its most common cause is left bundle branch block.

INCREASED INTENSITY OF THE PULMONIC COMPONENT OF S_2. When the pulmonic component of S_2 becomes equal to or louder than the aortic component or when splitting of S_2 can be heard at the apex, pulmonary hypertension may be suspected.

DECREASED INTENSITY OF THE PULMONIC COMPONENT OF S_2 is heard in pulmonic stenosis.

INCREASED INTENSITY OF S_2 IN THE AORTIC AREA (where S_2 is composed entirely of the aortic closure sound) occurs in arterial hypertension and aortic valve syphilis.

DECREASED INTENSITY OF S_2 IN THE AORTIC AREA is heard in aortic stenosis.

TABLE 9-7

TABLE 9-7. EXTRA HEART SOUNDS IN SYSTOLE

Extra sounds or clicks may be heard in early, mid, or late systole.

Early Systolic Ejection Clicks

S_1 E_j S_2

Early systolic ejection clicks occur shortly after the first heart sound.

Aortic ejection clicks are heard at both base and apex. They may be louder at the apex. They do not usually vary with respiration. They may occur with a dilated aorta and aortic valve disease.

Pulmonary ejection clicks are heard best in the second and third left interspaces. When the first heart sound, usually relatively soft in this area, appears to be loud, you may instead be hearing a pulmonary ejection click. Decreased intensity of the click during inspiration gives another clue. Causes include dilatation of the pulmonary artery, pulmonary hypertension or pulmonic stenosis.

Mid and Late Systolic Clicks

S_1 S_2

Most mid and late systolic clicks are related to deformity or ballooning of the mitral valve and are often associated with late systolic murmurs.

TABLE 9-8

TABLE 9-8. EXTRA HEART SOUNDS IN DIASTOLE

OPENING SNAP	S_1 $\quad$ S_2 $O.S.$ $\quad$ S_1	The opening snap is a very early diastolic sound produced by the opening of a stenotic mitral or, more rarely, tricuspid valve. When of mitral origin it is heard best inside the apex and radiates rather widely. It is earlier, sharper and higher in pitch than an S_3.
S_3	S_1 $\quad$ S_2 S_3 $\quad$ S_1	A *physiological third heart sound* is frequently heard in children and young adults. Occurring early in diastole during rapid ventricular filling, it is later than an opening snap, dull and low pitched and best heard at the apex in the left lateral decubitus position. The bell of the stethoscope should be used with very light pressure. A *pathological S_3 or ventricular gallop.* If an S_3 is heard in an older person it usually indicates myocardial failure. Less commonly it may be produced by conditions that create volume overloading of a ventricle, e.g., aortic, mitral or tricuspid regurgitation. The timing and quality of an S_3 are similar to those of a physiologic S_3. An S_3 secondary to left ventricular failure is usually best heard at the apex, in the left lateral decubitus position. A right-sided S_3 is best heard along the lower left sternal border, with the patient supine. It usually becomes louder on inspiration.
S_4	S_1 $\quad$ S_2 $\quad$ S_4 S_1	An S_4 (*atrial sound or atrial gallop*) occurs just before S_1. It is low pitched and best heard with the bell. An S_4 is occasionally heard in a normal person. More commonly it is related to increased resistance to ventricular filling following atrial contraction. When originating on the left side of the heart, it may be secondary to hypertensive cardiovascular disease, coronary artery disease, myocardiopathy or aortic stenosis. It is then heard at or medial to the apex. The less common right-sided S_4 is heard along the lower left sternal border. Causes include pulmonic stenosis and cor pulmonale. An S_4 may also be associated with delayed conduction between atria and ventricles. This delay separates the normally faint atrial sound from the louder S_1 and makes it audible. An S_4 is never heard in the absence of atrial contraction, e.g., in atrial fibrillation.

TABLE 9-9

TABLE 9-9. THREE CAUSES OF AN APPARENTLY SPLIT FIRST HEART SOUND

When you hear an apparently double first heart sound, there are three possibilities.

	S_4	SPLIT S_1	EJECTION CLICK
	$S_4\ S_1$ S_2	S_1 S_2	$S_1\ Ej$ S_2
Pitch	An S_4 is relatively low pitched; therefore, the split is better heard with the bell.	Both components of a split S_1 are relatively high pitched; therefore, the split is better heard with the diaphragm.	An ejection click is relatively high pitched, therefore the split is better heard with the diaphragm.
Location	Usually the apex, although an S_4 originating in the right ventricle may be best heard along the lower left sternal border	The tricuspid area, since the tricuspid component of S_1 is soft and does not radiate widely	An aortic ejection click is usually heard in the aortic area and at the apex. A pulmonic ejection click is usually best heard in the second or third left interspace.
Palpable Split	Sometimes a palpable extra impulse at the apex	No	No

TABLE 9-10

TABLE 9-10. MECHANISMS OF HEART MURMURS

Heart murmurs are of longer duration than heart sounds. They originate within the heart itself or in its great vessels and are usually caused by one of the following mechanisms.

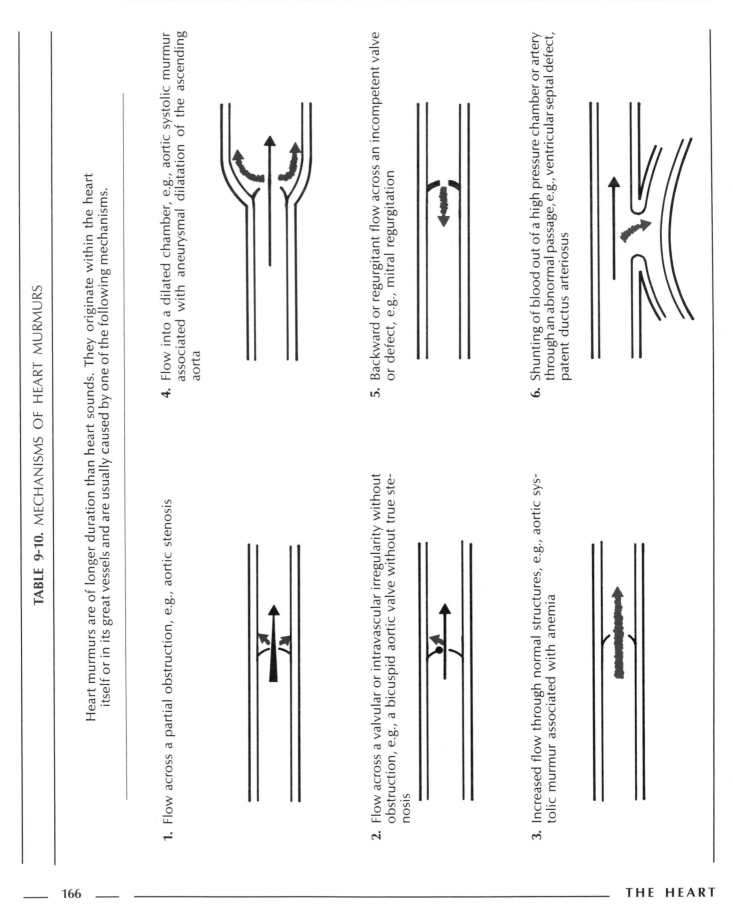

1. Flow across a partial obstruction, e.g., aortic stenosis

2. Flow across a valvular or intravascular irregularity without obstruction, e.g., a bicuspid aortic valve without true stenosis

3. Increased flow through normal structures, e.g., aortic systolic murmur associated with anemia

4. Flow into a dilated chamber, e.g., aortic systolic murmur associated with aneurysmal dilatation of the ascending aorta

5. Backward or regurgitant flow across an incompetent valve or defect, e.g., mitral regurgitation

6. Shunting of blood out of a high pressure chamber or artery through an abnormal passage, e.g., ventricular septal defect, patent ductus arteriosus

TABLE 9-11

TABLE 9-11. MIDSYSTOLIC EJECTION MURMURS

Midsystolic ejection murmurs constitute the most common kind of heart murmur. They may be (1) *organic*, i.e., secondary to structural cardiovascular abnormality; (2) *functional*, i.e., secondary to a physiologic alteration with or without heart disease; or (3) *innocent*, i.e., not associated with any functional or structural abnormality. Systolic ejection murmurs are relatively easy to identify but often hard to interpret. The entire cardiovascular examination, in fact a thorough evaluation of the whole patient, is frequently necessary.

Midsystolic ejection murmurs are associated with forward flow through the semilunar valves or outflow tracts. Constriction, structural irregularity, an increased rate of flow or flow into a dilated great vessel produces the systolic noise. The murmur has a crescendo-decrescendo (or diamond-shaped) pattern and is usually separated from the first and second heart sounds.

Organic causes of midsystolic ejection murmurs include aortic and pulmonic stenosis, i.e., failure of the aortic and pulmonic valves, respectively, to open as fully as they should during systole. Occasionally the constriction of flow occurs above or below the valve instead of in the valve itself. The murmurs of aortic and pulmonic valvular stenosis are contrasted below. Other causes of these murmurs are also discussed.

S_1 S_2

	AORTIC STENOSIS *Systole*	**PULMONIC STENOSIS** *Systole*
Location	Aortic area	Pulmonic area and third left interspace
Radiation	Into the neck, down the left sternal border and sometimes to the apex (Note: despite an apical location, an ejection type of murmur often originates in the aortic valve.)	Toward the left shoulder and upward toward the neck vessels, especially on the left.
Intensity	Variable. If loud, a thrill may be felt in the aortic area and neck.	Variable. If loud, a thrill may be felt in the pulmonic area.
Pitch	Medium	Medium
Quality	Often harsh	Often harsh
Associated Signs May Include	1. A diminished S_2 2. An early ejection click 3. A thrusting sustained apical impulse of left ventricular hypertrophy 4. A slowly rising carotid pulse contour 5. A narrow pulse pressure	1. A widely split S_2 and diminished to absent S_2P 2. An early ejection click 3. A left parasternal lift of right ventricular hypertrophy

TABLE 9-11

TABLE 9-11. (CONT'D)

OTHER CAUSES OF AORTIC SYSTOLIC MURMURS

Structural abnormality of the aortic valve without true stenosis may cause a midsystolic or early systolic ejection murmur indistinguishable from mild aortic stenosis. Two common examples are a congenitally *bicuspid but non-stenotic aortic valve* and the *somewhat sclerotic aortic valve associated with aging.* The lack of associated signs may help to make these diagnoses, but prolonged follow-up is often necessary.

Flow into an aorta dilated by syphilitic aortitis or by atherosclerosis may also cause this kind of systolic murmur.

Functional murmurs associated with increased blood flow across the aortic valve must also be considered in the differential diagnosis. Anemia and hyperthyroidism, for example, may cause such murmurs. If so, the murmur will disappear when the underlying condition is corrected. Aortic regurgitation increases left ventricular volume and, thus, augments systolic flow across the aortic valve. By this mechanism aortic regurgitation may produce an early or mid-systolic murmur (in addition to its own diastolic murmur) in the absence of true valvular stenosis.

OTHER CAUSES OF PULMONIC SYSTOLIC MURMURS

Increased blood flow across the pulmonic valve may produce a murmur that sounds like that of pulmonic stenosis. It is this mechanism, not flow through the defect, that produces the systolic murmur of *atrial septal defect.* Wide splitting of S_2 may accompany both atrial septal defect and pulmonic stenosis.

Increased blood flow from causes such as anemia or hyperthyroidism can also cause a pulmonic flow murmur.

Distinguishing the pulmonic murmurs of organic heart disease from the much more common *innocent murmurs* of children and young adults is a frequent and important problem. Innocent murmurs are usually (but not always) soft, i.e., Grade 1 or 2; they are usually short, i.e., early systolic, and are best heard in the left second and third interspaces. Splitting of the second sound is normal, no ejection click is heard and palpation of the right ventricle is normal. The character of an innocent murmur (intensity, duration) frequently changes with change in position, phase of respiration and heart rate. Chest x-ray and electrocardiogram may be needed to make sure of this diagnosis.

TABLE 9-12

TABLE 9-12. PANSYSTOLIC REGURGITANT MURMURS

Pansystolic regurgitant murmurs are heard when blood flows from a chamber of high pressure to one of lower pressure through a valve or other structure that should be closed. Regurgitation (also called incompetence or insufficiency) means there is a leak. Causes of pansystolic murmurs include mitral regurgitation (LV → LA), tricuspid regurgitation (RV → RA) and ventricular septal defect (LV → RV). The murmur begins immediately with the first heart sound and continues up to the second heart sound.

Three types of pansystolic murmurs are contrasted below.

	MITRAL REGURGITATION	TRICUSPID REGURGITATION	VENTRICULAR SEPTAL DEFECT
Location	Mitral area	Tricuspid area	Left sternal border in the 4th, 5th and 6th interspaces
Radiation	Into the left axilla	May radiate to the right of the sternum and to the left midclavicular line but not into the axilla	May radiate over the precordium but not into the axilla
Intensity	Variable, often loud; may be associated with an apical thrill; does not increase with inspiration	Variable; increases with inspiration	Often very loud and accompanied by a thrill
Pitch	High	High	High
Quality	Blowing	Blowing	Often harsh
Associated Signs May Include	Decreased S₁ An S₃ A thrusting sustained apical impulse displaced downward and to the left (left ventricular hypertrophy and dilatation)	A left parasternal lift of right ventricular hypertrophy Systolic pulsations in the jugular venous pulse and sometimes in the liver	Signs vary with the severity of the defect and with associated lesions.

A variant of the murmur of mitral regurgitation is confined to mid or late systole and is frequently preceded by a mid or late systolic click. Although the mitral valve is competent early in systole, a portion of it balloons into the left atrium later in ventricular contraction, allowing some regurgitation of blood.

TABLE 9-13

TABLE 9-13. DIASTOLIC MURMURS

Unlike systolic murmurs, diastolic murmurs are almost always indicative of heart disease. Two general types may be distinguished:

(1) the diastolic rumble originating in the atrioventricular valves and (2) the early diastolic murmurs of semilunar valve incompetence.

Diastolic rumbling murmurs are caused by (1) flow across distorted or stenotic mitral or tricuspid valves or by (2) increased blood flow across normal mitral or tricuspid valves. Because these valves open only after the aortic and pulmonic valves close, a short period of silence separates S_2 from the beginning of diastolic rumbles. These murmurs are low in pitch, rumbling in quality and heard best with the bell of the stethoscope in light skin contact. They tend to be loudest in the two phases of diastole when ventricular filling is most rapid: early in diastole immediately after valvular opening and again during atrial contraction (presystole).

Semilunar valve incompetence may result either from valvular deformity or from dilatation of the valvular ring. Murmurs of aortic regurgitation, together with most murmurs of pulmonic regurgitation, start immediately after the second sound and then diminish in intensity. They may be described therefore as *decrescendo diastolic murmurs* or immediate diastolic murmurs. In contrast to the rumbling atrioventricular valve murmurs, they are high pitched and blowing. They are best heard with the diaphragm pressed firmly on the chest.

The most common examples of these two types of diastolic murmurs are those of mitral stenosis and aortic regurgitation. They are contrasted on the next page.

TABLE 9-13

TABLE 9-13. (CONT'D)

	MITRAL STENOSIS	AORTIC REGURGITATION
	Diastole	*Diastole*
Location	Mitral (apical) area	Aortic area
Radiation	Very little; the murmur may be confined to a very small area and requires search.	Down the left sternal border, sometimes as far as the apex; also may radiate down the right sternal border
Intensity	Variable; may be brought out or accentuated in the left lateral decubitus position and by exercise	Variable, often faint; may be brought out by asking the patient to sit leaning forward with his breath exhaled
Pitch	Low (best heard with bell)	High (best heard with diaphragm)
Quality	Rumbling	Blowing
Associated Signs May Include	Increased S₁ in the mitral area Opening snap Increased S₂P and left parasternal lift of right ventricular hypertrophy if pulmonary hypertension has developed	Aortic systolic murmur from increased flow S₃ A sustained thrusting apical impulse displaced down and laterally (left ventricular hypertrophy and dilatation) Wide pulse pressure

TABLE 9-14

TABLE 9-14. DIFFERENTIATION OF CARDIOVASCULAR SOUNDS WITH BOTH SYSTOLIC AND DIASTOLIC COMPONENTS

Some cardiovascular sounds are not confined to one portion of the cardiac cycle.

Three examples are: (1) a pericardial friction rub, produced by inflammation of the pericardial sac; (2) patent ductus arteriosus, a congenital abnormality in which an open channel persists between aorta and pulmonary artery; and (3) a venous hum, a benign sound produced by turbulence of blood in the jugular veins (common in children). Their characteristics are contrasted below.

	PERICARDIAL FRICTION RUB	PATENT DUCTUS ARTERIOSUS	VENOUS HUM
Timing	May have three short components, each associated with cardiac movement: (1) atrial systole, (2) ventricular systole and (3) ventricular diastole. Usually the first two components are present; all three make diagnosis easy; only one invites confusion with a murmur.	Continuous murmur in both systole and diastole often with a silent interval late in diastole. Is loudest in late systole, obscures S_2 and fades in diastole.	Continuous murmur without a silent interval. Loudest in diastole
Location	Variable but usually best heard in the 3rd interspace to the left of the sternum	Left 2nd interspace	Above the medial ⅓ of the clavicles, especially on the right
Radiation	Little	Toward the left clavicle	1st and 2nd interspaces
Intensity	Variable. May increase when the patient leans forward and exhales	Usually loud, sometimes associated with a thrill	Soft to moderate. Can be obliterated by pressure on the jugular veins.
Quality	Scratchy, sounds close to the ear	Harsh, machinery-like	Humming, roaring
Pitch	High	Medium	Low

pressures and pulses: arterial and venous

ANATOMY AND PHYSIOLOGY

Arterial Blood Pressure and Pulse

Blood Pressure in the arterial system varies with the cardiac cycle, reaching a systolic peak and a diastolic trough, the levels of which are measured by sphygmomanometry. The difference between systolic and diastolic pressures is known as the pulse pressure.

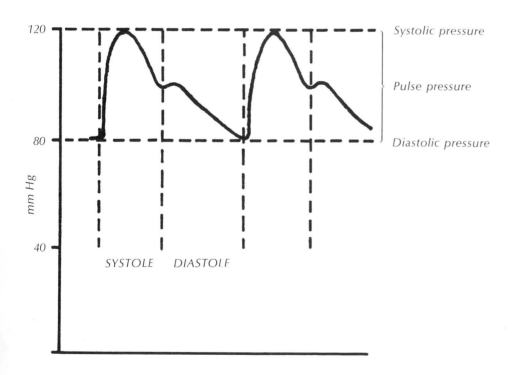

Several factors influence arterial pressure:

1. *Cardiac Output.* The pumping action of the left ventricle is of course essential to the maintenance of blood pressure. It affects chiefly the systolic pressure.

2. *Elastic Recoil of the Aorta and Large Arteries.* As the left ventricle forces blood into the aorta and large arteries, it distends their elastic walls. Recoil of the vessel walls during diastole advances the blood down the arterial tree and helps to maintain diastolic pressure. A competent aortic valve is also necessary to assure forward flow.

3. *Peripheral Resistance.* Peripheral resistance to blood flow depends primarily on the caliber of the arterioles, under control of the autonomic nervous system. It is the chief determinant of diastolic blood pressure.

4. *Volume of Blood in the Arterial System*

5. *Viscosity of the Blood*

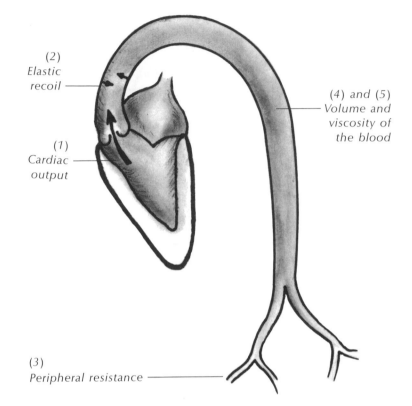

Changes in any of these five factors alter systolic pressure, diastolic pressure or both.

With each ventricular contraction a pressure wave is transmitted through the arterial system. The contour of this *arterial pulse* can be estimated by palpation. This pressure wave travels about 10 times faster than the blood itself. Because of the proximity of the carotid artery to the heart, the carotid arterial pulse is especially useful in timing cardiac events. The more peripheral pulses should not be used for this purpose since their slight delay is confusing. The pulse wave normally reaches the femoral artery very slightly before it reaches the radial—a useful clinical point in detecting coarctation of the aorta (see p. 180).

Jugular Venous Pressure and Pulse

Pressure on the venous side of the circulatory system is much lower than on the arterial side. It is ultimately dependent upon left ventricular contraction, but much of this force is dissipated as the blood passes through the arterial tree and capillary bed. Other important determinants of venous pressure include: (1) blood volume and (2) the capacity of the right heart to receive blood and to eject it onward into the pulmonary arterial system. When any of these variables is altered pathologically, abnormalities in venous pressure result. For example, the venous pressure falls when left ventricular output or blood volume is significantly reduced; it rises when the right heart fails or when increased pressure in the pericardial sac impedes the return of blood to the right atrium.

In the laboratory, venous pressure is measured from a zero point in the right atrium. Since it is difficult to establish this point reliably during physical examination, a stable and reproducible landmark is substituted— the sternal angle. In most positions, whether upright or supine, the sternal angle is roughly 5 to 7 cm above the right atrium.

Although it is possible to measure venous pressure elsewhere in the venous system, the best estimate of right atrial pressure, and therefore of right heart function, can be made from the internal jugular veins. If these are impossible to see, the external jugular veins can be used but they are less reliable. The level of venous pressure is determined by finding the highest point of oscillation in the internal jugular veins or, if necessary, the point above which the external jugular veins appear collapsed. The vertical distance in centimeters between either of these points and the sternal angle is recorded as the venous pressure. The zero point, i.e., the sternal angle should also be stated.

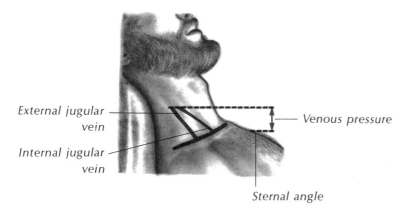

External jugular vein

Internal jugular vein

Venous pressure

Sternal angle

In order to see the venous pressure level, it may be necessary to alter the patient's position. When the pressure is relatively low, for example, the jugular veins may be visible only at or below the level of the sternal angle. To see them you should elevate the patient's head and trunk only slightly. Were this patient sitting up, his venous pulsations would be well below his clavicles and therefore invisible. In contrast, a high venous pressure may distend the supine patient's neck veins throughout their course in the neck; the level may then be well above the jaw and therefore obscured.

Pressures more than 3 cm above the sternal angle are considered elevated.

Careful observation reveals that the internal jugular pulse is composed of two or sometimes three waves. These are called *a*, *c* and *v* waves. Their analysis gives important information about the cardiac events and pressures in the right atrium.

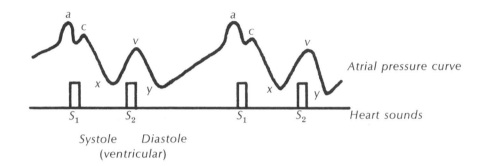

The *a wave* represents a slight rise in atrial pressure that occurs with atrial contraction, just before ventricular systole. With the beginning of ventricular systole, the tricuspid valve closes and the atrium relaxes. The resulting fall in right atrial pressure is reflected in the jugular venous pulse as a fall in the height of the blood column—a trough known as the x *descent*. As the venous return to the right atrium continues and the chamber begins to fill, there is another rise in right atrial pressure, seen as the *v wave*. This wave begins during the latter part of ventricular systole. With the beginning of diastole and the opening of the tricuspid valve, the right atrium empties rapidly into the right ventricle. The right atrial pressure again falls, forming a second trough or y *descent*. Sometimes a *c wave* is visible. It is a reflected wave from the nearby carotid artery.

TECHNIQUES OF EXAMINATION

The Arterial Pulse

Although one may observe the pulse in a number of locations, the radial artery is most frequently examined. The carotid artery is more satisfactory, however, for assessing the pulse contour and for timing cardiovascular events. Use the following techniques:

1. *Radial Artery.* With the pads of your index and middle fingers, compress the radial artery at the wrist until a maximum pulsation is detected.

2. *Carotid Artery.* Examine one side at a time. With your index and middle fingers at or hooked around the medial edge of the sternomastoid, press gently on the carotid artery in the lower half of the neck. Avoid the carotid sinus, which may respond to pressure by producing an undesirable decrease in pulse or blood pressure. Turning the patient's head slightly toward the side being examined may be helpful.

Decreased or absent carotid pulse suggests arterial narrowing or occlusion.

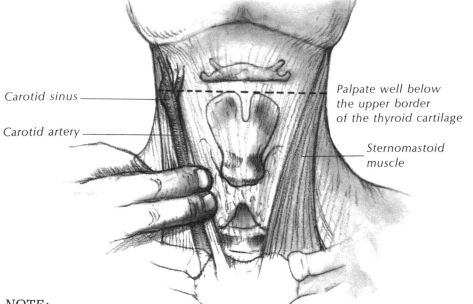

Carotid sinus

Carotid artery

Palpate well below the upper border of the thyroid cartilage

Sternomastoid muscle

NOTE:

1. The rate and rhythm of the pulse. If you detect abnormalities here, they are best evaluated by cardiac auscultation.

   See Table 10-1, Abnormalities of the Arterial Pulse (p. 185).

2. The amplitude of the pulse.

3. The contour of the pulse, i.e., the speed of its apparent expansion or upstroke, the duration of its peak and the speed of its collapse.

4. Any variation in amplitude—
   a. From beat to beat
   b. With respiration

If the patient is elderly, or if you suspect cerebrovascular disease, listen to the carotid arteries with the diaphragm of your stethoscope.

A bruit here suggests narrowing of the carotid artery or radiation of a systolic murmur from the aortic area.

Blood Pressure

Choice of Sphygmomanometer. Blood pressure may be satisfactorily measured with a sphygmomanometer of either the aneroid or mercury type. It is essential, however, to select a cuff of the proper size. The inflatable bag encased in the cuff should be about 20 percent wider than the diameter of the limb on which it is to be used. It should be long enough to encircle the limb. For an average adult, a bag 12 to 14 cm wide and 30 cm long is suitable. Wider cuffs (e.g., 18 to 20 cm) should be used on thighs and obese arms; narrower cuffs on children or adults with very thin arms.

Cuffs that are too small may give falsely high readings; cuffs that are too large may give falsely low readings.

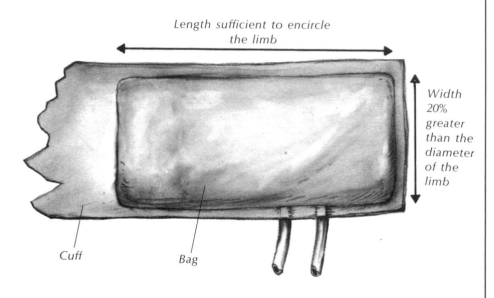

Length sufficient to encircle the limb

Width 20% greater than the diameter of the limb

Cuff

Bag

Technique. The patient should be as comfortable as possible, his arm free and slightly flexed at the elbow, his brachial artery approximately at heart level. Center the inflatable bag over the brachial artery on the inside of the arm. Its lower border should be about 2.5 cm above the antecubital crease. Secure the cuff snugly.

Inflate the cuff to about 30 mm Hg above the level at which the radial pulse disappears. Lower the cuff pressure slowly until the radial pulse is again detectable. This is the palpatory systolic pressure and helps you avoid being misled by an auscultatory gap (see the diagram on p. 181). Deflate the cuff completely.

Place a stethoscope firmly, but without undue pressure, over the brachial artery in the antecubital space. This point is usually found just medial to the biceps tendon. The stethoscope should touch neither cuff nor clothing.

If the brachial artery is much below heart level, the blood pressure will appear falsely high. Conversely, if the artery is much above heart level, the blood pressure will appear falsely low. A 13.6 cm difference between arterial and cardiac levels produces a blood pressure error of 10 mm Hg.

Inflate the cuff again, to about 30 mm Hg above the palpatory systolic pressure. Then deflate the cuff slowly, allowing the pressure to drop at a rate of about 3 mm Hg per second. Note the level at which you hear the sounds of at least two consecutive beats. This is the systolic pressure.

Continue to lower the pressure slowly until the sounds become suddenly muffled. This point is the most reliable measure of diastolic pressure, although usually somewhat above that found by intra-arterial measurement.

Continue decreasing the pressure and note the point at which all sounds disappear. Record all three points, e.g., 120/80/70.* When using a mercury sphygmomanometer, make all readings at eye level with the meniscus.

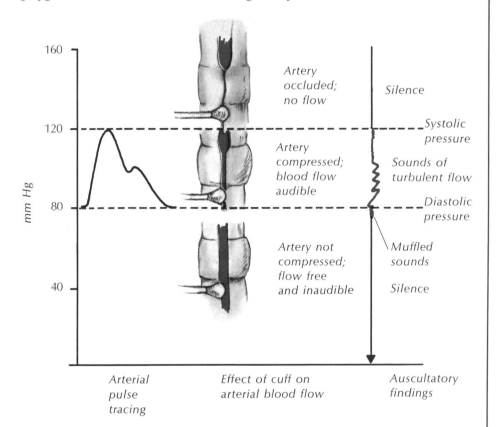

Blood pressure should be taken in both arms, at least when evaluating the patient initially. Normally there may be a difference in pressure of 5 mm Hg, sometimes up to 10 mm Hg. Subsequent readings should be made on the arm with the higher pressure.

When the patient is taking antihypertensive medications, when he has a history of fainting or postural dizziness or when you suspect depletion of

Pressure difference of over 10 mm Hg suggests arterial compression or obstruction on the side with the lower pressure.

A substantial drop in diastolic pressure is abnormal. Causes include drugs, depletion of blood volume, and disease of the peripheral autonomic nervous system.

*Recording of diastolic pressures has never been satisfactorily standardized. A committee of the American Heart Association (1967) recommended recording both muffling and disappearance points, but suggested that the muffling point was the better index of diastolic pressure. The disappearance point is recommended, however, by the Joint National Commission on Detection, Evaluation, and Treatment of High Blood Pressure (1977).

blood volume, take his blood pressure in three positions—supine, sitting and standing (unless, of course, these positions are contraindicated). Normally, as the patient rises from the horizontal, his systolic pressure drops slightly or remains unchanged while his diastolic pressure rises slightly.

Upper limits of normal blood pressure in adults have been traditionally set between 140/90 and 150/95. Even the lower of these two criteria would be suspiciously high, however, in a young adult. Blood pressure readings on at least three separate visits should usually be taken and averaged before making a diagnosis of hypertension.

Lower limits of normal blood pressure, sometimes estimated at 90/60 in adults, should always be interpreted in the light of past readings and the patient's present clinical state.

A pressure of 110/70 might well be normal, for example, but could also indicate significant hypotension in a patient whose past pressures have been high.

Special Problems

1. *The Apprehensive Patient.* Anxiety is a frequent cause of high blood pressure, especially on a first visit. Make repeated measurements before concluding that the patient has persistent hypertension.

2. *The Obese Arm.* Use a wider cuff that completely encircles the arm. Be sure that the bag does not balloon out from under the cuff.

3. *Leg Pulses and Pressures.* In order to rule out coarctation of the aorta, two observations should be made at least once on every hypertensive patient: (1) Compare the volume and timing of the radial and femoral pulses. (2) Compare blood pressures in the arm and leg.

To determine blood pressure in the leg, use a wide cuff on the lower third of the thigh. Center the bag over the posterior surface, wrap it securely and listen over the popliteal artery. If possible the patient should be prone. If he cannot lie on his abdomen, flex his leg slightly. By sphygmomanometry, systolic pressure in the legs is usually found to be substantially higher than in the brachial artery. This does not reflect true intra-arterial pressure differences. A systolic pressure lower in the legs than the arms is abnormal.

A diminished, delayed femoral pulse in relation to the radial pulse suggests coarctation of the aorta or occlusive aortic disease. Blood pressure lower in the legs than in the arms is confirmatory.

4. *Inaudible Blood Pressure.* Consider these possibilities; act accordingly.
   a. Erroneous placement of your stethoscope. Search again for the brachial artery.
   b. Venous engorgement of the arm from repeated inflation of the cuff. Remove the cuff. Elevate the patient's arm over his head for one or two minutes, then reapply the cuff and try again.
   c. Shock. It may be impossible to measure the blood pressure of a patient in shock without direct arterial puncture.

5. *Arrhythmias.* Irregular rhythms produce variations in pressure and therefore unreliable measurements. Ignore the effects of an occasional premature contraction. With frequent premature contractions and in atrial fibrillation, take an average of several observations and note that your measurements are approximate.

6. *Auscultatory Gap.* In some patients, usually those who are hypertensive, there is a silent interval part way between systolic and diastolic pressures. If this is not recognized, it may lead to serious underestimation of systolic pressure or overestimation of diastolic pressure.

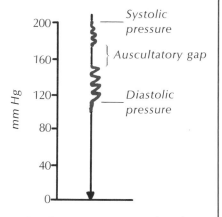

Record your findings completely , e.g., "blood pressure is 200/110/100 with an auscultatory gap from 170 to 150."

7. *Pulsus Alternans* and *Pulsus Paradoxus.* See Table 10-1.

See Table 10-1, Abnormalities of the Arterial Pulse (p. 185).

Jugular Venous Pressure

Examination of the jugular veins and their pulsations allows quite accurate estimation of the central venous pressure and therefore gives important information about cardiac compensation. The internal jugular pulsations, although somewhat harder to see than the external jugulars, give a more accurate reading.

Position the patient so that he is relaxed and comfortable, with his head slightly elevated on a pillow and his sternomastoid muscles relaxed. Adjust the head of the bed so as to maximize the jugular venous pulsations and make them visible above the clavicles but well below the jaw. Usually the head of the bed needs slight elevation, e.g., 15 degrees to 30 degrees from the horizontal. When the patient's venous pressure is increased, however, an elevation to 45 degrees or even to 90 degrees may be required.

Use tangential (oblique) lighting and examine *both sides* of the neck. Unilateral distention, especially of an external jugular vein, may be deceptive: it can be caused by local factors in the neck.

Identify the external jugular vein on each side. Then *find the pulsations of the internal jugular vein.* Since this vein lies deep to muscle, you will not see the vein itself. Watch instead for the pulsations transmitted through the surrounding soft tissues. Look for them in the suprasternal notch, between the attachments of the sternomastoid on the sternum and clavicle, or just posterior to the sternomastoid. Distinguish these pulsations from those of the adjacent carotid artery by the following points.

INTERNAL JUGULAR PULSATIONS	CAROTID PULSATIONS
Rarely palpable	Palpable
Soft undulating quality usually with 2 or 3 outward components (a, c and v waves)	A more vigorous thrust with a single outward component
Pulsation eliminated by light pressure on the vein just above the sternal end of the clavicle	Pulsation not eliminated
Level of pulsation usually descends with inspiration	Pulsation not affected by inspiration
Pulsations vary with position	Pulsations are unchanged by position

Identify the highest point at which pulsations of the internal jugular vein can be seen. With a centimeter ruler measure the vertical distance between this point and the sternal angle. A sturdy square-cornered piece of paper helps establish the horizontal and vertical relationships that underlie this measurement. A second observer at some distance from you can help establish a truly horizontal line.

Increased pressure suggests right-sided heart failure or, less commonly, constrictive pericarditis or superior vena cava obstruction. In patients with obstructive lung disease, venous pressure may appear elevated on expiration only; the veins collapse on inspiration. This finding does not indicate congestive heart failure.

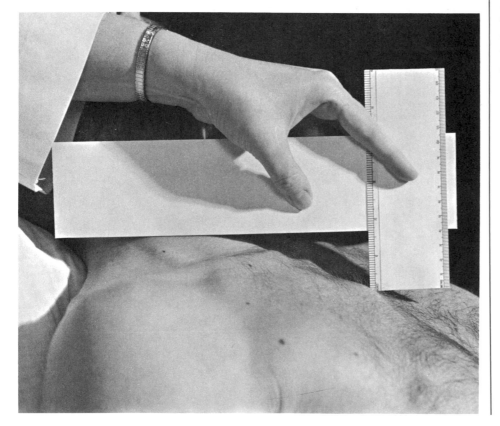

If the highest point of venous pulsation is below the sternal angle, hold the ruler at the neck rather than at the sternal angle.

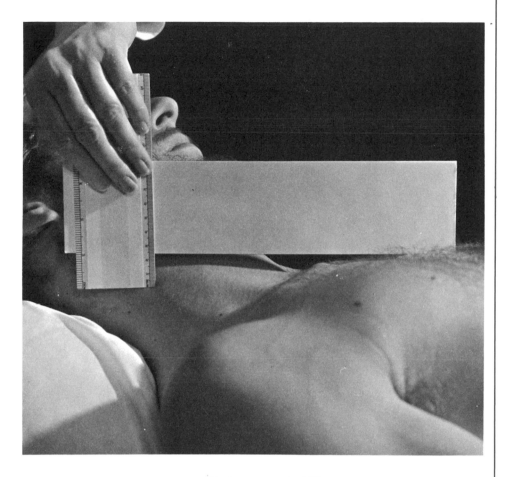

If you are unable to visualize the internal jugular pulsations, identify *the point above which the external jugular veins appear to be collapsed.* Make this observation on each side of the neck. Measure the vertical distance of this point from the sternal angle.

Unilateral distention of the external jugular vein is usually due to local kinking or obstruction. Occasionally even bilateral distention has a local cause.

By either technique, record the distance in centimeters above or below the sternal angle together with the angle at which the patient was lying, e.g., "the internal jugular venous pulse is 6 cm above the sternal angle, with the head of the bed elevated to 45 degrees." Venous pressure greater than 3 cm above the sternal angle is abnormal.

If congestive heart failure is suspected, whether or not the jugular venous pressure appears elevated, *check for a hepatojugular reflux.* Adjust the position of the patient so that the highest level of pulsation is readily identifiable in the lower half.of the neck. Exert firm and sustained pressure with your hand over the patient's right upper quadrant for 30 to 60 seconds. Be sure the patient remains relaxed and continues to breathe easily. If a tender

A rise in jugular venous pressure with this maneuver (a positive hepatojugular reflux) suggests congestive heart failure.

right upper quadrant prevents this, press on another part of the abdomen. Watch for an increase in the jugular venous pressure during this maneuver. A rise of more than 1 cm is abnormal.

Observe the amplitude and timing of the jugular venous pulsations. In order to time these pulsations, listen to the heart simultaneously. The a wave is approximately synchronous with S_1. The x descent can be seen as a systolic collapse between S_1 and S_2. The v wave coincides approximately with S_2. Look for absent or unusually prominent waves.

The a waves disappear in atrial fibrillation.

Giant a waves are seen in tricuspid stenosis and severe cor pulmonale.

Large v waves characterize tricuspid regurgitation.

TABLE 10-1

TABLE 10-1. ABNORMALITIES OF THE ARTERIAL PULSE

NORMAL

mm Hg

The pulse pressure is about 30-40 mm Hg. The pulse contour is smooth and rounded. (The notch on the descending slope of the pulse wave is not palpable.)

SMALL, WEAK PULSES

The pulse pressure is diminished. The pulse contour may show a slowed upstroke and prolonged peak. Causes include: (1) decreased stroke volume as in heart failure, shock; (2) mechanical obstruction to left ventricular output as in aortic stenosis.

LARGE, BOUNDING PULSES

The pulse pressure is increased. The pulse contour frequently shows a rapid rise, brief peak and rapid fall. Causes include: (1) hyperkinetic states, e.g., anxiety, exercise, fever, anemia, hyperthyroidism; (2) abnormally rapid runoff of blood as in aortic regurgitation, patent ductus arteriosus; and (3) increased aortic rigidity as in aging and atherosclerosis.

PULSUS ALTERNANS

To make this observation the rhythm must be regular. The pulse alternates in amplitude from beat to beat. When the variation is slight, it can be detected only by sphygmomanometry: lower the cuff pressure slowly toward the systolic level; note alternating loud and soft sounds or a sudden doubling of the rate as the cuff pressure declines. Pulsus alternans is evidence of left-sided heart failure.

BIGEMINAL PULSE

This is really a disorder of rhythm that may masquerade as pulsus alternans. Do not confuse them. A bigeminal rhythm is usually produced by a normal beat alternating with a premature contraction. The stroke volume of the latter is diminished and the pulse varies in its amplitude, alternating between strong and weak. The rhythm here is irregular.

Premature contractions

PULSUS PARADOXUS

The pulse diminishes perceptibly in amplitude on inspiration. This is frequently detectable only by sphygmomanometry. As the patient breathes quietly, lower the cuff pressure slowly toward the systolic level. Note the pressure reading when the first sounds can be heard. Drop the cuff pressure very slowly until sounds can be heard throughout the respiratory cycle. Again note the pressure reading. If the readings are 10 mm Hg or more apart, a paradoxical pulse is present. A paradoxical pulse, an exaggeration of the normal response to respiration, is found in severe obstructive lung disease and constrictive pericardial disease.

Inspiration

Expiration

the breasts and axillae

ANATOMY AND PHYSIOLOGY

The female breast lies between the second and sixth ribs, between the sternal edge and midaxillary line. About two-thirds of it is superficial to the pectoralis major, about one-third to the serratus anterior. The nipple is located centrally where it is surrounded by the areola. Sebaceous glands on the areola present as small round elevations.

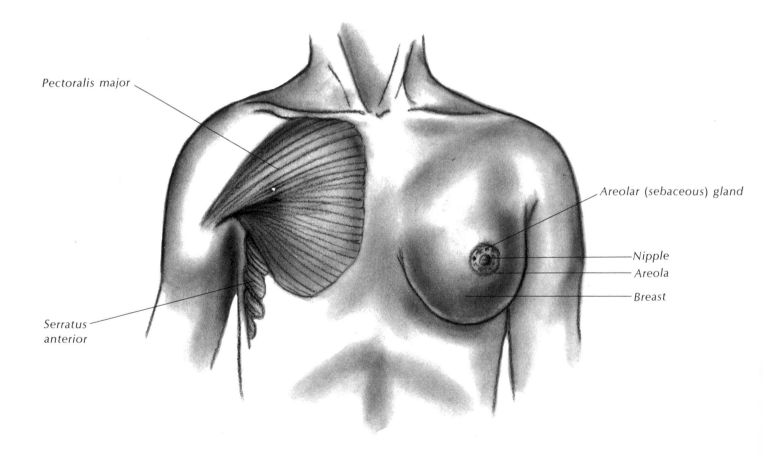

Pectoralis major

Serratus anterior

Areolar (sebaceous) gland

Nipple

Areola

Breast

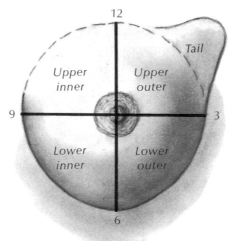

LEFT BREAST

For purposes of description, the breast may be divided into four quadrants by horizontal and vertical lines crossing at the nipple. In addition a tail of breast tissue frequently extends toward or into the axilla. An alternative method of localizing findings visualizes the breast as the face of a clock. A lesion may be located by the "time," e.g., 4 o'clock, and by the distance in centimeters from the nipple.

Breast tissue has three principal components. (1) The *glandular tissue* is organized into 12 to 20 lobes, each of which terminates in a duct that opens on the surface of the nipple. (2) This glandular tissue is supported by *fibrous tissue,* including suspensory ligaments that are connected both to the skin and to fascia underlying the breast. (3) *Fat* surrounds the breast and predominates both superficially and peripherally. The proportions of these components vary with age, the general state of nutrition, pregnancy and other factors.

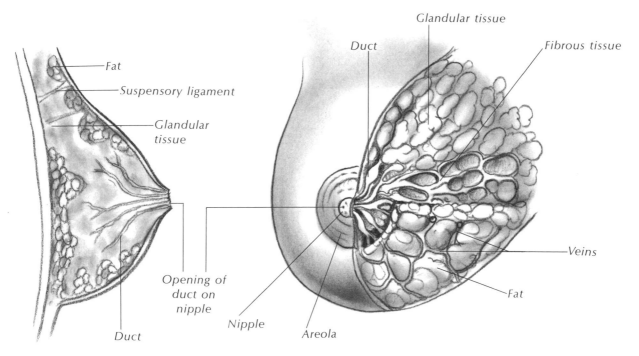

CROSS SECTION, LATERAL VIEW

The male breast consists chiefly of a small nipple and areola. These overlie a thin disc of undeveloped breast tissue that is not usually distinguishable clinically from the surrounding tissues.

Since the lymphatics of much of the breast drain toward the axilla, axillary anatomy is considered at this time. The axilla can be visualized as a pyramidal space the base of which is formed by the skin of the axilla or arm pit. The apex of the pyramid lies between the clavicle and first rib. The anterior border of the axilla is formed by the pectoral muscles; the posterior border by muscles including the latissimus dorsi and subscapularis; the medial border by the rib cage and serratus anterior muscle; and the lateral border by the upper arm.

The central axillary nodes are located high in the axilla close to the ribs and serratus anterior. Into them drain channels from three other groups of lymph nodes:
1. The pectoral (or anterior) group of nodes is located along the lower border of the pectoralis major inside the anterior axillary fold. These nodes drain the anterior chest wall and most of the breasts.
2. The subscapular (or posterior) group is located along the lateral border of the scapula and is felt deep in the posterior axillary fold. These nodes drain the posterior chest wall and a portion of the arm.
3. The lateral group is felt along the upper humerus. These nodes drain most of the arm.

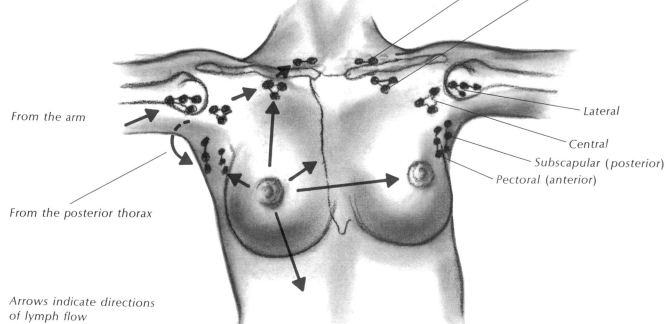

Supraclavicular

Infraclavicular

From the arm

Lateral

Central

Subscapular (posterior)

Pectoral (anterior)

From the posterior thorax

Arrows indicate directions of lymph flow

Lymph drains from the central axillary nodes to the infraclavicular and supraclavicular nodes.

Note that the lymphatics of the breast do not all drain into the axilla. Depending upon the location of a lesion in the breast, spread may occur directly to the infraclavicular nodes, into deep channels within the chest or abdomen and even to the opposite breast.

The Female Breast

While examining a woman's breasts, you have an ideal opportunity to explain what you are doing and to instruct her in self-examination. If she is unfamiliar with this procedure, help her to repeat it after you.

INSPECTION

With the patient in the sitting position, disrobed to the waist and with her arms at her sides—

Inspect the breasts, noting:

1. Their size and symmetry. Some difference in size is common and usually normal.

2. Their contour, with special reference to masses, dimpling or flattening.

3. The appearance of the skin, including:
   a. Color
   b. Thickening or edema
   c. Venous pattern

See Table 11-1, Visible Signs of Breast Cancer (p. 196).

Redness in infection or inflammatory carcinoma

Edema or increased venous prominence in carcinoma

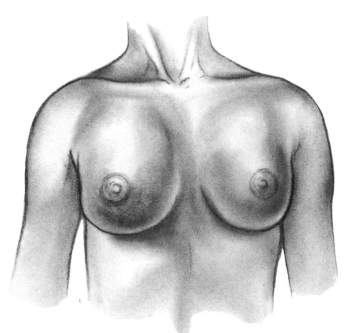

ARMS AT SIDE

Inspect the nipples, noting:
1. Their size and shape. Simple inversion of long standing is common and usually normal.
2. The direction in which they point.
3. Rashes or ulcerations.
4. Discharge.

See Table 11-2, Abnormalities of Nipple and Areola (p. 197).

In order to bring out dimpling or retraction that may otherwise be over-looked, ask the patient (1) to raise her arms over her head and (2) to press her hands against her hips. Again inspect the breast contour carefully.

Dimpling or retraction of the breast suggests an underlying cancer.

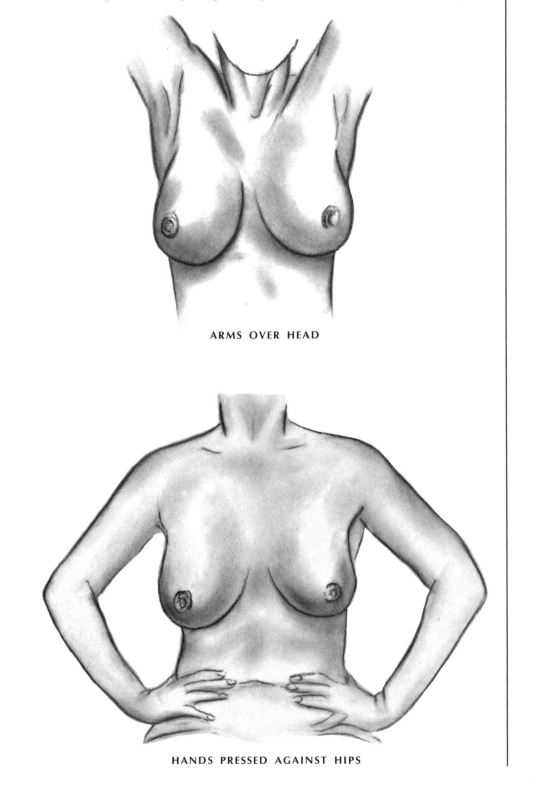

ARMS OVER HEAD

HANDS PRESSED AGAINST HIPS

Occasionally, other maneuvers may be useful.

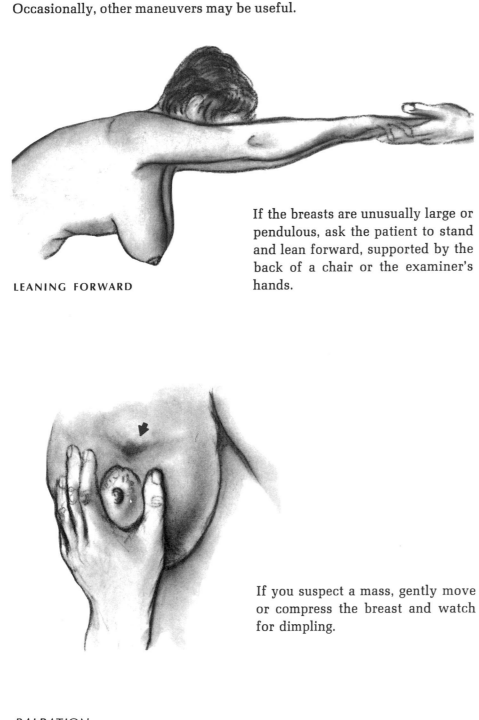

LEANING FORWARD

If the breasts are unusually large or pendulous, ask the patient to stand and lean forward, supported by the back of a chair or the examiner's hands.

If you suspect a mass, gently move or compress the breast and watch for dimpling.

PALPATION

Ask the patient to lie down. Unless the breasts are quite small, place a small pillow under the patient's shoulder on the side you are examining. This maneuver helps to spread the breast more evenly across the chest and makes it easier to find nodules.

Use the pads of your three fingers in a rotary motion to compress the breast tissue gently against the chest wall. Proceed systematically, examining the entire breast, including the periphery, tail and areola.

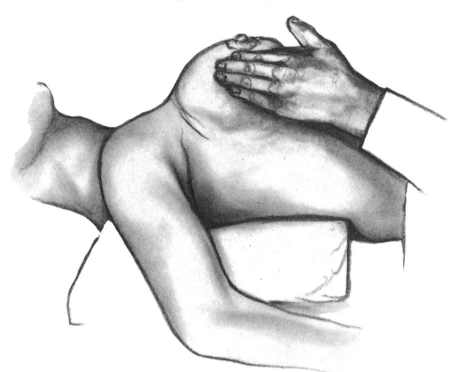

A uniform pattern of examination, as in the following diagram, helps to assure a complete assessment.

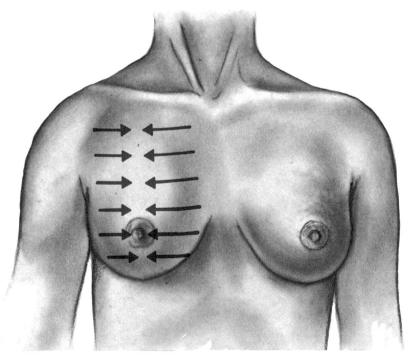

NOTE:

The consistency or elasticity of the tissues. Normal variations include the firm elasticity of the young breast, the lobular feel of glandular tissue, and the somewhat stringy or granular feel of the older breast. Premenstrual fullness, nodularity and tenderness are common. Especially in large breasts a firm transverse ridge of compressed tissue may be present along the lower edge of the breast. This is the normal inframammary ridge and should not be confused with a tumor.

Induration

Tenderness

Nodules. If present, describe:
1. Their location, by quadrant or the clock method, with centimeters from the nipple
2. The size in centimeters
3. Shape, e.g., round or discoid, regular or irregular
4. Consistency, e.g., soft, firm or hard
5. Delimitation in relationship to surrounding tissues, e.g., well circumscribed or not
6. Mobility, with special reference to the skin and underlying tissues
7. Tenderness

See Table 11-3, Differentiation of Common Breast Nodules (p. 198).

Hard, poorly circumscribed nodules, fixed to the skin or underlying tissues, strongly suggest cancer.

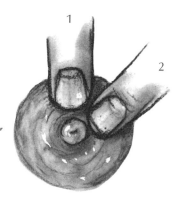

Palpate each nipple, noting its elasticity. Compress it between your thumb and index finger. Inspect for discharge. If there is a history or physical evidence of nipple discharge, try to determine its origin by compressing the areola with your index finger placed in radial positions around the nipple. Watch for discharge appearing through one of the duct openings on the nipple's surface.

Loss of elasticity in cancer. Bloody discharge of intraductal papilloma.

The tactile stimulation of examination may produce temporary erection of the nipple and wrinkling or puckering of the areola. These normal phenomena should not be confused with signs of cancer.

Inversion, flattening or retraction of the nipple and edema of the areola suggest cancer.

The Male Breast

Examination of the male breast can be brief but should not be omitted.

Inspect the nipple and areola for nodules, swelling or ulceration.

See Table 11-4, Abnormalities of the Male Breast (p. 199).

Palpate the areola for nodules. If the breast appears enlarged, distinguish between the soft fatty enlargement that may accompany obesity and the firm disc of glandular enlargement.

The Axillae

Although the axillae may be examined with the patient lying down, a sitting position is preferable.

INSPECTION

Inspect the skin of each axilla, noting evidence of:
  Rash
  Infection

  Unusual Pigmentation

PALPATION

To examine the patient's left axilla, ask him to relax with his left arm down. Help him by supporting his left wrist or hand with your left hand. Cup together the fingers of your right hand and reach as high as you can toward the apex of his axilla. Bringing your fingers down over the surface of the ribs

A firm disc of glandular enlargement in a male is called gynecomastia.

Deodorant and other rashes
Sweat gland infections (hidradenitis suppurativa)
Deeply pigmented, velvety axillary skin suggests the rare acanthosis nigricans, one form of which is associated with internal malignancy.

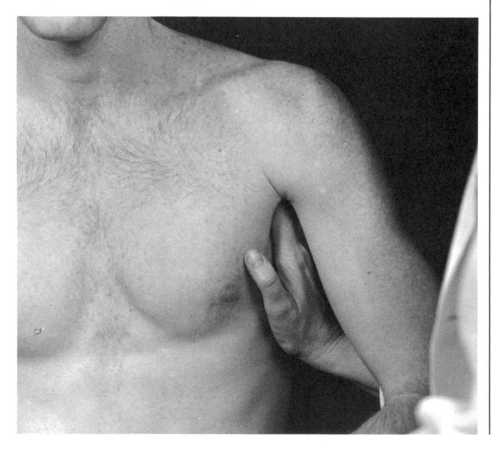

and serratus anterior, try to feel the central nodes by compressing them against the chest wall. Of the axillary nodes, the central nodes are most often palpable.

Feel inside the anterior and posterior axillary folds and against the humerus for the pectoral, subscapular and lateral axillary nodes respectively. The subscapular and lateral nodes may be more easily identified by standing behind the patient.

Reverse the procedure to examine the right axilla.

Axillary metastases of breast cancer; lymphadenitis from infection of hand or arm.

TABLE 11-1

TABLE 11-1. VISIBLE SIGNS OF BREAST CANCER

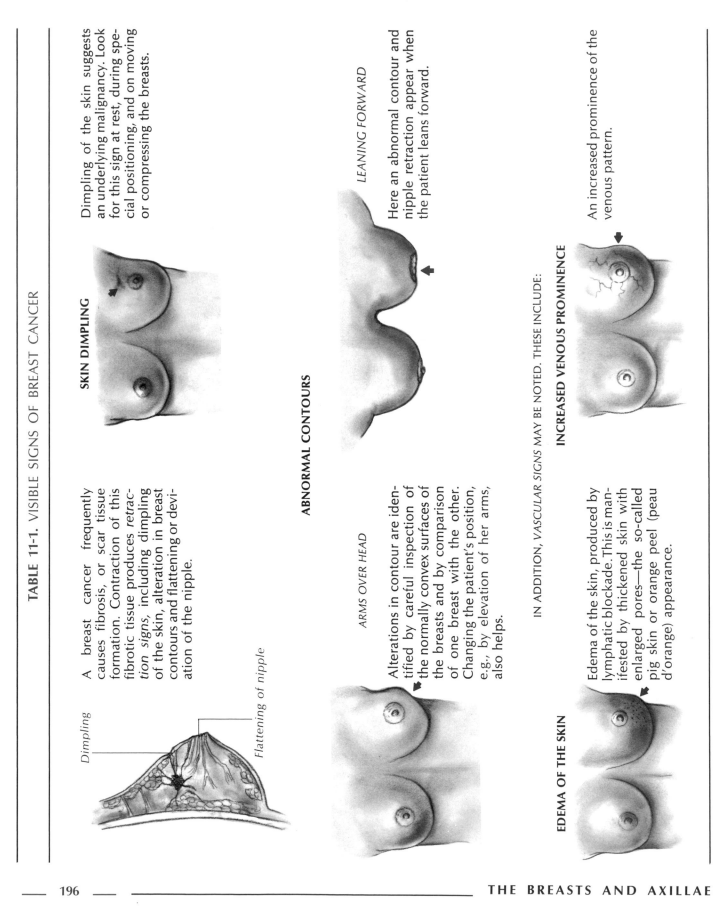

A breast cancer frequently causes fibrosis, or scar tissue formation. Contraction of this fibrotic tissue produces *retraction signs*, including dimpling of the skin, alteration in breast contours and flattening or deviation of the nipple.

Dimpling

Flattening of nipple

SKIN DIMPLING

Dimpling of the skin suggests an underlying malignancy. Look for this sign at rest, during special positioning, and on moving or compressing the breasts.

ABNORMAL CONTOURS

ARMS OVER HEAD

Alterations in contour are identified by careful inspection of the normally convex surfaces of the breasts and by comparison of one breast with the other. Changing the patient's position, e.g., by elevation of her arms, also helps.

LEANING FORWARD

Here an abnormal contour and nipple retraction appear when the patient leans forward.

IN ADDITION, *VASCULAR SIGNS* MAY BE NOTED. THESE INCLUDE:

INCREASED VENOUS PROMINENCE

An increased prominence of the venous pattern.

EDEMA OF THE SKIN

Edema of the skin, produced by lymphatic blockade. This is manifested by thickened skin with enlarged pores—the so-called pig skin or orange peel (peau d'orange) appearance.

TABLE 11-2

TABLE 11-2. ABNORMALITIES OF NIPPLE AND AREOLA

NIPPLE INVERSION

Simple nipple inversion is a common variant of normal and is usually of long standing. It may be unilateral or bilateral. The nipple can usually be pulled out of the sulcus in which it lies. Flattening, broadening and true retraction are absent. The recent development of inversion in a previously erect nipple, however, is highly suspicious of malignancy.

NIPPLE FLATTENING OR RETRACTION

The fibrosis associated with a cancer behind the nipple pulls the nipple inward and may broaden and flatten it.

NIPPLE DEVIATION OR POINTING

The fibrosis associated with cancer may deviate the axis in which the nipple points. The nipple deviates toward the cancer.

EDEMA OF NIPPLE AND AREOLA

The pig skin or orange peel appearance produced by lymphatic blockade often affects the areola first. It strongly suggests cancer.

PAGET'S DISEASE

A form of breast cancer, Paget's disease progresses slowly from a smooth redness to rough thickening to erosion or ulceration of the nipple and areola. In any dermatitis of nipple and areola, cancer must be suspected.

NIPPLE DISCHARGE

There are many causes of nipple discharge, most of them non-malignant. Note the color of the discharge and if possible identify its source.

SUPERNUMERARY BREASTS

One or more extra breasts may be located along the "milk line," most commonly in the axillae or below the normal breasts. A supernumerary breast usually consists of a small nipple and areola and may be mistaken for a mole. Less commonly glandular tissue is present.

TABLE 11-3

TABLE 11-3. DIFFERENTIATION OF COMMON BREAST NODULES

Despite the classic differences listed below, definitive diagnosis usually depends on aspiration of cysts or surgical biopsy. Differentiation is most difficult in cases where it is most desirable—the early small nodule.

	CYSTIC DISEASE	ADENOFIBROMA	CANCER
PATHOLOGY	*Single or Multiple Cysts*	*A Benign Neoplasm*	*A Malignant Neoplasm*
Findings by palpation (The illustrations do not imply visibility to inspection.)			
Usual age	30-55, regresses after menopause	Puberty and young adulthood, up to 55	30-80, most common in middle-aged and elderly
Number	Single or multiple	Usually single, may be multiple	Usually single although may coexist with other nodular lesions
Shape	Round	Round, discoid or lobular	Irregular or stellate
Consistency	Soft to firm, usually elastic	May be soft, usually firm	Firm or hard
Delimitation	Well delineated	Well delineated	Not clearly delineated from surrounding tissues
Mobility	Mobile	Very mobile	May be fixed to skin or underlying tissues
Tenderness	Often tender	Usually non-tender	Usually non-tender
Retraction signs	Absent	Absent	Often present

TABLE 11-4

TABLE 11-4. ABNORMALITIES OF THE MALE BREAST

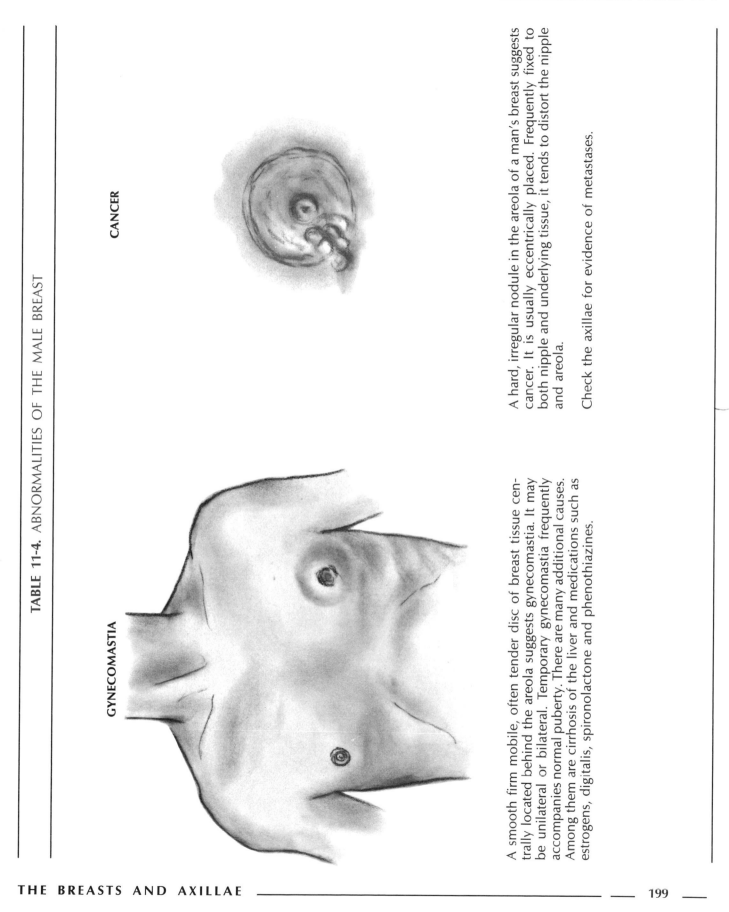

GYNECOMASTIA

CANCER

A smooth firm mobile, often tender disc of breast tissue centrally located behind the areola suggests gynecomastia. It may be unilateral or bilateral. Temporary gynecomastia frequently accompanies normal puberty. There are many additional causes. Among them are cirrhosis of the liver and medications such as estrogens, digitalis, spironolactone and phenothiazines.

A hard, irregular nodule in the areola of a man's breast suggests cancer. It is usually eccentrically placed. Frequently fixed to both nipple and underlying tissue, it tends to distort the nipple and areola.

Check the axillae for evidence of metastases.

the abdomen

ANATOMY AND PHYSIOLOGY

Review the anatomy of the abdominal wall, identifying the illustrated landmarks. The rectus abdominis muscles can be identified by asking the patient to raise his head from a supine position.

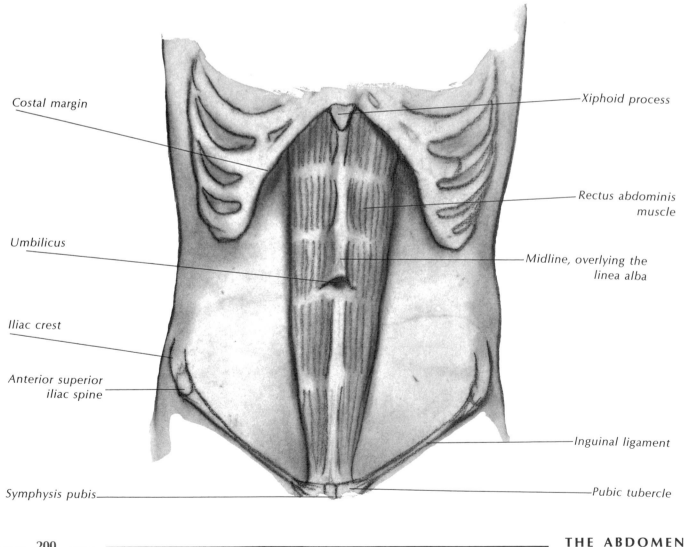

For descriptive purposes the abdomen is generally divided into four quadrants by imaginary lines crossing at the umbilicus: right upper, right lower, left upper and lower quadrants. Another system divides the abdomen into nine sections. Terms for three of them are commonly used: epigastric, umbilical, and hypogastric or suprapubic.

Several structures may normally reveal themselves to the palpating hand although they frequently do not. These include the liver edge, portions of the large bowel, the pulsating aorta and iliac arteries, and the lower pole of the right kidney. The left kidney, usually slightly higher than the right, is rarely palpable. The sacral promontory can be felt occasionally, especially in thin and well-relaxed abdomens. It presents as a bony mass deep in the abdomen below the level of the umbilicus and can be mistaken for a tumor. Other "tumors" that may mislead the examiner are a distended bladder and pregnant uterus.

The abdomen extends up under the rib cage to the dome of the diaphragm. When organs are confined to this region they are examined chiefly by percussion. They include the liver, spleen and stomach, as shown in the figure below at the left.

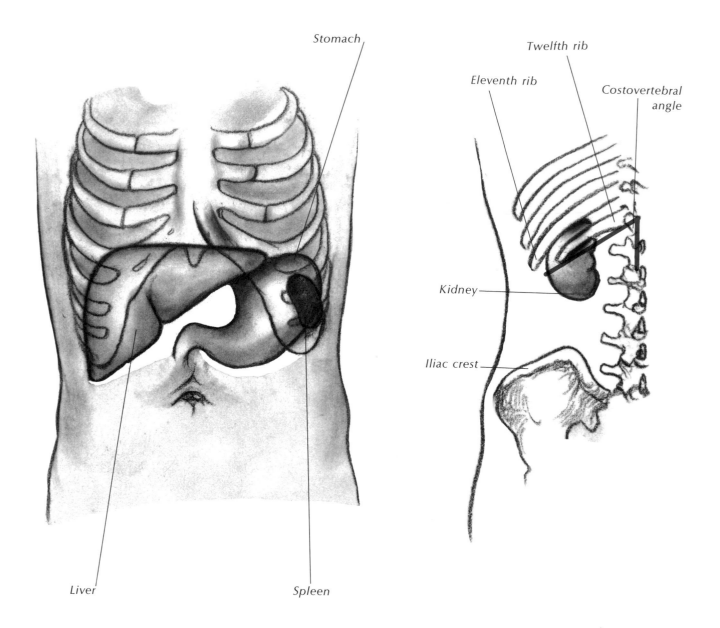

The kidneys are posterior organs, protected above by the ribs and below by the heavy back muscles. The costovertebral angles, formed by rib cage and vertebral column, are clinically useful landmarks. (See the figure above at the right.)

General Approach

Essential conditions for a good abdominal examination include (1) good lighting, tangential to the abdomen for best observation; (2) full exposure of the abdomen; and (3) a relaxed patient. To achieve relaxation:

1. The patient should *not* have a full bladder.

2. Make him comfortable in a supine position with a pillow for his head, perhaps also under his knees. You can ascertain whether or not he is relaxed flat on the table by trying to insert your hand underneath his low back.

3. He should keep his arms at his sides or folded across the chest. Although patients commonly put their arms over their heads, this move should be discouraged since it stretches and tightens the abdominal wall and makes palpation difficult.

4. Have warm hands, a warm stethoscope and short fingernails. Rubbing your hands together or running hot water over them may help to warm them.

5. Approach slowly, with your examining hand and forearm on a horizontal plane.

6. Distract him if necessary with conversation or questions.

7. If he is very frightened or very ticklish, begin palpation with the patient's hand beneath your own.

8. Ask the patient to point to any areas of pain and examine tender areas last.

9. Monitor your examination by watching the patient's face.

Make a habit of visualizing each organ in the region you are examining. From the patient's right side proceed in an orderly fashion: inspection, auscultation, percussion, palpation.

INSPECTION

From the right side of the bed, inspect the abdomen, noting:

1. The skin, including:

   Scars. Describe their location.

   Striae. Describe their size and color.

   Dilated veins. A fine venous network may normally be present.

   Rashes and lesions.

   Old silver striae of stretching; pink-purple striae of Cushing's syndrome

   Dilated veins of inferior vena cava obstruction

2. The umbilicus—its contour, location, signs of inflammation or hernia.

   See Table 12-1, Abdominal Hernias and Bulges (p. 213).

3. Contour of the abdomen, e.g., flat, rounded, protuberant or scaphoid (concave); local bulges. Include in this survey the inguinal and femoral areas. The techniques of examining for inguinal and femoral hernias, however, are described in Chapter 13.

4. Symmetry.

5. Masses.

6. Peristalsis. Peristalsis is best seen by looking across the patient's abdomen. Observation over several minutes may be required. Peristalsis may be visible normally in very thin people.

7. Pulsations. A normal aortic pulsation is frequently visible in the epigastrium.

See Table 12-2, Protuberant Abdomens (p. 214).

Suprapubic bulge of distended bladder or pregnant uterus

Increased peristaltic waves of intestinal obstruction

Increased pulsation of aortic aneurysm

AUSCULTATION

Auscultation prior to percussion and palpation is recommended since the latter maneuvers may alter the frequency of bowel sounds.

Listen in all four quadrants and the epigastrium.
   Note the frequency and character of bowel sounds. These are clicks and gurgles, the frequency of which has been estimated at from 5 to 34 per minute. Occasionally you may hear borborygmi—loud prolonged gurgles of hyperperistalsis—the familiar "stomach growling."

   Listen for bruits—vascular sounds resembling systolic heart murmurs.

   If indicated by the suspicion of liver tumor, gonococcal infection or splenic infarction, listen over the liver and spleen for friction rubs.

See Table 12-3, Sounds in the Abdomen (p. 215).

PERCUSSION

Percussion is useful for general orientation to the abdomen, for measurement of the liver and sometimes of the spleen, and for identification of air in the stomach and bowel. Although percussion for all these purposes is described in this section, some practitioners prefer to alternate percussion with palpation as they examine liver, spleen and other areas of the abdomen. Either approach is satisfactory.

For General Orientation. Percuss the abdomen lightly in all four quadrants to assess the general proportions and distribution of tympany and dullness. Tympany usually predominates. Check for the suprapubic dullness of a distended bladder.

See Table 12-2, Protuberant Abdomens (p. 214).

The Liver. In the right midclavicular line, starting at a level below the umbilicus (in an area of gas, not dullness), lightly percuss upward toward the liver. Ascertain the lower border of liver dullness in the midclavicular line.

Next identify the upper border of liver dullness in the midclavicular line. Lightly percuss from lung resonance down toward liver dullness. Now measure in centimeters the vertical span, or height, of liver dullness. If the liver appears enlarged, you may wish to outline the boundaries of liver dullness in other locations also, for example, the midsternal line and the right anterior axillary line.

The span of liver dullness is increased when the liver is enlarged.

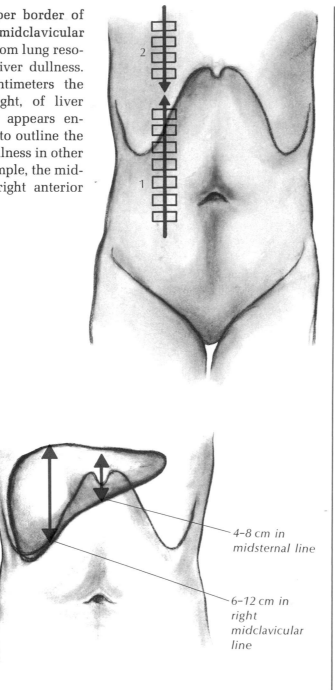

4–8 cm in midsternal line

6–12 cm in right midclavicular line

CAUTION
Dullness of a right pleural effusion or consolidated lung, if adjacent to liver dullness, may falsely increase the estimated liver size.

CAUTION
Gas in the colon may produce tympany in the right upper quadrant, obscure liver dullness and falsely decrease the estimated liver size.

Liver dullness may be decreased or absent when free air is present below the diaphragm, as from a perforated hollow viscus.

Normal liver heights are shown above. They are generally greater in men than in women, in tall people than in short. Although percussion is probably the most accurate clinical method of estimating liver size, it provides only a gross estimate. Furthermore, each border of liver dullness is sometimes obscured.

Ask the patient to take a deep breath and hold it. Again percuss the lower border of liver dullness in the midclavicular line, always percussing from tympany to dullness. Estimate its descent. This maneuver will help guide subsequent palpation.

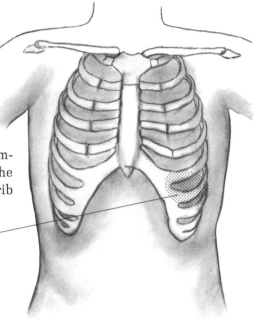

The Stomach. Identify the tympany of the gastric air bubble, in the area of the left lower anterior rib cage. Its size is variable.

Tympany of gastric air bubble

Increase in the size of the gastric air bubble, together with upper abdominal distention, suggests gastric dilatation.

The Spleen. Identify if possible the small oval area of splenic dullness near the left tenth rib just posterior to the midaxillary line. This finding is often obscured by gastric or colonic air. Describe any enlargement in this area of dullness. As another method of identifying slight degrees of splenic enlargement, percuss the lowest interspace in the left anterior axillary line. This area is usually tympanitic. Ask the patient to take a deep breath. When spleen size is normal, the percussion note usually remains tympanitic.

Midaxillary line

Percuss here

Splenic dullness

Anterior axillary line

A change in percussion note from tympany to dullness on inspiration suggests splenic enlargement.

THE ABDOMEN

LIGHT PALPATION

Light palpation is especially helpful in identifying muscular resistance, abdominal tenderness and some superficial organs and masses. Its gentleness helps also to reassure and relax the patient.

Use the pads of your fingertips, with fingers together, in a light, gentle, dipping motion. Avoid short quick jabs. Moving smoothly, feel in all quadrants. Identify any organs or masses, any area of tenderness or increased resistance. If resistance is present, try to determine whether it is voluntary resistance or involuntary spasm: **(1)** Try all the maneuvers to relax the patient (p. 203). **(2)** Feel for the relaxation of the rectus muscles that normally accompanies expiration. If the rigidity remains unaltered by all these maneuvers, it is probably involuntary.

Involuntary rigidity or spasm of the abdominal muscles indicates peritoneal inflammation.

DEEP PALPATION

Deeper palpation is usually required to delineate abdominal organs and masses.

Again using the palmar surfaces of the fingers, feel in all four quadrants.

Identify any masses and note their location, size, shape, consistency, tenderness, pulsations, mobility (for example, with respiration or with the examining hand).

Identify any tender areas. If tenderness is present, check for rebound tenderness by firmly and slowly pressing in, then quickly withdrawing your fingers. Rebound tenderness is elicited when pain is noted during the withdrawal maneuver.

See Table 12-4, Tender Abdomens (pp. 216–217).

Rebound tenderness suggests peritoneal inflammation.

When deep palpation is difficult, for example, because of obesity or muscular resistance, use two hands, one on top of the other. Exert pressure with the outside hand while concentrating on feeling with the inside hand.

The Liver. Place your left hand behind the patient, parallel to and supporting his right eleventh and twelfth ribs. Remind the patient to relax on your hand if necessary. By pressing your left hand forward, the patient's liver is more easily felt in front.

Place your right hand on the patient's right abdomen lateral to the rectus muscle, with your fingertips well below the lower border of liver dullness and pointing toward the right costal margin. Press gently in and up.

Ask the patient to take a deep breath. Teaching him to "breathe with his abdomen" rather than with his chest may aid in bringing the liver, as well as spleen and kidneys, into a palpable position. Try to feel the liver edge as it comes down to meet your fingertips. When palpable, a normal liver edge presents a firm, sharp, regular ridge with a smooth surface, although sometimes only a sense of increased resistance can be perceived. If unsuccessful, exert more pressure inward and repeat. Readjust the position of your right hand closer to the right costal margin and repeat.

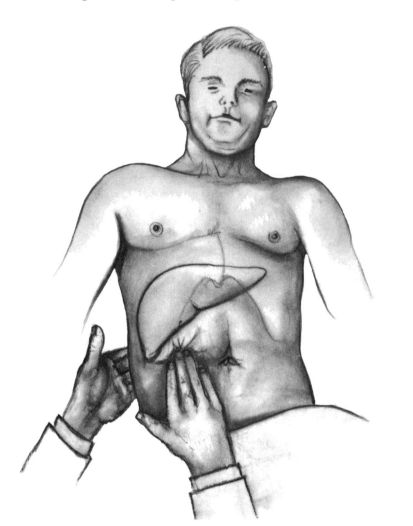

Toward the peak of inspiration it may be helpful to release the pressure of your right hand slightly and let it ride up and over the descending liver edge. It is primarily the descending liver and not your hand, however, that moves in this maneuver.

If palpable, trace the liver edge both medially and laterally by repeating your maneuvers. The edge may extend over into the left upper quadrant. Describe the contour and surface of the liver and note any tenderness.

See Table 12-5, Liver Enlargement: Apparent and Real (pp. 218–219).

The liver may also be felt by the "hooking technique." Stand to the right of the patient and face his feet. Place both hands, side by side, on his right abdomen below the border of liver dullness. Press in with your fingers and up toward the costal margin. Ask him to take a deep breath.

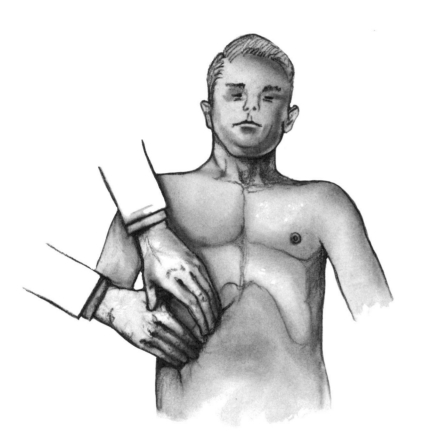

To check for liver tenderness when the organ is not palpable, place your left hand flat on the lower right rib cage, then strike your hand with the ulnar surface of your right fist. Ask the patient to compare the sensation with that produced by a similar maneuver on the left side.

Tenderness suggests inflammation, as in hepatitis.

The Spleen. With your left hand reach over and around the patient to support and press forward his lower left rib cage. With your right hand below the left costal margin, press in toward the spleen. Begin palpation low enough to be sure that you are below a possibly enlarged spleen. Furthermore, if your hand is too close to the costal margin it is not sufficiently mobile to reach up under the rib cage. Ask the patient to take a deep breath. Try to feel the tip or edge of the spleen as it comes down to meet your fingertips.

See Table 12-6, Steps in Splenic Enlargement (p. 220).

If the spleen of an adult is palpable, it is probably considerably larger than normal.

Repeat with the patient lying on his right side and his legs somewhat flexed at hips and knees. In this position, gravity may bring the spleen forward and to the right into a palpable location.

The Right Kidney. Place your left hand behind and supporting the patient's right loin, between rib cage and iliac crest. Place your right hand below the right costal margin with your fingertips pointing to the left. Press your hands firmly together. Because of the posterior location of the kidneys, palpation should be deeper than when searching for the liver. As the patient takes a deep breath, try to feel the lower pole of the right kidney come down between your fingers.

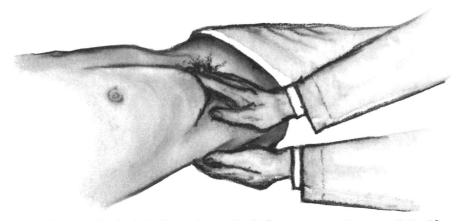

As another method of feeling the right kidney, try to "capture" it. Place your hands as before. At the peak of inspiration, press your fingers together quickly, exerting slightly more pressure above than below. Ask the patient to breathe out and then to stop breathing briefly. Slowly release the pressure of your fingers. Feel for the kidney as it slips between your fingers back up into place.

Causes of kidney enlargement include hydronephrosis, neoplasm and polycystic disease.

If the kidney is palpable describe its size, contour and tenderness.

The Left Kidney. Use the same maneuvers. From the patient's right side support his left loin with your left hand while your right hand palpates his anterior abdominal wall. The capture technique is more easily done from the patient's left: place your right hand behind the patient, your left in front. A normal left kidney is rarely palpable.

Although *kidney tenderness* is usually looked for posteriorly during examination of the back, thus saving the patient needless exertion, the technique will be mentioned here. Place the palm of your left hand over each costovertebral angle in turn. Strike it with the ulnar surface of your right fist. Normally the patient should perceive a jar or thud, but not pain.

Costovertebral angle tenderness suggests kidney infection.

The Aorta. Press firmly deep into the upper abdomen, slightly to the left of the midline. Identify the aortic pulsation. If the pulsation is prominent, try to place your thumb along one side of the aorta, your fingers along the other. If the abdominal wall is thick and palpation difficult, use the index and middle fingers of both hands, one hand on each side of the aorta. Feel for an expansile pulsation of the aorta.

A prominent pulsation with lateral expansion suggests an aortic aneurysm. A normal aorta or an aorta covered by a mass transmits the pulsation forward without lateral expansion.

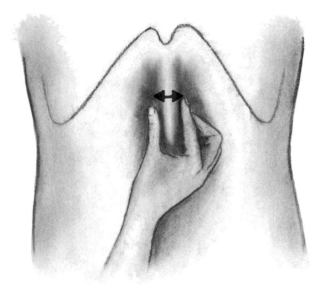

SPECIAL MANEUVERS

To Assess Possible Appendicitis. When the history suggests appendicitis, evaluate the patient carefully.

1. Ask the patient to point to where the pain began and where it is now.

2. Search carefully for an area of local tenderness.

3. Feel for muscular rigidity.

4. Perform a rectal examination and compare tenderness high on both sides.

   If you are still in doubt about the diagnosis, some additional maneuvers may be helpful.

5. Check the tender area for rebound tenderness. (If other signs are typically positive, you can save the patient unnecessary pain by omitting this test).

6. Press deeply and evenly in the left lower quadrant.

7. Check abdominal sensitivity to pin prick. Lightly and evenly touch the patient's skin with a pinpoint, testing in lines down both sides of the abdomen.

8. Place your hand just above the patient's right knee and ask him to flex his leg against it. Alternatively, ask him to turn on to his left side. Then extend his right leg at the hip.

9. Flex the patient's right thigh at the hip, with his knee bent, and rotate the leg internally at the hip.

To Distinguish an Abdominal Mass from a Mass in the Abdominal Wall. An occasional mass is in the abdominal wall rather than inside the abdominal cavity. Ask the patient to tighten his muscles by raising his head and shoulders or by straining.

---

1. The patient with appendicitis classically points to the umbilicus, then to the right lower quadrant.

2. Localized tenderness anywhere in the right lower quadrant, even in the right flank, may indicate appendicitis.

3. Rigidity (involuntary muscular spasm that persists during expiration) suggests local peritoneal inflammation.

4. Right-sided rectal tenderness suggests pelvic appendicitis and is also helpful in detecting masses or tubo-ovarian disease.

5. Rebound tenderness suggests peritoneal inflammation, as from appendicitis.

6. Pain felt in the right lower quadrant may accompany appendicitis (a positive Rovsing's sign).

7. An increased sensitivity to pin prick (hyperaesthesia) in the right lower quadrant may accompany appendicitis.

8. Increased abdominal pain on either maneuver constitutes a positive psoas sign, suggesting irritation of the psoas muscle by an inflamed appendix.

9. Right hypogastric pain constitutes a positive obturator sign, suggesting irritation of the obturator muscle.

A mass in the abdominal wall remains palpable; an intra-abdominal mass is obscured by muscular tension.

TABLE 12-1

TABLE 12-1. ABDOMINAL HERNIAS AND BULGES

UMBILICAL HERNIA

INFANT

These are almost always made more evident when the patient stands or when he raises his head and shoulders from a supine position.

ADULT

In young children an umbilical hernia is centrally located. In adults it is usually partially above the umbilicus.

INCISIONAL HERNIA

A defect in the abdominal muscles may develop after a surgical incision.

DIASTASIS RECTI

Palpable separation

Ridge when head and shoulders are elevated

Not a true hernia, a diastasis recti is a separation of the two rectus abdominis muscles often caused by pregnancy or obesity. The increased intra-abdominal pressure produced by the patient's elevating his head and shoulders causes a midline ridge-like bulge. It is of no clinical consequence.

HERNIA OF THE LINEA ALBA

This is a small, often tender, midline nodule usually located in the epigastrium and best discovered with the patient standing up. Its pain may mimic an ulcer. To find it, run the pad of your index finger down the linea alba.

TABLE 12-2 _____

TABLE 12-2. PROTUBERANT ABDOMENS

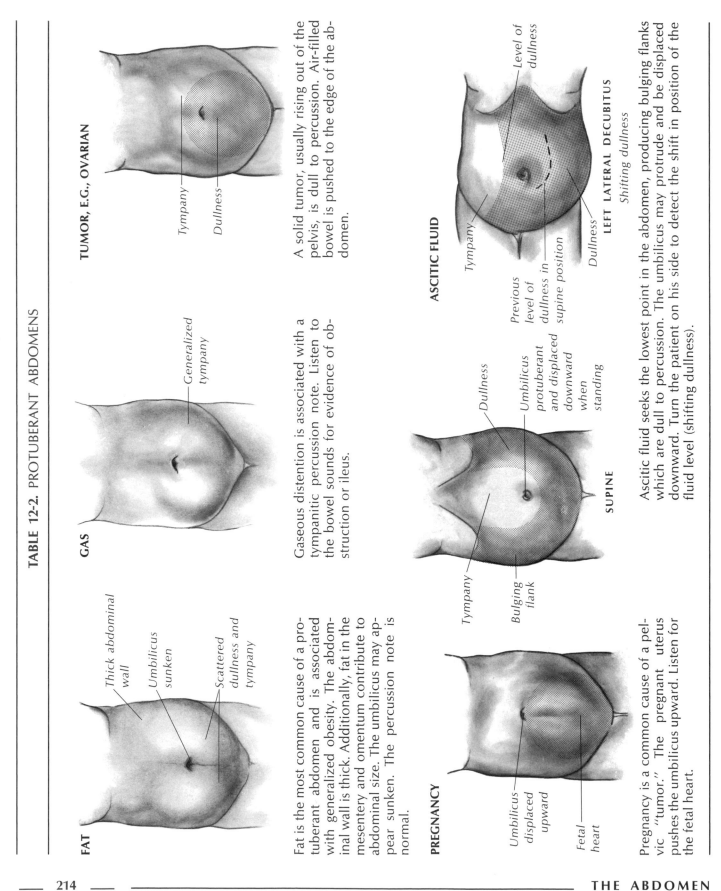

FAT

Thick abdominal wall

Umbilicus sunken

Scattered dullness and tympany

Fat is the most common cause of a protuberant abdomen and is associated with generalized obesity. The abdominal wall is thick. Additionally, fat in the mesentery and omentum contribute to abdominal size. The umbilicus may appear sunken. The percussion note is normal.

GAS

Generalized tympany

Gaseous distention is associated with a tympanitic percussion note. Listen to the bowel sounds for evidence of obstruction or ileus.

TUMOR, E.G., OVARIAN

Tympany

Dullness

A solid tumor, usually rising out of the pelvis, is dull to percussion. Air-filled bowel is pushed to the edge of the abdomen.

PREGNANCY

Umbilicus displaced upward

Fetal heart

Pregnancy is a common cause of a pelvic "tumor." The pregnant uterus pushes the umbilicus upward. Listen for the fetal heart.

ASCITIC FLUID

Level of dullness

Tympany

Previous level of dullness in supine position

Dullness

LEFT LATERAL DECUBITUS
Shifting dullness

Dullness

Umbilicus protuberant and displaced downward when standing

Tympany

Bulging flank

SUPINE

Ascitic fluid seeks the lowest point in the abdomen, producing bulging flanks which are dull to percussion. The umbilicus may protrude and be displaced downward. Turn the patient on his side to detect the shift in position of the fluid level (shifting dullness).

TABLE 12-3

TABLE 12-3. SOUNDS IN THE ABDOMEN

BOWEL SOUNDS

Bowel sounds may be:
1. Increased, as from diarrhea or early intestinal obstruction.
2. Decreased, then absent, as in paralytic ileus and peritonitis. Before deciding bowel sounds are absent, sit down and listen where shown for two minutes or even longer.

High-pitched tinkling sounds suggest intestinal fluid and air under tension in a dilated bowel. Rushes of high pitched sounds coinciding with an abdominal cramp indicate intestinal obstruction.

SYSTOLIC BRUITS

Renal artery
Aorta
Iliac artery

Systolic bruits are vascular sounds resembling cardiac murmurs. They suggest partial arterial obstruction or turbulent flow, as in an aneurysm. Do not be misled by a cardiac murmur radiating to the abdomen.

VENOUS HUM

Epigastric and umbilical

A venous hum is rare. It is a continuous noise that may have systolic accentuation. It is indicative of increased collateral circulation between portal and systemic venous systems, as in hepatic cirrhosis.

FRICTION RUBS

Hepatic
Splenic

Friction rubs are rare. They are grating sounds with respiratory variation. They indicate inflammation of the peritoneal surface of an organ as from a liver tumor, gonococcal perihepatitis or splenic infarct.

TABLE 12-4

TABLE 12-4. TENDER ABDOMENS

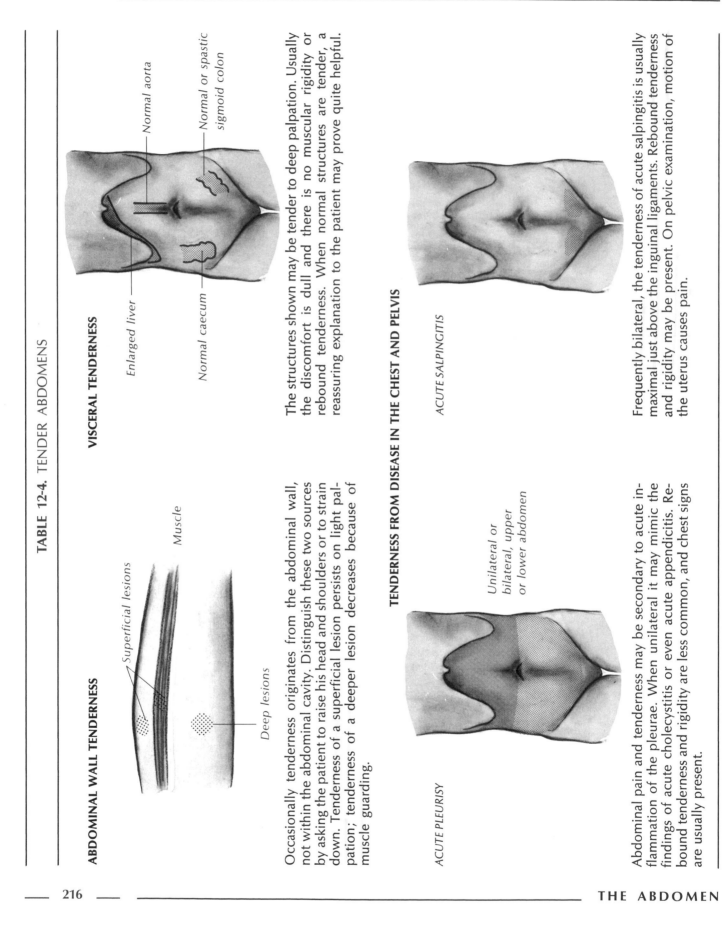

ABDOMINAL WALL TENDERNESS

Superficial lesions

Muscle

Deep lesions

Occasionally tenderness originates from the abdominal wall, not within the abdominal cavity. Distinguish these two sources by asking the patient to raise his head and shoulders or to strain down. Tenderness of a superficial lesion persists on light palpation; tenderness of a deeper lesion decreases because of muscle guarding.

VISCERAL TENDERNESS

Normal aorta

Normal or spastic sigmoid colon

Enlarged liver

Normal caecum

The structures shown may be tender to deep palpation. Usually the discomfort is dull and there is no muscular rigidity or rebound tenderness. When normal structures are tender, a reassuring explanation to the patient may prove quite helpful.

TENDERNESS FROM DISEASE IN THE CHEST AND PELVIS

ACUTE PLEURISY

Unilateral or bilateral, upper or lower abdomen

Abdominal pain and tenderness may be secondary to acute inflammation of the pleurae. When unilateral it may mimic the findings of acute cholecystitis or even acute appendicitis. Rebound tenderness and rigidity are less common, and chest signs are usually present.

ACUTE SALPINGITIS

Frequently bilateral, the tenderness of acute salpingitis is usually maximal just above the inguinal ligaments. Rebound tenderness and rigidity may be present. On pelvic examination, motion of the uterus causes pain.

TABLE 12-4 (CONT'D)

TENDERNESS OF PERITONEAL INFLAMMATION

Tenderness associated with peritoneal inflammation is usually more severe than visceral tenderness. Muscular rigidity and rebound tenderness are frequently but not necessarily present. Examples include:

ACUTE CHOLECYSTITIS

Signs are maximal in the right upper quadrant. Press your left thumb just under the right costal margin and ask the patient to take a deep breath. A sharp increase in tenderness with a sudden stop in inspiratory effort constitutes a positive Murphy's sign of acute cholecystitis.

ACUTE APPENDICITIS

Just below the middle of a line joining the umbilicus and the anterior superior iliac spine

Right rectal tenderness

Right lower quadrant signs are typical of acute appendicitis but may be absent early in the course. The typical area of tenderness is illustrated. Explore other portions of the right lower quadrant also, as well as the right flank. A suspicion of appendicitis always indicates a rectal examination. See p. 212 for further maneuvers.

ACUTE PANCREATITIS

In acute pancreatitis epigastric tenderness and rebound are usually present but the abdominal wall may be soft.

ACUTE DIVERTICULITIS

Acute diverticulitis resembles a left-sided appendicitis.

TABLE 12-5

TABLE 12-5. LIVER ENLARGEMENT: APPARENT AND REAL

Estimates of liver size should be based upon full evaluation by both percussion and palpation. A palpable liver edge does not necessarily indicate hepatomegaly.

NORMAL VARIATIONS IN LIVER SHAPE

Elongated right lobe

In some individuals, especially those with a lanky build, the liver tends to be somewhat elongated so that its right lobe is easily palpable as it projects downward toward the iliac crest. Such an elongation represents a variation in shape, not an increase in liver volume or size. This variant illustrates the basic limitations of assessing liver size. We can only estimate the upper and lower borders of an organ that has three dimensions and differing shapes. Some error is unavoidable.

DOWNWARD DISPLACEMENT OF THE LIVER BY A LOW DIAPHRAGM

Upper border low

Height by percussion normal

This is a common finding, e.g., in emphysema, where the diaphragm is low. The liver edge may be readily palpable well below the costal margin. Percussion, however, reveals a low upper edge also, and the total span or height is normal.

TABLE 12-5 (CONT'D)

TABLE 12-5 (CONT'D)

SMOOTH NON-TENDER LIVER

Cirrhosis may produce an enlarged liver with a firm non-tender edge. The liver is not always enlarged in this condition, however, and many other diseases may produce similar findings.

IRREGULAR LIVER

An enlarged liver that is firm or hard and that presents an irregular edge or surface suggests malignancy. There may be a single or multiple nodules. The liver may or may not be tender.

SMOOTH TENDER LIVER

An enlarged liver with a smooth tender edge suggests inflammation, as in hepatitis, or venous congestion, as in right-sided heart failure.

TABLE 12-6

TABLE 12-6. STEPS IN SPLENIC ENLARGEMENT

1. Normal splenic dullness (10th rib posterior to the midaxillary line). This may enlarge—or

2. The first sign of splenomegaly may be a change from normal tympany to splenic dullness as an enlarged spleen descends toward the costal margin on deep inspiration. For this sign percuss in the lowest interspace in the anterior axillary line.

3. The spleen tip then becomes palpable on inspiration below the left costal margin.

4. A markedly enlarged spleen descends into the left lower quadrant. A notch can frequently be felt along its medial border and may be helpful in distinguishing this organ from an enlarged left kidney.

5. A massively enlarged spleen may extend across the midline.

male genitalia and hernias

ANATOMY AND PHYSIOLOGY

Review the anatomy of the male genitalia.

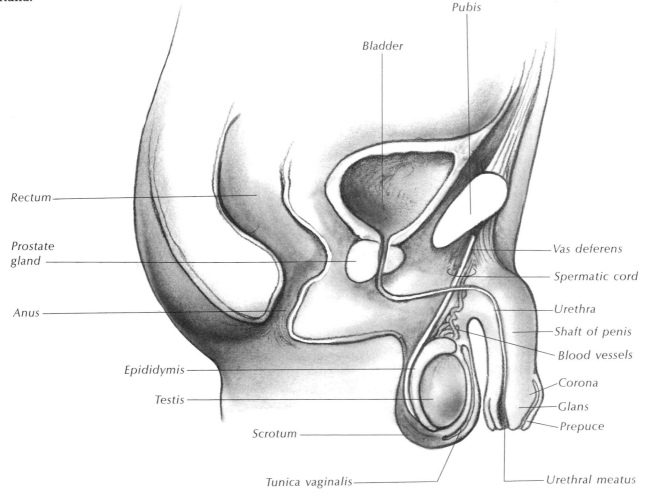

At the end of the penis is the cone-shaped glans with its expanded base, or corona, and the urethral meatus at its tip. Note that the urethra is located ventrally in the shaft of the penis.

The testes are ovoid, somewhat rubbery structures, about 5 cm long in the adult. The left is usually somewhat lower than the right. On the posterolateral surface of each testis is the softer comma-shaped epididymis. It is most prominent along the superior margin of the testis.

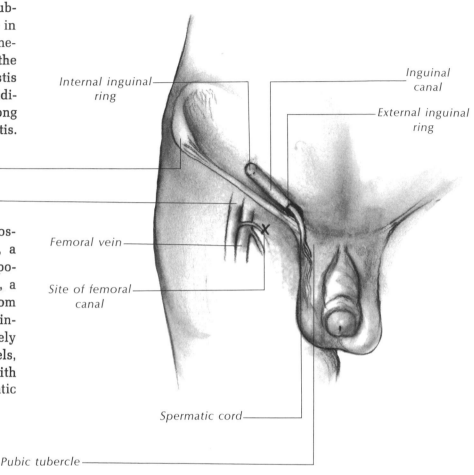

Internal inguinal ring

Inguinal canal

External inguinal ring

Anterior superior iliac spine

Femoral artery

Femoral vein

Site of femoral canal

Spermatic cord

Pubic tubercle

Surrounding the testis, except posteriorly, is the tunica vaginalis, a serous membrane enclosing a potential cavity. The vas deferens, a cord-like structure, travels up from the epididymis to the external inguinal ring. In its course it is closely associated with blood vessels, nerves and muscle fibers, with which it makes up the spermatic cord.

The external inguinal ring is a triangular slit-like structure palpable just above and lateral to the pubic tubercle. The inguinal canal forms a passage through the abdominal wall. Its internal ring is about 1 cm above the midpoint of the inguinal ligament, between pubic tubercle and the anterior superior iliac spine. Neither canal nor internal ring are palpable through the abdominal wall. Through the inguinal canal passes the vas deferens on its way into the abdominal cavity toward the seminal vesicle.

The femoral canal is not identifiable by palpation but its location is important since femoral hernias may protrude here. It is a potential space medial to the femoral artery, below the inguinal ligament, and lateral to the pubic tubercle.

Its location can be estimated by placing your right index finger from below on the patient's right femoral artery. Your middle finger will then overlie the femoral vein, your ring finger, the femoral canal.

TECHNIQUES OF EXAMINATION

Cover the chest and abdomen. Expose the genitalia and groins.

Penis

INSPECTION

Observe:
1. The skin

2. The prepuce or foreskin. If present, retract it or ask the patient to retract it. This step is essential for the detection of many chancres and carcinomas.

   Phimosis: prepuce cannot be retracted.

3. The glans

   See Table 13-1, Abnormalities of the Penis (p. 225).

4. The urethral meatus

Note any ulcers, scars or nodules. Note the location of the urethral meatus and any discharge from it.

Gonorrhea is a common cause of urethral discharge.

PALPATION

If inflammatory lesions are present, use gloves.

Palpate any abnormality, noting tenderness, induration, size and contour.

Palpate the shaft of the penis between your thumb and first two fingers, noting any induration.

Scrotum

See Table 13-2, Abnormalities in the Scrotum (pp. 226–227).

INSPECTION

Inspect the skin of the scrotum, noting any nodules, inflammation or ulcers. Lift up the scrotum so that you can see its posterior surface as well. Observe the contour of the scrotum and its contents, noting any evidence of swelling.

Pubic or genital excoriations suggest the possibility of lice. Look for nits or lice at the bases of the pubic hairs.

PALPATION

Between your thumb and first two fingers palpate each testis and epididymis. Note their size, shape, consistency and tenderness. Pressure on the testis normally produces a deep visceral pain. Identify each spermatic cord with its vas deferens and palpate along its course from epididymis to the superficial inguinal ring. Note any nodules or swellings. Any swelling in the scrotum other than the testicle should be evaluated by trans-illumination. After darkening the room, shine the beam of a penlight from behind the scrotum through the mass. Look for transmission of the light as a red glow.

Swellings containing serous fluid trans-illuminate, those containing blood or tissue do not.

Hernias

This examination is best done with the patient standing, the observer sitting.

INSPECTION

Inspect the inguinal and femoral areas carefully for bulges. While you continue your observation, ask the patient to strain down.

A bulge that appears on straining suggests a hernia

PALPATION

Using in turn your right hand for the patient's right side and your left hand for the patient's left side, invaginate loose scrotal skin with your index finger. Start at a point low enough to ensure full mobility of your finger. This may be the bottom of the scrotal sac. Follow the spermatic cord upward to the triangular slit-like opening of the external inguinal ring. This is just above and lateral to the pubic tubercle. If the ring is somewhat enlarged, it may admit your index finger. If possible, gently follow the inguinal canal laterally in its oblique course. With your finger located either at the external ring or within the canal, ask the patient to strain down and cough. Note any palpable herniating mass as it touches your finger.

See Table 13-3, Course and Presentation of Hernias in the Groin (p. 228).

See Table 13-4, Differentiation of Hernias in the Groin (p. 229).

A hernia is *incarcerated* when it cannot be reduced, i.e. its contents cannot be returned to the abdominal cavity.

A hernia is *strangulated* when the blood supply to the entrapped contents is compromised. Suspect strangulation in the presence of tenderness, nausea and vomiting.

Anterior superior spine

linguinal ligament

External inguinal ring

Palpate the anterior thigh in the region of the femoral canal. Ask the patient to strain down again and cough. Note any swelling or tenderness.

TABLE 13-1

TABLE 13-1. ABNORMALITIES OF THE PENIS

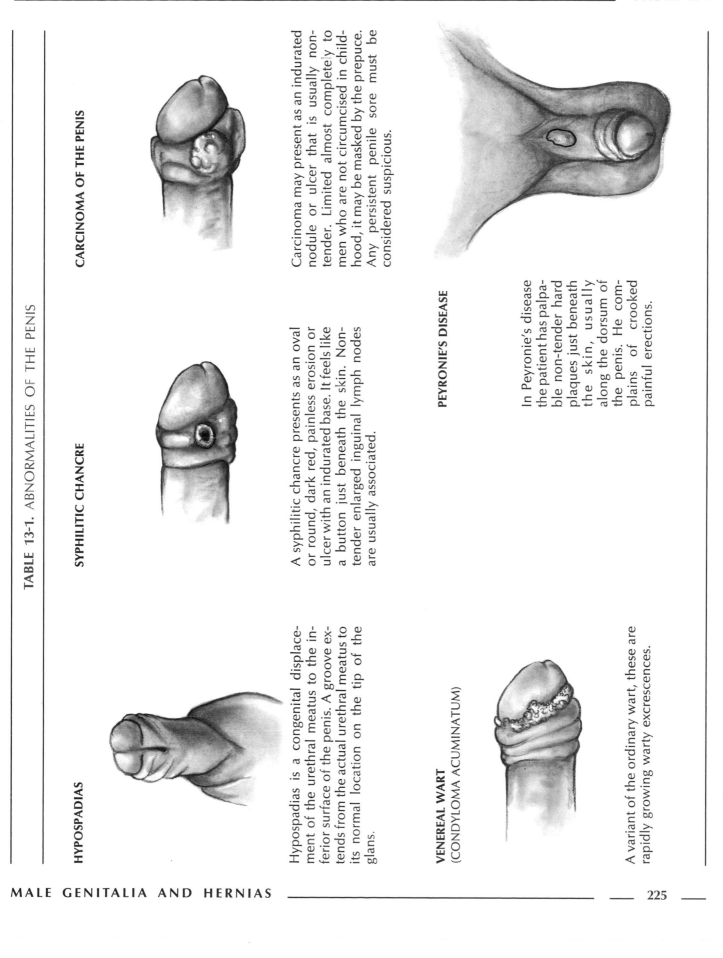

SYPHILITIC CHANCRE

CARCINOMA OF THE PENIS

A syphilitic chancre presents as an oval or round, dark red, painless erosion or ulcer with an indurated base. It feels like a button just beneath the skin. Non-tender enlarged inguinal lymph nodes are usually associated.

Carcinoma may present as an indurated nodule or ulcer that is usually non-tender. Limited almost completely to men who are not circumcised in child-hood, it may be masked by the prepuce. Any persistent penile sore must be considered suspicious.

HYPOSPADIAS

PEYRONIE'S DISEASE

Hypospadias is a congenital displacement of the urethral meatus to the inferior surface of the penis. A groove extends from the actual urethral meatus to its normal location on the tip of the glans.

In Peyronie's disease the patient has palpable non-tender hard plaques just beneath the skin, usually along the dorsum of the penis. He complains of crooked painful erections.

VENEREAL WART
(CONDYLOMA ACUMINATUM)

A variant of the ordinary wart, these are rapidly growing warty excrescences.

TABLE 13-2

TABLE 13-2. ABNORMALITIES IN THE SCROTUM

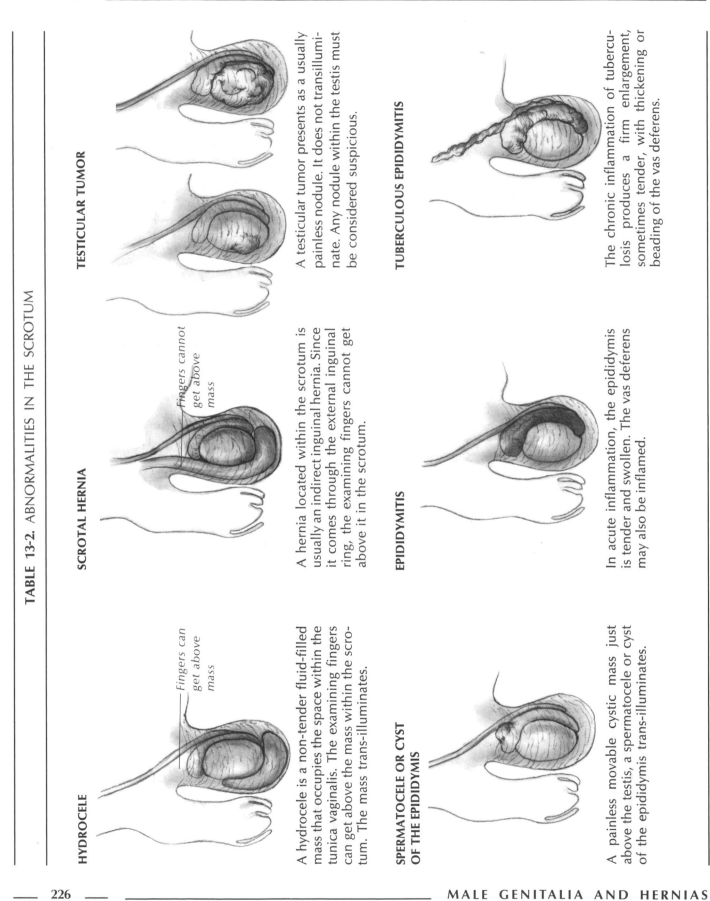

HYDROCELE

Fingers can get above mass

A hydrocele is a non-tender fluid-filled mass that occupies the space within the tunica vaginalis. The examining fingers can get above the mass within the scrotum. The mass trans-illuminates.

SPERMATOCELE OR CYST OF THE EPIDIDYMIS

A painless movable cystic mass just above the testis, a spermatocele or cyst of the epididymis trans-illuminates.

SCROTAL HERNIA

Fingers cannot get above mass

A hernia located within the scrotum is usually an indirect inguinal hernia. Since it comes through the external inguinal ring, the examining fingers cannot get above it in the scrotum.

EPIDIDYMITIS

In acute inflammation, the epididymis is tender and swollen. The vas deferens may also be inflamed.

TESTICULAR TUMOR

A testicular tumor presents as a usually painless nodule. It does not transilluminate. Any nodule within the testis must be considered suspicious.

TUBERCULOUS EPIDIDYMITIS

The chronic inflammation of tuberculosis produces a firm enlargement, sometimes tender, with thickening or beading of the vas deferens.

MALE GENITALIA AND HERNIAS

TABLE 13-2 (CONT'D)

TABLE 13-2 (CONT'D)

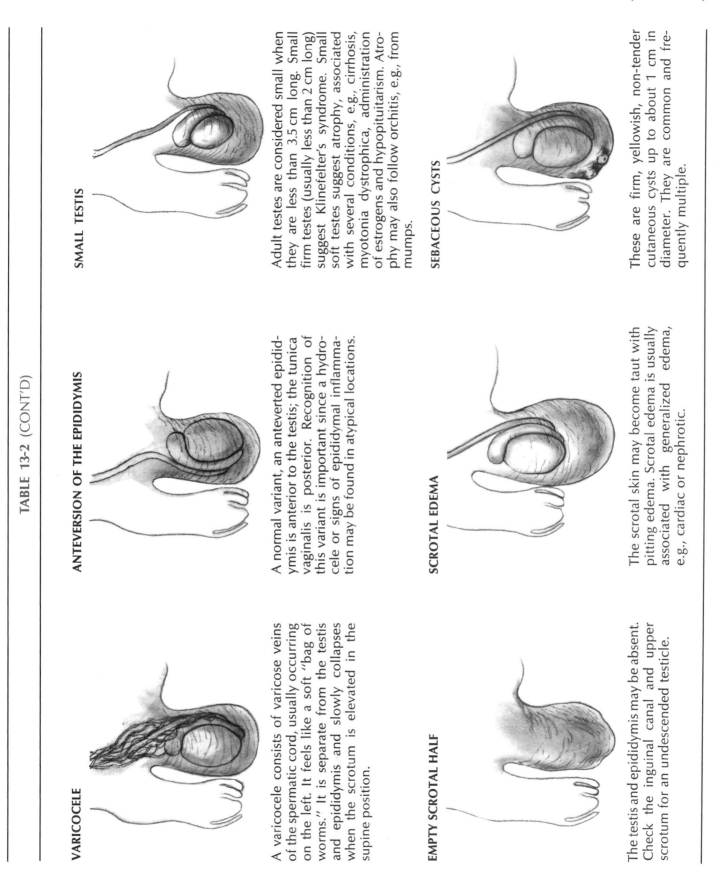

SMALL TESTIS

Adult testes are considered small when they are less than 3.5 cm long. Small firm testes (usually less than 2 cm long) suggest Klinefelter's syndrome. Small soft testes suggest atrophy, associated with several conditions, e.g., cirrhosis, myotonia dystrophica, administration of estrogens and hypopituitarism. Atrophy may also follow orchitis, e.g., from mumps.

SEBACEOUS CYSTS

These are firm, yellowish, non-tender cutaneous cysts up to about 1 cm in diameter. They are common and frequently multiple.

ANTEVERSION OF THE EPIDIDYMIS

A normal variant, an anteverted epididymis is anterior to the testis; the tunica vaginalis is posterior. Recognition of this variant is important since a hydrocele or signs of epididymal inflammation may be found in atypical locations.

SCROTAL EDEMA

The scrotal skin may become taut with pitting edema. Scrotal edema is usually associated with generalized edema, e.g., cardiac or nephrotic.

VARICOCELE

A varicocele consists of varicose veins of the spermatic cord, usually occurring on the left. It feels like a soft "bag of worms." It is separate from the testis and epididymis and slowly collapses when the scrotum is elevated in the supine position.

EMPTY SCROTAL HALF

The testis and epididymis may be absent. Check the inguinal canal and upper scrotum for an undescended testicle.

TABLE 13-3

TABLE 13-3. COURSE AND PRESENTATION OF HERNIAS IN THE GROIN

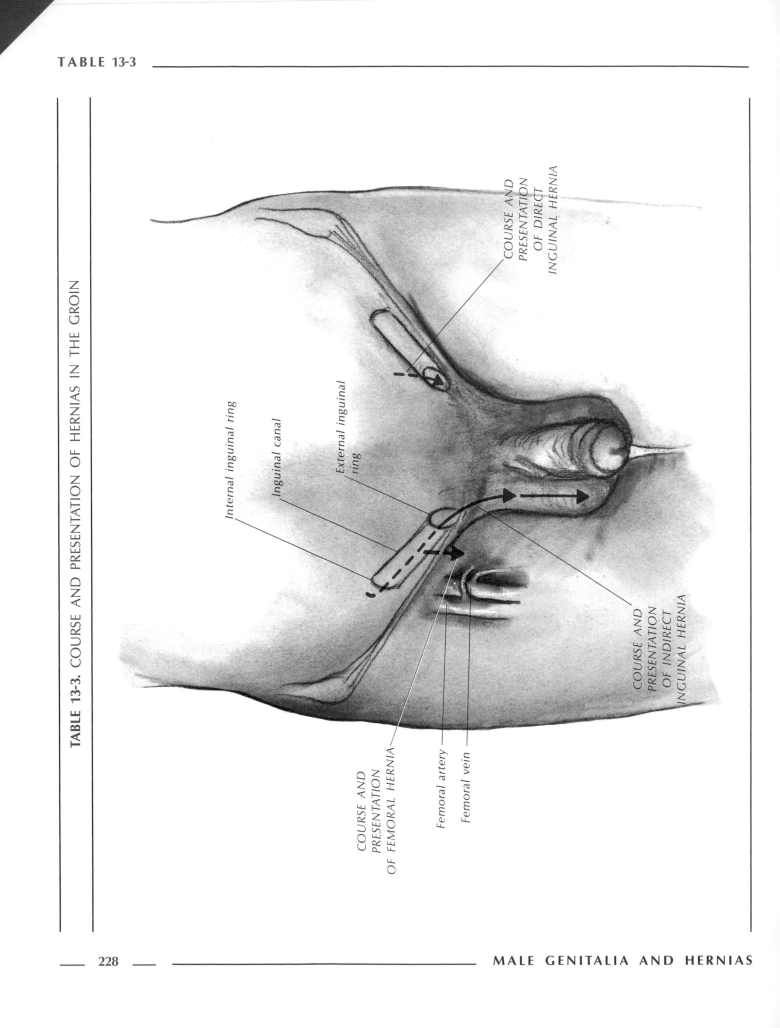

COURSE AND PRESENTATION OF DIRECT INGUINAL HERNIA

Internal inguinal ring

Inguinal canal

External inguinal ring

COURSE AND PRESENTATION OF INDIRECT INGUINAL HERNIA

COURSE AND PRESENTATION OF FEMORAL HERNIA

Femoral artery

Femoral vein

TABLE 13-4

TABLE 13-4. DIFFERENTIATION OF HERNIAS IN THE GROIN

Differentiation between these hernias is not always clinically possible. Understanding of their features, however, improves your observation.

FEATURES	INGUINAL		FEMORAL
	INDIRECT	DIRECT	
Frequency	Most common, all ages, both sexes	Less common	Least common
Age and Sex	Often in children, may be in adults	Usually men over 40, rare in women	More common in women than in men
Point of Origin	Above inguinal ligament, near its midpoint (the internal inguinal ring)	Above inguinal ligament, close to the pubic tubercle (near the external inguinal ring)	Below the inguinal ligament, appears more lateral than an inguinal hernia and may be hard to differentiate from lymph nodes
Course	Often into the scrotum	Rarely into the scrotum	Never into the scrotum
(With the examining finger in the inguinal canal during straining or cough)	Hernia comes down the inguinal canal and touches the fingertip.	Hernia bulges anteriorly and pushes the side of the finger forward.	The inguinal canal is empty.

female genitalia

ANATOMY AND PHYSIOLOGY

Review the anatomy of the external female genitalia, or vulva, including:

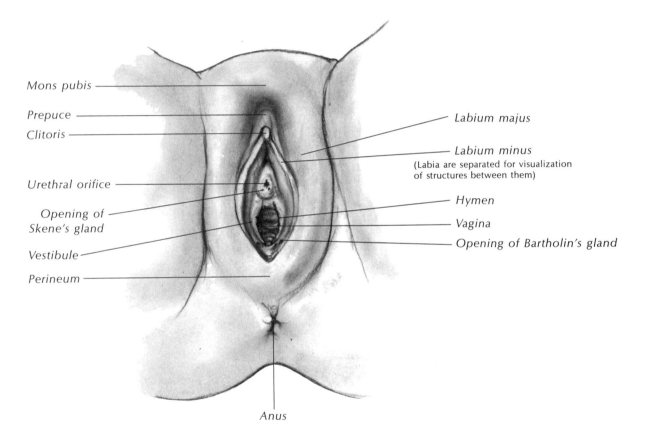

Mons pubis

Prepuce

Clitoris

Urethral orifice

Opening of Skene's gland

Vestibule

Perineum

Labium majus

Labium minus
(Labia are separated for visualization of structures between them)

Hymen

Vagina

Opening of Bartholin's gland

Anus

the mons pubis, a hair-covered fat pad overlying the symphysis pubis; the labia majora, rounded folds of adipose tissue; the labia minora, thinner pinkish-red folds that extend anteriorly to form the prepuce; and the clitoris. The vestibule refers to the boat-shaped fossa between the labia minora. In its posterior portion lies the vaginal opening or introitus, which in virgins may be hidden by the hymen. The term perineum, as commonly used clinically, refers to the tissues between the introitus and anus.

The urethral orifice opens into the vestibule between the clitoris and vagina. Just posterior to it on either side can sometimes be discerned the openings of the paraurethral or Skene's glands. The openings of Bartholin's glands are located posteriorly, on either side of the vaginal opening, but are not usually visible. Bartholin's glands themselves are situated more deeply.

The vagina is a hollow tube extending between urethra and rectum upward and back. It terminates in the cup-shaped fornix. At almost right angles to it sits the uterus, a flattened pear-shaped fibromuscular structure. Its cervix protrudes into the vagina, dividing the fornix into anterior, posterior and lateral fornices. A round or slit-like depression, the external os of the cervix, marks the opening into the endocervical canal and uterine cavity.

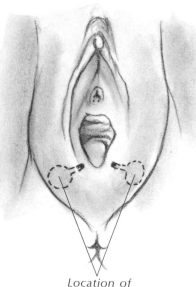

Location of Bartholin's gland

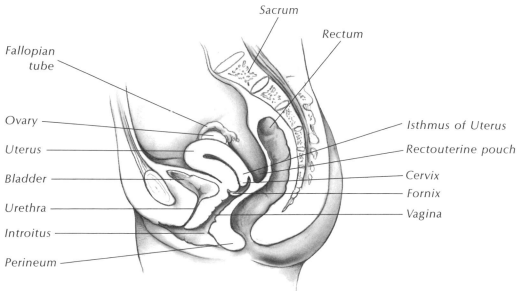

CROSS SECTION, SIDE VIEW

The upper part of the uterus is called the body or fundus; the area between the body and cervix is the isthmus. From each side of the fundus extends a Fallopian tube. The fringed funnel-shaped end of each tube curves toward the ovary. Each ovary is an almond-shaped structure, varying considerably in size, but averaging about 3.5 × 2 ×1.5 cm.

Both ovaries and tubes are supported by peritoneal folds called ligaments. Neither these ligaments nor the tubes, however, are normally palpable. The term adnexa refers to the ovaries, tubes and supporting tissues.

As in the male (see p. 250) the peritoneal surface becomes accessible to the examining finger just anterior to the rectum—beyond the posterior fornix of the vagina in the rectouterine pouch (also called the pouch of Douglas or cul-de-sac).

The patient should be lying in the lithotomy position, her thighs flexed and abducted, her feet resting in stirrups, and her buttocks extending slightly beyond the edge of the examining table. A pillow should support her head.

Relaxation is essential for an adequate examination. To achieve it:
1. The patient should be given an opportunity to empty her bladder.
2. Drape her appropriately. Some patients are more comfortable when the drape is extended well over thighs and knees. Others prefer to watch both the practitioner and the examination itself and object to drapes that obscure their view. Ask the patient which method she prefers.
3. The patient's arms should be at her sides or folded across her chest.
4. Explain in advance each step in the examination, avoiding any sudden or unexpected movements.
5. Have warm hands and a warm speculum.
6. Monitor your examination when possible by watching the patient's face.

Equipment within reach should include a good light, a vaginal speculum of appropriate size, and materials for bacteriologic cultures and Papanicolaou smears. Wear gloves. Male examiners are customarily attended by female assistants. Female examiners may or may not prefer to work alone but should be similarly attended if the patient is emotionally disturbed.

Inspect the Patient's External Genitalia.   *Seat yourself* comfortably and inspect the mons pubis, the labia and perineum. With your gloved hand, separate the labia and inspect:

Itchy, small, red maculopapules suggest pediculosis pubis. Look for nits and lice at the bases of the pubic hairs.

Enlarged clitoris in masculinizing conditions

See Table 14-1, Lesions of the Vulva (p. 239).

> The labia minora
> The clitoris
> The urethral orifice
> The vaginal opening or introitus

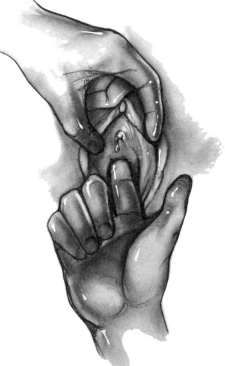

Note any inflammation, ulceration, discharge, swelling or nodules. If there are any lesions, palpate them.

Syphilitic chancre, sebaceous cyst

If urethritis or inflammation of Skene's glands (e.g., from gonorrhea) is suspected, insert your index finger into the vagina and milk the urethra gently from inside outward. Note any discharge from or about the urethral orifice. If present, culture it.

If there is a history or appearance of labial swelling, check Bartholin's glands. Insert your index finger into the vagina near the posterior end of the introitus. Place your thumb outside the posterior part of the labium majus. On each side in turn palpate between your finger and thumb for swelling or tenderness. Note any discharge exuding from the duct opening of the gland. If present, culture it.

Assess the Support of the Vaginal Outlet. With the labia separated by your middle and index finger, ask the patient to strain down. Note any bulging of the vaginal walls.

Inspect the Vagina and Cervix. Select a speculum of appropriate size, lubricate and warm it with warm water. (Other lubricants may interfere with cytological or other studies but may be used if no such tests are planned.) By having your speculum ready during assessment of the vaginal outlet, you can ease speculum insertion and increase your efficiency by proceeding to the next maneuver while the patient is still straining down.

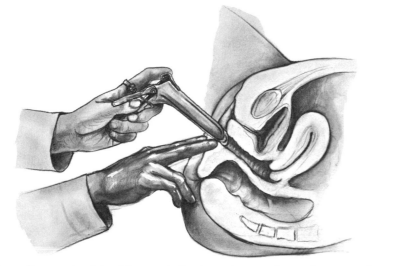

Place two fingers just inside or at the introitus and gently press down on the perineal body. With your other hand introduce the closed speculum past your fingers at a 45-degree angle downward. The blades should be held obliquely and the pressure exerted toward the posterior vaginal wall in order to avoid the more sensitive anterior wall and urethra. Be careful not to pull on the pubic hair or to pinch the labia with the speculum.

See Table 14-2, Bulges and Swellings of Vulva and Vagina (p. 240).

Cystocele and rectocele

After the speculum has entered the vagina, remove your fingers from the introitus. Rotate the blades of the speculum into a horizontal position, maintaining the pressure posteriorly.

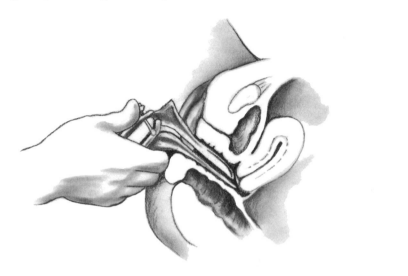

Open the blades after full insertion and maneuver the speculum so that the cervix comes into full view.

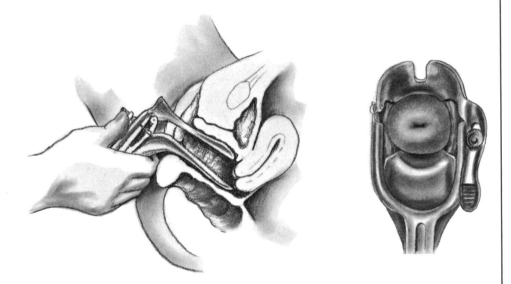

When the uterus is retroverted, the cervix points more anteriorly than diagrammed. Position the speculum more anteriorly, i.e., more horizontally, in order to bring the cervix into view.

Inspect the cervix and its os. Note the color of the cervix, its position, any ulcerations, nodules, masses, bleeding or discharge.

Purplish color in pregnancy

See Table 14-3, Variations and Abnormalities of the Cervix (pp. 241–242).

Secure the speculum with the blades open by tightening the thumb screw.

Obtain Specimens for Cervical Cytology (Papanicolaou smears). Take three specimens in order:

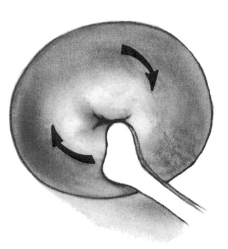

1. *The Endocervical Swab.* Moisten the end of a cotton applicator stick with saline and insert it into the os of the cervix. Roll it between your thumb and index finger, clockwise and counterclockwise. Remove it. Smear a glass slide with the cotton swab, gently in a painting motion. (Rubbing hard on the slide will destroy the cells.) Place the slide into the ether-alcohol fixative at once.

2. *Cervical Scrape.* Place the longer end of the scraper on the os of the cervix. Press, turn and scrape. Smear on a second slide as before.

3. *Vaginal Pool.* Roll a cotton applicator stick on the floor of the vagina below the cervix. Prepare a third slide as before.

If the cervix has been removed, do a vaginal pool and a scrape from the cuff of the vagina.

Inspect the Vagina. Withdraw the speculum slowly while observing the vagina. As the speculum clears the cervix, release the thumb screw and maintain the speculum in its open position with your thumb. Close the blades as the speculum emerges from the introitus, avoiding both excessive stretching and pinching of the mucosa. During withdrawal, inspect the vaginal mucosa, noting its color, inflammation, discharge, ulcers or masses.

See Table 14-4, Inflammations of and Around the Vagina (pp. 243–244).

Cancer of the vagina

Perform a Bimanual Examination. From a *standing position* introduce the index and middle finger of your gloved and lubricated hand into the vagina, again exerting pressure primarily posteriorly. Your thumb should be abducted, your ring and little fingers flexed into your palm. Note any nodularity or tenderness in the vaginal wall, including the region of the urethra and bladder anteriorly.

Identify the cervix, noting its position, shape, consistency, regularity, mobility and tenderness. Palpate the fornix around the cervix.

See Table 14-5, Changes in Pregnancy (p. 245).

Place your abdominal hand about midway between the umbilicus and symphysis pubis and press downward toward the pelvic hand. Your pelvic hand should be kept in a straight line with your forearm, and inward pressure exerted on the perineum by your flexed fingers. Support and stabilize your arm by resting your elbow either on your hip or on your knee which is elevated by placing your foot on a stool. Identify the uterus between your hands and note its size, shape, consistency, mobility, tenderness and masses.

See Table 14-6, Abnormalities and Displacements of the Uterus (pp. 246–247).

Uterine enlargement suggests pregnancy, benign or malignant tumors.

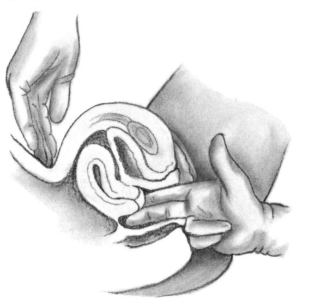

Place your abdominal hand on the right lower quadrant, your pelvic hand in the right lateral fornix. Maneuver your abdominal hand downward, and using your pelvic hand for palpation, identify the right ovary and any masses in the adnexa.

Three to five years after menopause the ovaries have usually atrophied and are no longer palpable. If you can feel an ovary in a post-menopausal woman, suspect an ovarian tumor.

VIEW FROM THE RIGHT SIDE

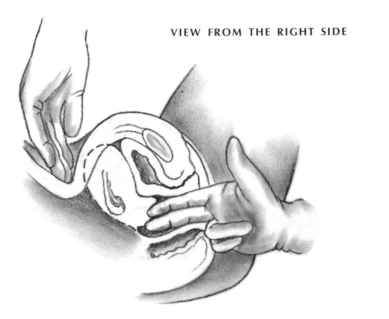

Note the size, shape, consistency, mobility and tenderness of any palpable organs or masses. (The normal ovary is somewhat tender.) Repeat the procedure on the left side.

See Table 14-7, Adnexal Masses (p. 243).

Withdraw you fingers, lubricate your gloves again if necessary. (See note below on using lubricant). Then slowly reintroduce your index finger into the vagina, your middle finger into the rectum. Ask the patient to strain down as

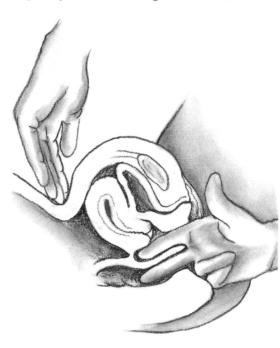

you do this so that her anal sphincter will relax. Tell her that this examination may make her feel as if she has to move her bowels—but she won't. Repeat the maneuvers of the bimanual examination, giving special attention to the region behind the cervix which may be accessible only to the rectal finger. In addition, try to push the uterus backward with your abdominal hand so that your rectal finger can explore as much of the posterior uterine surface as possible.

Proceed to the rectal examination (see Chapter 15). After your examination, wipe off the external genitalia and anus or offer the patient some tissue with which to do it herself.

A Note on Examining Virgins. Many virginal vaginal orifices will readily admit a single examining finger. The technique can be modified so that the index finger alone is used. Special small specula or a nasal speculum may make inspection possible also. When the orifice is even smaller, a fairly good bimanual examination can be performed with one finger in the rectum.

Similar techniques may be indicated in elderly women in whom the introitus has become tight.

A Note on Using Lubricant. When performing either a pelvic or rectal examination, you should never contaminate the tube of lubricant by touching it with your gloved hand after touching the patient. Develop the following habit: Always allow the lubricant to drop onto your gloved fingers without actually touching them.

If you should accidentally contaminate the lubricant tube, discard it.

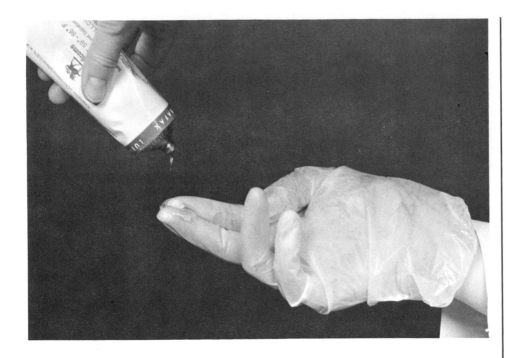

The Risk of Spreading Infection Between Vagina and Rectum. Gonorrhea may infect the rectum as well as the female genitalia. This fact, together with the rising prevalence of gonorrhea, has led to the recommendation that gloves be changed between vaginal and rectal examination in order to avoid spreading gonococcal infection. In order to avoid fecal soiling, gloves should always be changed if for some reason the practitioner examines the vagina after the rectum.

TABLE 14-1

TABLE 14-1. LESIONS OF THE VULVA

SEBACEOUS CYST

Cystic nodule in skin

Small, firm, round cystic nodules in the labia suggest sebaceous cysts. They are sometimes yellowish in color. Look for the dark punctum marking the blocked opening of the gland.

VENEREAL WART (CONDYLOMA ACUMINATUM)

Warts

Warty lesions on the labia and within the vestibule suggest condylomata acuminata. Like warts elsewhere, they are reactions to a viral infection.

SECONDARY SYPHILIS (CONDYLOMA LATUM)

Flat, gray papules

Slightly raised, flat, round or oval papules, covered by a gray exudate, suggest condylomata lata. These constitute one manifestation of secondary syphilis and are contagious.

SYPHILITIC CHANCRE

Firm ulcer

A firm painless ulcer suggests the chancre of primary syphilis. Since most chancres in women develop internally, they often go undetected.

HERPES INFECTION

Shallow ulcers on red bases

Shallow, small painful ulcers on red bases suggest a herpes infection. Initial infection may be extensive, as illustrated here. Recurrent infections are usually confined to a small local patch.

CARCINOMA OF THE VULVA

Raised and red or ulcerated

An ulcerated or raised, red vulvar lesion in an elderly woman may indicate vulvar carcinoma.

TABLE 14-2

TABLE 14-2. BULGES AND SWELLINGS OF VULVA AND VAGINA

CYSTOCELE

A cystocele is present when the anterior wall of the vagina, together with the bladder above it, bulges into the vagina and sometimes out the introitus. Look for the bulging vaginal wall as the patient strains down.

Bulge

RECTOCELE

A rectocele is formed by the anterior and downward bulging of the posterior vaginal wall together with the rectum behind it. To identify it, spread the patient's labia and ask her to strain down.

Bulge

INFLAMMATION OF BARTHOLIN'S GLAND

Inflammation of Bartholin's glands may be acute or chronic. It is commonly but not necessarily caused by gonococcal infection. Acutely, it presents as a tense, hot, very tender abscess. Look for pus coming out of the duct or erythema around the duct opening. Chronically, a non-tender cyst occupies the posterior labium. It may be large or small.

Labial swelling

URETHRAL CARUNCLE

A urethral caruncle is a bright red, polypoid growth that protrudes from the urethral meatus. Most cause no symptoms. A caruncle may be confused with simple outward pouting of the posterior aspect of the urethral mucosa, which is often visible in post-menopausal women.

Red, bulging

TABLE 14-3

TABLE 14-3. VARIATIONS AND ABNORMALITIES OF THE CERVIX

NORMAL NULLIPAROUS CERVIX

Round or oval

The nulliparous cervical os is small and either round or oval. The cervix is covered by smooth pink epithelium.

NORMAL PAROUS CERVIX

Slit-like

After childbirth, the cervical os presents a slit-like appearance.

LACERATIONS OF THE CERVIX

UNILATERAL TRANSVERSE *BILATERAL TRANSVERSE* *STELLATE*

The trauma of difficult deliveries may tear the cervix, producing permanent transverse or stellate lacerations.

TABLE 14-3 (CONT'D)

TABLE 14-3. (CONT'D)

ECTROPION (EROSION)

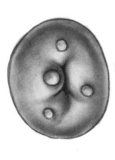

The mucosa around the central os is at times a plush red rather than the usual shiny pink. It may bleed easily when touched. This appearance is usually due to an ectropion, i.e., the presence of columnar epithelium like that lining the cervical canal. An ectropion is not abnormal but may be difficult to distinguish from early carcinoma without further study, e.g., by cytology, colposcopy or biopsy. The term erosion is also used for this condition but is misleading since the mucosa has not actually been eroded away.

NABOTHIAN OR RETENTION CYSTS

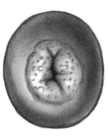

Retention or Nabothian cysts may accompany or follow chronic cervicitis. Variable in size, single or multiple, they appear as translucent nodules on the cervical surface.

CERVICAL POLYP

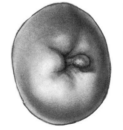

Cervical polyps usually arise from the endocervical canal, becoming visible when they protrude through the cervical os. They are bright red, soft and rather fragile. When only the tips are seen they cannot be clinically differentiated from polyps originating in the endometrium.

CARCINOMA OF THE CERVIX

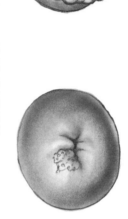

Carcinoma of the cervix usually begins at or near the cervical os. It presents a hard granular surface which bleeds easily, proceeding later to an extensive irregular cauliflower type of growth. Early carcinomas are clinically indistinguishable from ectropions and may even be present in a cervix that appears normal.

TABLE 14-4

TABLE 14-4. INFLAMMATIONS OF AND AROUND THE VAGINA

TRICHOMONAS VAGINITIS*

Red spots

Inflamed mucosa

MONILIA (CANDIDA) VAGINITIS*

White patches

Inflamed mucosa

	TRICHOMONAS VAGINITIS*	MONILIA (CANDIDA) VAGINITIS*
Discharge	Thin or thick; white, yellowish or green; often bubbly; often pooled in the vaginal fornix; profuse	May be thin but is characteristically thick, white and curdy; not so profuse as in Trichomonas vaginitis.
Vulva	Often inflamed	Often inflamed
Urethritis	Usually absent, but a Trichomonas cystitis occurs occasionally.	Absent
Bartholin's gland infection	Absent	Absent
Vaginal mucosa	Red, inflamed, with red granular or petechial spots in the fornix	Red, inflamed, with white or grayish often tenacious patches of discharge. May bleed when plaques. of discharge are scraped off.
Cervix	May show red spots ("strawberry spots").	May show patches of discharge.

*Many patients present less typical signs. Definitive diagnosis depends on identification of the causative organism.

TABLE 14-4 (CONT'D)

TABLE 14-4. (CONT'D)

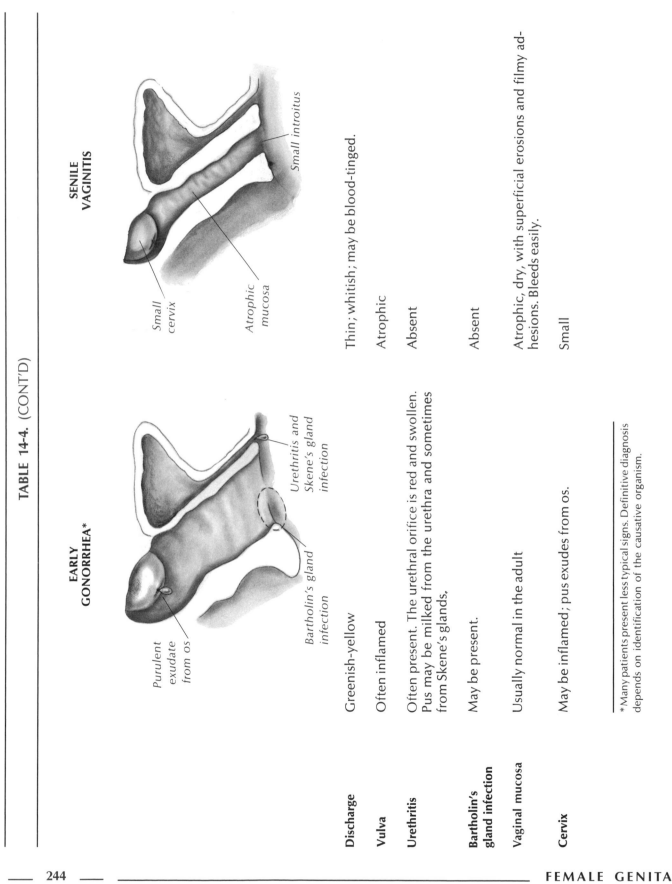

	EARLY GONORRHEA*	SENILE VAGINITIS
Discharge	Greenish-yellow	Thin; whitish; may be blood-tinged.
Vulva	Often inflamed	Atrophic
Urethritis	Often present. The urethral orifice is red and swollen. Pus may be milked from the urethra and sometimes from Skene's glands.	Absent
Bartholin's gland infection	May be present.	Absent
Vaginal mucosa	Usually normal in the adult	Atrophic, dry, with superficial erosions and filmy adhesions. Bleeds easily.
Cervix	May be inflamed; pus exudes from os.	Small

*Many patients present less typical signs. Definitive diagnosis depends on identification of the causative organism.

TABLE 14-5

TABLE 14-5. CHANGES IN PREGNANCY

3rd THROUGH 10th MONTHS

(Read from the bottom up.)

The height of the fundus drops slightly during the 10th month as the fetus settles deeper into the pelvis in preparation for labor and delivery.

Fetal movements become palpable after the 5th month and fetal parts may be discernible.

By the 5th month the fundus is at the level of the umbilicus. The fetal heart becomes audible, giving the first absolute proof of pregnancy obtainable by physical examination. Listen for it at this stage just above the symphysis pubis.

By the 3rd month, the uterus has become globular in shape and first rises above the symphysis pubis.

6th WEEK FROM THE LAST MENSTRUAL PERIOD

The isthmus of the uterus softens. Its soft consistency contrasts with the firm cervix below and the somewhat doughy or elastic uterus above. This phenomenon is called Hegar's sign. It is the first clinical manifestation of pregnancy but is not absolutely diagnostic. The uterine fundus tends to feel more globular and may become asymmetrical at the site of fetal implantation.

2nd MONTH

The cervix itself softens. In consistency it begins to resemble lips rather than a nose. Its color and that of the adjacent vaginal mucosa become purplish.

Soft and purplish

TABLE 14-6

TABLE 14-6. ABNORMALITIES AND DISPLACEMENTS OF THE UTERUS

PROLAPSE OF THE UTERUS

Normal position

Prolapse of the uterus results from weakness of the supporting structures of the pelvic floor and is often associated with a cystocele and rectocele. In progressive stages the uterus becomes retroverted and descends down the vaginal canal to the outside. In first degree prolapse, the cervix is still well within the vagina. In second degree, it is at the introitus. In third degree prolapse, also called procidentia uteri, the cervix and vagina are outside the introitus.

MYOMAS OF THE UTERUS (FIBROIDS)

Myomas

Myomas are very common, benign uterine tumors. They may be single or multiple and vary greatly in size, occasionally reaching massive proportions. They present as firm irregular nodules in continuity with the uterine surface. Occasionally a myoma projecting laterally can be confused with an ovarian mass; a nodule projecting posteriorly can be mistaken for a retroflexed fundus. Submucous myomas project toward the endometrial cavity and are not themselves palpable although they may be suspected because of an enlarged uterus.

TABLE 14-6 (CONT'D)

TABLE 14-6. (CONT'D)

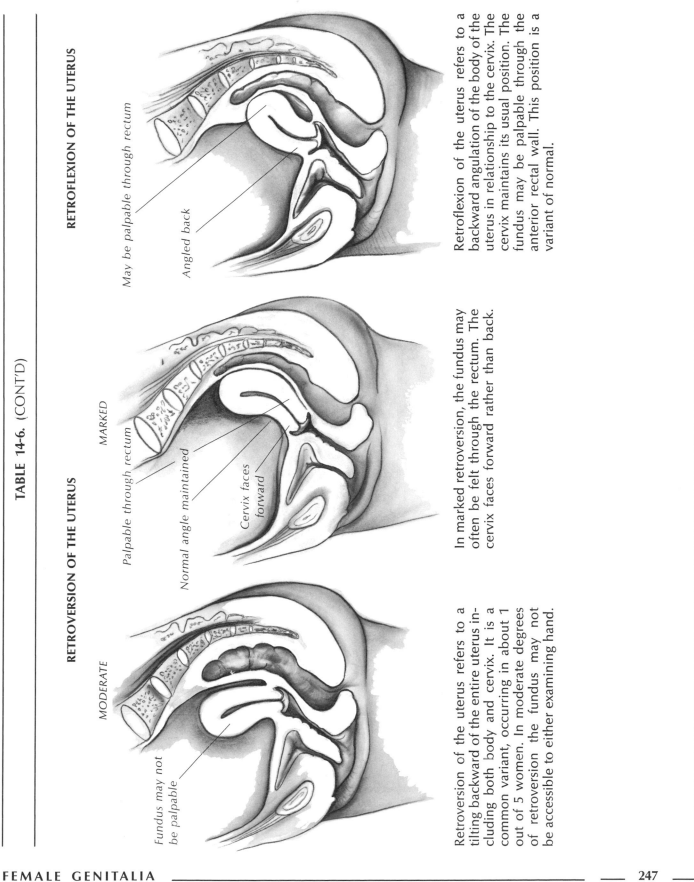

RETROVERSION OF THE UTERUS

MODERATE

Fundus may not
be palpable

MARKED

Palpable through rectum

Normal angle maintained

Cervix faces
forward

RETROFLEXION OF THE UTERUS

May be palpable through rectum

Angled back

Retroversion of the uterus refers to a tilting backward of the entire uterus including both body and cervix. It is a common variant, occurring in about 1 out of 5 women. In moderate degrees of retroversion the fundus may not be accessible to either examining hand.

In marked retroversion, the fundus may often be felt through the rectum. The cervix faces forward rather than back.

Retroflexion of the uterus refers to a backward angulation of the body of the uterus in relationship to the cervix. The cervix maintains its usual position. The fundus may be palpable through the anterior rectal wall. This position is a variant of normal.

TABLE 14-7

TABLE 14-7. ADNEXAL MASSES

One or both sides, usually non-tender

Bilateral, tender

Bilateral tender

Movement of cervix painful

Unilateral, tender

Movement of cervix painful

OVARIAN CYSTS AND TUMORS

Ovarian cysts and tumors may be detected as adnexal masses on one or both sides. Later they may grow up out of the pelvis. Cysts tend to be smooth and compressible, tumors more solid and often nodular. They are not usually tender.

PELVIC INFLAMMATORY DISEASE

Acute pelvic inflammatory disease is associated with very tender bilateral adnexal masses although pain and muscle spasm usually make it impossible to delineate them. Movement of the cervix produces pain. *Chronic pelvic in-flammatory disease* is manifested by bilateral, tender, usually irregular and fairly fixed adnexal masses.

RUPTURED TUBAL PREGNANCY

Typically a ruptured tubal pregnancy presents with signs of hemorrhage into the peritoneal cavity: marked pelvic tenderness, and tenderness and rigidity of the lower abdomen. Motion of the cervix produces pain. A tender unilateral adnexal mass may indicate the site of the pregnancy. Tachycardia and shock reflect the hemorrhage.

anus and rectum

ANATOMY AND PHYSIOLOGY

The gastrointestinal tract terminates in a short segment, the anal canal. Its external margin is poorly demarcated, but generally the skin of the anal canal can be distinguished from the surrounding perianal skin by its moist, hairless appearance. The anal canal is normally held in a closed position by action of the voluntary external muscular sphincter and the involuntary internal sphincter, the latter an extension of the muscular coat of the rectal wall.

The direction of the anal canal on a line roughly between anus and umbilicus should be carefully noted. Unlike the rectum above it the canal is liberally supplied by somatic sensory nerves, so that a poorly directed finger or instrument will produce pain.

The anal canal is demarcated from the rectum superiorly by a serrated line marking the change from skin to mucous membrane. This anorectal junction (often called the pectinate or dentate line) also denotes the boundary between somatic and visceral nerve supplies. It is readily visible on proctoscopic examination but is not palpable.

Above the anorectal junction, the rectum balloons out and turns posteriorly into the hollow of the coccyx and sacrum, forming almost a right angle with the anal canal. In the male, the prostate gland is palpable anteriorly as a rounded heart-shaped structure about 2.5 cm in length. Its two lateral lobes are separated by a shallow median sulcus or groove. The seminal vesicles, shaped like rabbit ears above the prostate, are not normally palpable.

Through the anterior wall of the female rectum the uterine cervix can usually be felt.

The rectal wall contains three inward foldings called valves of Houston. The lowest of these can sometimes be felt, usually on the patient's left.

Although most of the rectum accessible to the examining finger does not have a peritoneal surface, the anterior rectum, which the tip of the examining finger reaches, usually does. This relationship makes it possible to identify the tenderness of peritoneal inflammation or the nodularity of peritoneal metastases by rectal examination.

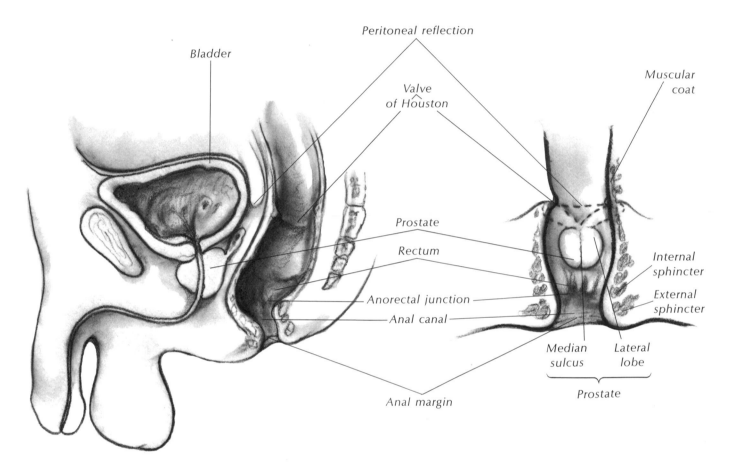

CROSS SECTION, SIDE VIEW

ANTERIOR WALL

ANUS AND RECTUM—MALE

ANUS AND RECTUM

Male

Many examiners prefer to do a rectal examination on an ambulatory patient when he is standing, with hips flexed and upper body resting across the examining table. This position tends to flatten the buttocks and make the anal canal and rectum more accessible to the examining finger.

For the non-ambulatory patient, the lateral position is necessary and some examiners may prefer to use it routinely. In this situation, ask the patient to lie on his left side with his right hip and knee somewhat flexed, his buttocks close to the edge of the examining table near you.

Adjust the lighting for good visualization of the anus and surrounding area. Put a glove on your right hand and lubricate the index finger. With your left hand, spread the buttocks apart.

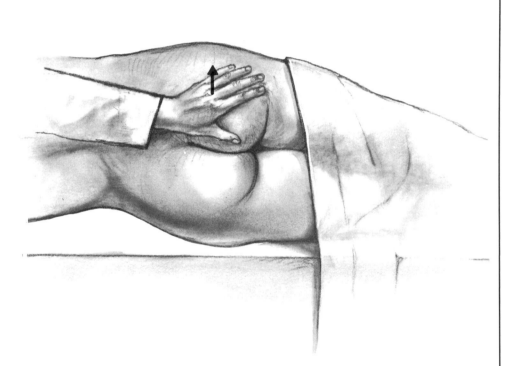

Inspect the sacrococcygeal and perianal areas for lumps, inflammation, rashes or excoriations. Palpate any abnormal areas, noting lumps or tenderness.

Swollen, thickened, fissured skin with excoriations in pruritus ani

Ask the patient to strain down. Inspect the anus, noting any lesions.

As the patient strains, place the pad of your lubricated and gloved index finger over the anus. As the sphincter relaxes, gently insert your fingertip into the anal canal, in a direction pointing toward the umbilicus.

See Table 15-1, Abnormalities of the Anus, Surrounding Skin and Rectum (pp. 254–255).

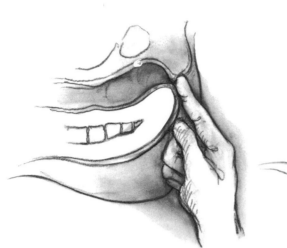

Instruct the patient to relax. Explain that this examination will make him feel as if he is moving his bowels.

Note:
    The sphincter tone of the anus
    Tenderness
    Irregularities or nodules

Sphincter tightness in anxiety, inflammation or scarring; laxity in some neurological disease and with habitual anal intercourse.

Insert your finger further into the rectum so that you can examine as much of the rectal wall as possible. Palpate in sequence the right lateral, posterior and left lateral surfaces, noting any nodules or irregularities. Then turn your hand so that your finger can examine the anterior surface. Identify the lateral lobes of the prostate and the median sulcus between them. Note the size, shape and consistency of the prostate and any nodularity or tenderness.

See Table 15-2, Abnormalities of the Prostate (p. 256).

If possible, extend your finger above the prostate to the region of the seminal vesicles and peritoneal cavity. Note nodules or tenderness.

Rectal lesions just beyond your fingertip can sometimes be felt by asking the patient again to strain down. Use this maneuver if there is any suspicion of cancer.

Gently withdraw your finger and test any fecal material adherent to it for occult blood.

Female

The rectum is usually examined after the female genitalia, while the patient is in the lithotomy position. This position is essential for bimanual palpation. If a rectal examination alone is indicated, the lateral position offers a satisfactory alternative and affords much better visualization of the perianal and sacrococcygeal areas.

The technique is basically similar. The cervix is usually readily felt through the anterior rectal wall. Sometimes a retroverted uterus is also palpable. Neither of these, nor a tampon, should be mistaken for a tumor.

TABLE 15-1

TABLE 15-1. ABNORMALITIES OF THE ANUS, SURROUNDING SKIN AND RECTUM

PILONIDAL CYST AND SINUS

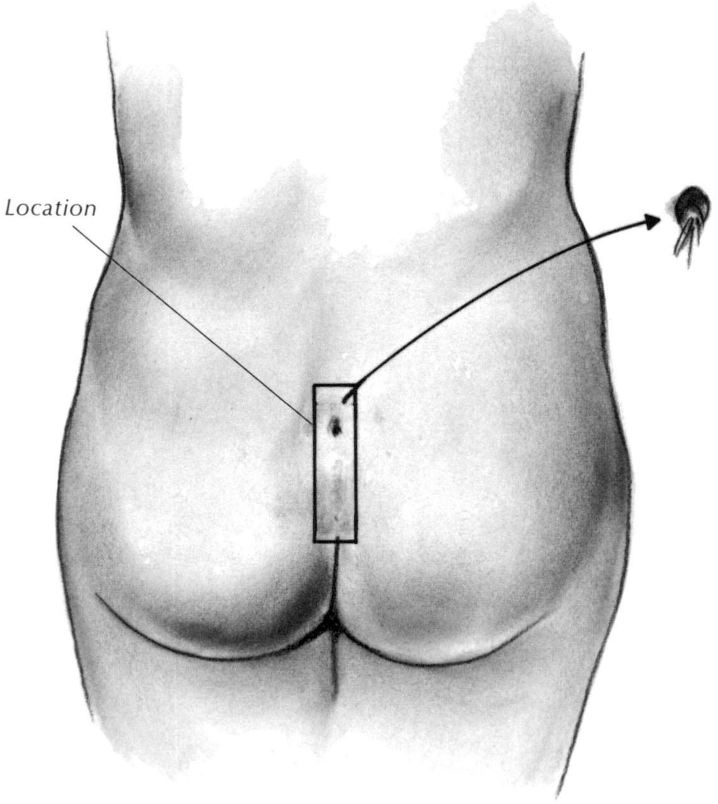

Location

A pilonidal cyst is a fairly frequent, probably congenital abnormality located in the midline superficial to the coccyx or lower sacrum. It is clinically identified by the opening of a sinus tract. This opening may exhibit a small tuft of hair and be surrounded by a halo of erythema. Although generally asymptomatic except perhaps for slight drainage, abscess formation and secondary sinus tracts may complicate the picture.

ANORECTAL FISTULA

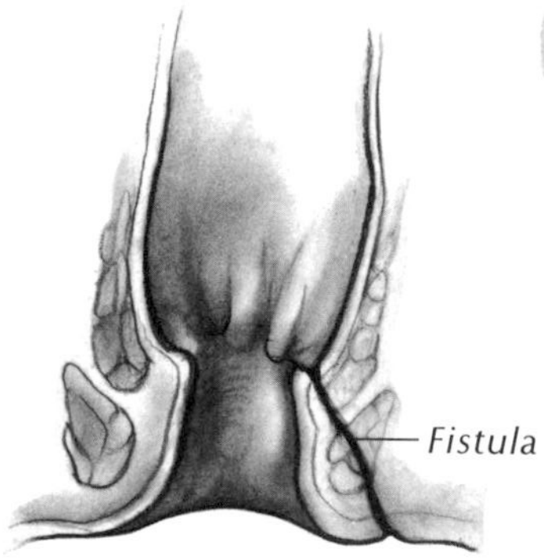

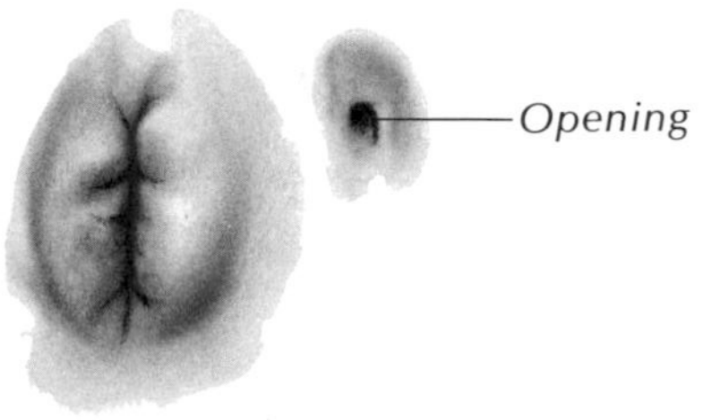

Opening

Fistula

An anorectal fistula is an inflammatory tract or tube, one end of which opens into the anus or rectum, while the other end opens onto the skin surface, as shown here, or into another viscus. An abscess usually antedates such a fistula. Look for the fistulous opening or openings anywhere in the skin around the anus.

ANAL FISSURE

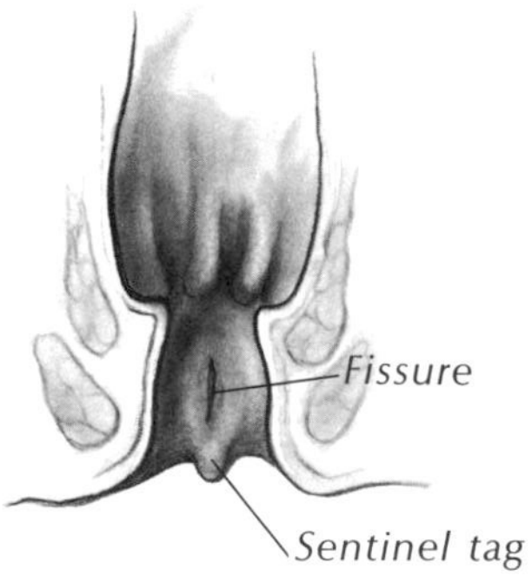

Fissure

Sentinel tag

An anal fissure is a very painful oval ulceration of the anal canal, most commonly found in the midline posteriorly, less commonly in the midline anteriorly. Its long axis lies longitudinally. Inspection may reveal a "sentinel" skin tag just below it, and gentle separation of the anal margins may reveal the lower edge of the fissure. The sphincter is spastic; the examination painful. Local anesthesia may be required.

TABLE 15-1 (CONT'D)

POLYPS OF THE RECTUM

Polyps of the rectum are fairly common. Varying considerably in size and number, they can develop on a stalk (pedunculated) or may lie close to the mucosal surface (sessile). They are soft and may be difficult or impossible to feel even when in reach of the examining finger. Proctoscopy is usually required for diagnosis, as is biopsy for the differentiation of benign from malignant lesions.

Sessile

Pedunculated

CARCINOMA OF THE RECTUM

Asymptomatic carcinoma of the rectum makes routine rectal examination mandatory for virtually all adults. As noted above, polypoid masses may be malignant. Another common form of presentation is the firm nodular rolled edge of an ulcerated malignancy.

Rolled nodular edge

PERITONEAL METASTASES

SIDE VIEW   ANTERIOR WALL

Palpable rectal shelf

Widespread peritoneal metastases from any source may develop in the area of the peritoneal reflection anterior to the rectum. A firm to hard nodular rectal "shelf" may be just palpable with the tip of the examining finger.

EXTERNAL HEMORRHOID

Hemorrhoids are varicose veins. External hemorrhoids originate below the anorectal line and are covered by anal skin. When uncomplicated they may not be visible at rest, but a thrombosed hemorrhoid presents as a painful, bluish, shiny, ovoid mass at the anal margin. Flabby or fibrotic skin tags may mark the location of previously thrombosed or inflamed hemorrhoids.

Thrombosed

INTERNAL HEMORRHOID

Internal hemorrhoids originate above the anorectal junction and are covered by mucous membrane, not skin. They are not visible unless they prolapse through the anus, nor are the soft swellings normally identifiable by palpation. Proctoscopic examination is usually required for diagnosis.

Soft

PROLAPSE OF THE RECTUM

On straining for a bowel movement, the rectal mucosa, with or without its muscular wall, may prolapse through the anus, presenting as a doughnut or rosette of red mucosa. A prolapse involving only mucosa is shown here. When the entire bowel wall is involved, the prolapse is larger; and circular rather than radiating folds are seen.

TABLE 15-1. (CONT'D)

TABLE 15-2

TABLE 15-2. ABNORMALITIES OF THE PROSTATE

THE NORMAL PROSTATE GLAND

Smooth, elastic, symmetrical

As palpated through the anterior rectal wall, the normal prostate is a rounded heart-shaped structure about 2.5 cm in length, projecting less than 1.0 cm into the rectal lumen. The median sulcus can be felt between the two lateral lobes. Only the posterior surface of the prostate is palpable. Anterior lesions, including those that may obstruct the urethra, may not be detectable by physical examination.

CARCINOMA OF THE PROSTATE

SINGLE NODULE — *irregular, hard*

ADVANCED — *Hard, irregular, fixed*

A hard irregular nodule, producing asymmetry of the gland and a variation in its consistency, is especially suggestive of carcinoma. Prostatic stones and chronic inflammation can produce similar findings, and differential diagnosis often depends upon biopsy. Later in its course, the carcinoma grows in size, obliterates the median sulcus and may extend beyond the confines of the gland, producing a fixed, hard irregular mass.

BENIGN PROSTATIC HYPERTROPHY

Smooth, elastic, symmetrical

A very common condition in men over 50 years of age, benign prostatic hypertrophy presents as a firm smooth symmetrical and slightly elastic enlargement of the gland. It may bulge more than a centimeter into the rectal lumen. The hypertrophied tissue tends to obliterate the median sulcus.

PROSTATITIS

ACUTE — *Swollen, tender*

The acutely inflamed prostate gland is swollen, tender and often somewhat asymmetrical.

The gland of chronic prostatitis is variable: it may (1) feel normal, (2) be somewhat enlarged, tender and boggy, or (3) contain scattered firm areas of fibrosis.

the peripheral vascular system

ANATOMY AND PHYSIOLOGY

Arteries

The anatomy of the carotid arteries and abdominal aorta have been described in Chapters 7 and 12, respectively. This section will focus on the arteries supplying the arms and legs.

In the arms, arterial pulses are clinically accessible in two or perhaps three locations: **(1)** the *brachial artery* just medial to the biceps muscle above the elbow, **(2)** the *radial artery* and **(3)** the less easily felt *ulnar artery* at the wrist.

The radial and ulnar arteries are interconnected by two vascular arches within the hand. Circulation to the hand and fingers is thereby doubly protected against possible arterial occlusion.

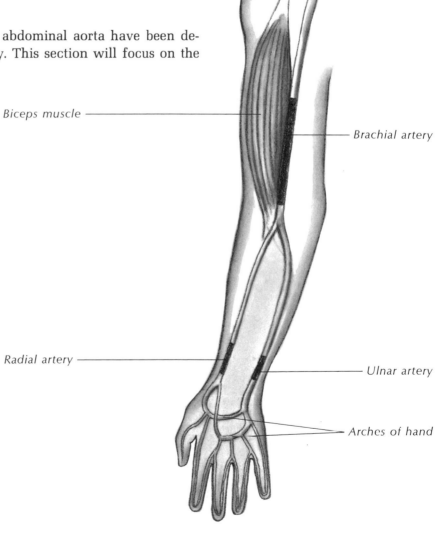

RIGHT ARM

Biceps muscle ———

——— Brachial artery

Radial artery ———

——— Ulnar artery

——— Arches of hand

RIGHT LEG

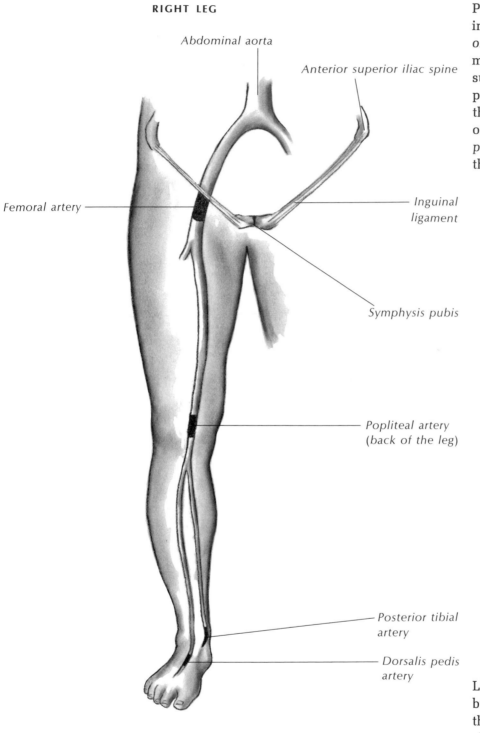

Abdominal aorta

Anterior superior iliac spine

Femoral artery

Inguinal ligament

Symphysis pubis

Popliteal artery (back of the leg)

Posterior tibial artery

Dorsalis pedis artery

Pulses in the legs can be identified in the following locations: the *femoral artery* below the inguinal ligament midway between the anterior superior iliac spine and symphysis pubis; the *popliteal artery*, behind the knee; the *dorsalis pedis artery* on the dorsum of the foot; and the *posterior tibial artery*, just behind the medial malleolus.

Like the hand, the foot is protected by an interconnecting arch between the two chief arterial branches supplying it.

Veins

The jugular veins have been discussed in Chapter 7. They are the principal veins of the head and together with veins from the arms and upper trunk drain into the superior vena cava. Veins from the legs and lower trunk drain into the inferior vena cava. Since venous disease most commonly affects the legs, special attention should be paid to the structure and function of the leg veins.

The *deep veins* of the legs are responsible for about 90 percent of the venous return from the lower extremities. They are well supported by surrounding tissues and are further aided in their work against gravity by valves that normally allow blood to flow only toward the heart. The deep veins are not visible clinically.

In contrast, the *superficial veins* are located subcutaneously and are supported relatively poorly. They include: **(1)** the *great saphenous vein* which originates on the dorsum of the foot, passes just in front of the medial malleolus and then up the medial aspect of the leg to join the deep venous system (the femoral vein) below the inguinal ligament; **(2)** the *small saphenous vein* which begins at the side of the foot and passes upward along the back of the leg to join the deep system in the popliteal space. The several tributaries and anastomoses between the two saphenous veins are not illustrated. From the superficial to the deep systems run short *communicating veins*.

Normally both saphenous and communicating veins are also supplied with valves, thus ensuring the proper direction of flow.

FRONT   BACK   LEFT SIDE

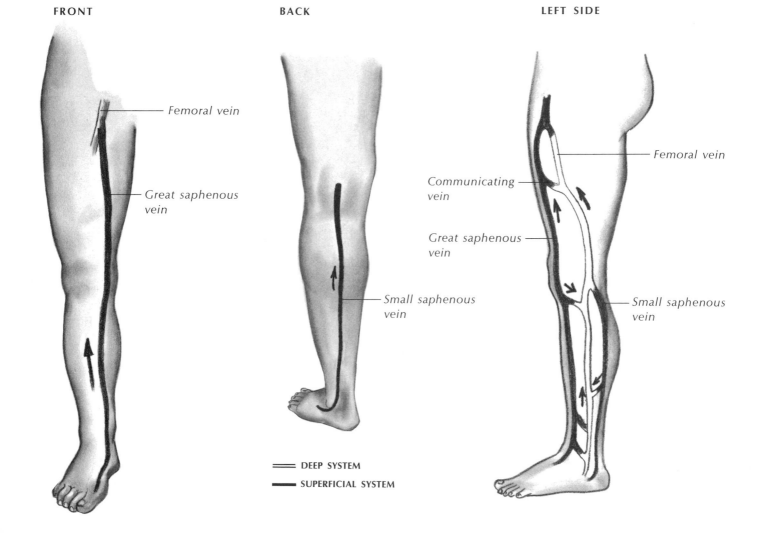

Femoral vein

Great saphenous vein

Small saphenous vein

Communicating vein

Great saphenous vein

Femoral vein

Small saphenous vein

═══ DEEP SYSTEM
▬▬▬ SUPERFICIAL SYSTEM

The Lymphatic System and Lymph Nodes

The lymphatic system consists of a series of channels that begin peripherally in blind lymphatic capillaries. These capillaries remove excess fluid from the tissues. The lymph so formed is carried centrally through lymphatic vessels and collecting ducts to empty into the venous system at the root of the neck. In its passage, lymph is filtered through lymph nodes that are interposed along the way.

The lymphatics draining the head and neck have been described in Chapter 7, the lymph nodes of the axilla in Chapter 11.

Recall that the axillary lymph nodes drain most of the arm. Lymphatics from the ulnar surface of the forearm, the little and ring fingers, and the adjacent surface of the middle finger drain first into the *epitrochlear node*. This node is located on the medial surface of the arm above the elbow. Most of the rest of the arm sends lymphatics directly to the axillary nodes. Some lymphatics may go directly to the infraclaviculars.

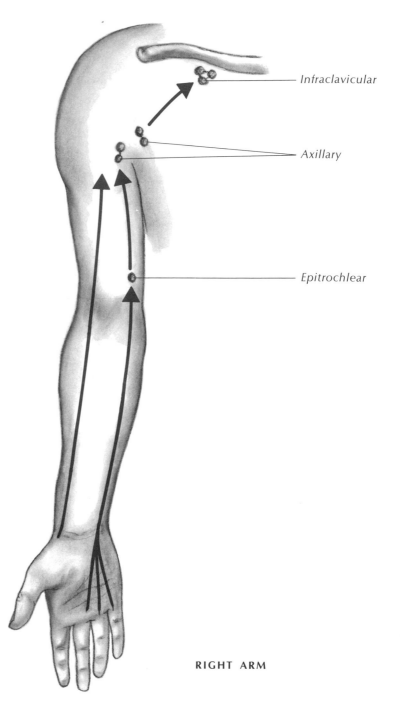

Infraclavicular

Axillary

Epitrochlear

RIGHT ARM

The lymphatic drainage of the lower extremity parallels the venous supply, consisting of both superficial and deep systems. Only the superficial system is accessible to physical examination. There are two groups of *superficial inguinal nodes.* The *vertical group* lies close to the upper portion of the great saphenous vein and has a similar drainage area from the leg. That portion of the leg drained by the small saphenous, i.e., the heel and outer aspect of the foot, sends lymphatics via the popliteal space into the deep system.

A *horizontal group* of superficial nodes lies just below the inguinal ligament. This group drains the skin of the lower abdominal wall, the external genitalia (excluding the testes), the anal canal and gluteal area.

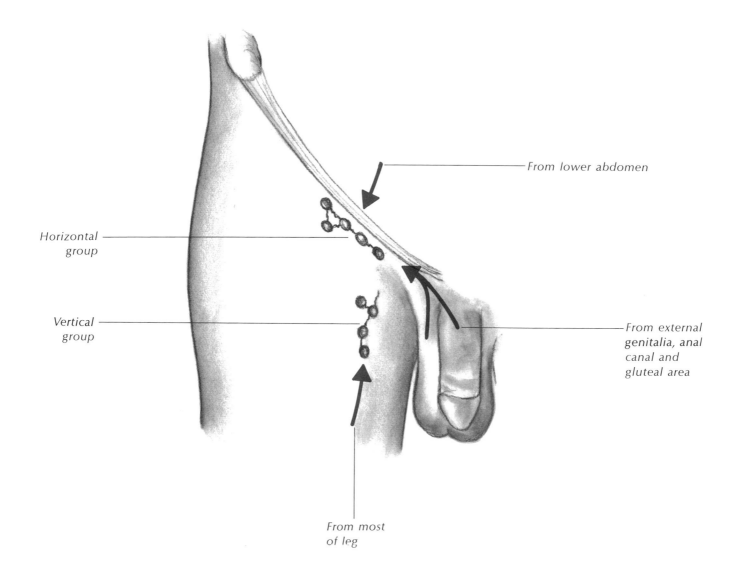

From lower abdomen

Horizontal group

Vertical group

From external genitalia, anal canal and gluteal area

From most of leg

Although described separately here, the examination of the peripheral vascular system should be integrated with your assessment of the skin, the musculoskeletal and the neurological systems. See Chapter 3 for a survey approach to the extremities.

Arms

Inspect both arms from the fingertips to the shoulders. Note:

Their size and symmetry
The color and texture of the skin and nail beds
The venous pattern
Edema

With the pads of your index and middle fingers, *palpate the radial pulse* on the flexor surface of the wrist laterally. Compare the volume of the pulses on each side.

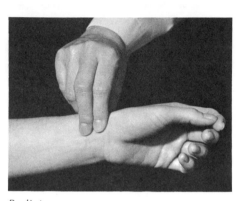

Radial pulse

Pallor or cyanosis of the fingers in Raynaud's phenomenon

Edema and prominent veins in venous obstruction

Pulses may be described as normal, diminished or absent. A finer numerical classification is based on a 0 to 4 scale:

    0—completely absent
    1—markedly impaired
    2—moderately impaired
    3—slightly impaired
    4—normal

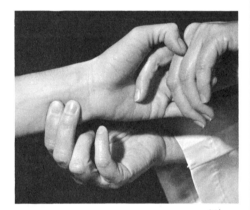

Ulnar pulse

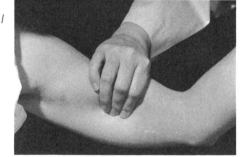

Brachial pulse

If arterial insufficiency is suspected, palpate also (1) for the *ulnar pulse,* on the flexor surface of the wrist medially and (2) for the *brachial pulse* in the groove between the biceps and triceps muscle above the elbow.

Since the normal ulnar artery is frequently not palpable, another maneuver is useful—the *Allen test*—for patency of the radial and ulnar arteries. Ask the patient to rest his hands in his lap. Place your thumbs over his radial arteries and ask him to clench his fists tightly. Compress the radial arteries firmly, then ask the patient to open his hands into a relaxed position. Observe the color of the palms. They normally should turn pink promptly. Repeat, occluding the ulnar arteries.

Persistence of pallor when one artery (e.g., the radial) is manually compressed indicates occlusion of the other (e.g., the ulnar).

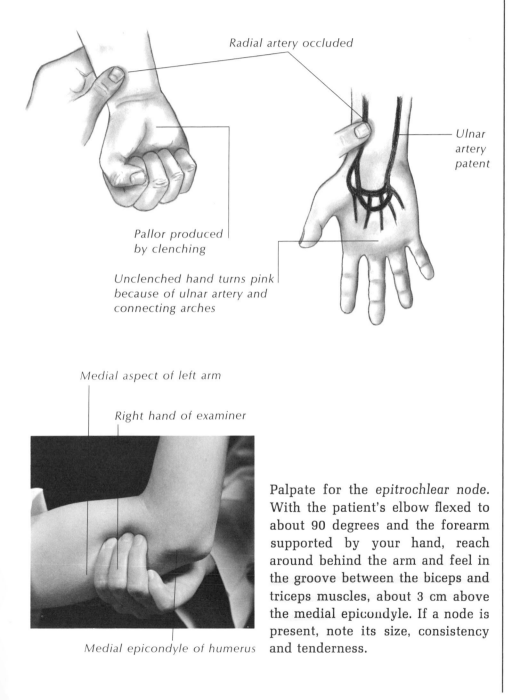

Radial artery occluded

Ulnar artery patent

Pallor produced by clenching

Unclenched hand turns pink because of ulnar artery and connecting arches

Medial aspect of left arm

Right hand of examiner

Medial epicondyle of humerus

Palpate for the *epitrochlear node*. With the patient's elbow flexed to about 90 degrees and the forearm supported by your hand, reach around behind the arm and feel in the groove between the biceps and triceps muscles, about 3 cm above the medial epicondyle. If a node is present, note its size, consistency and tenderness.

Legs

Drape the patient so that the external genitalia are covered and the legs fully exposed. A good examination is impossible through stockings or socks!

Inspect both legs from the groin and buttocks to the feet. Note:
   Their size and symmetry
   The color and texture of the skin and nail beds, and the hair distribution on the lower legs, feet and toes
   Pigmentation, rashes, scars and ulcers
   The venous pattern and evidence of venous enlargement
   Edema

See Table 16-1, Chronic Insufficiency of Arteries and Veins (p. 268).

See Table 16-2, Common Ulcers of Feet and Ankles (p. 269).

Palpate the superficial inguinal lymph nodes, both the horizontal and vertical groups. Note their size, consistency and tenderness. (Small mobile nontender inguinal nodes are frequently present).

Tenderness suggests lymphadenitis.

Note any tenderness in the region of the femoral vein.

Venous tenderness suggests phlebitis.

Palpate the pulses:
   1. *The Femoral Pulse.* Press deeply, below the inguinal ligament and about midway between the anterior superior iliac spine and the symphysis pubis. As in deep abdominal palpation, the use of two hands, one on top of the other, may facilitate this examination, especially in obese patients.

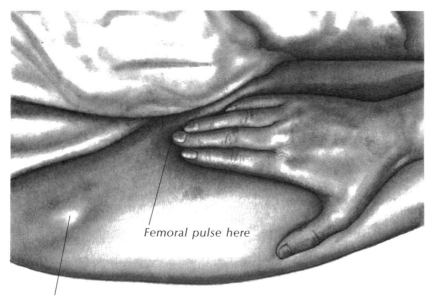

Femoral pulse here

Anterior superior iliac spine

   2. *The Popliteal Pulse.* The patient's knee should be slightly flexed, the leg relaxed. Press the fingertips of both hands deeply into the popliteal fossa, slightly lateral to the midline. The popliteal pulse is frequently more difficult to find than other pulses. It is deeper and feels more diffuse.

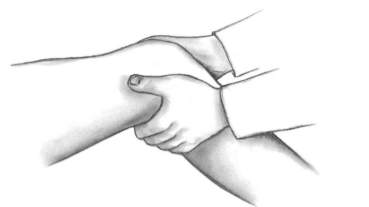

If you cannot feel the popliteal pulse with this approach, ask the patient to roll onto his abdomen. With the patient's leg flexed to 90 degrees at the knee, palpate deeply for the popliteal pulse.

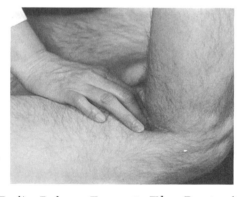

3. *The Dorsalis Pedis Pulse.* For this pulse feel the dorsum of the foot (not the ankle) usually just lateral to the extensor tendon of the great toe. (This pulse is sometimes congenitally absent.)

4. *The Posterior Tibial Pulse.* Curve your fingers behind and slightly below the medial malleolus of the ankle. (This pulse may also be congenitally absent.)

Diminished or absent pulses suggest arterial insufficiency.

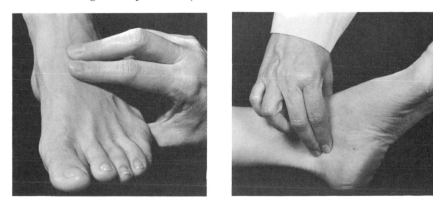

Note: Some pulses may be difficult to feel. As aids: (1) Keep your own body and examining hand comfortable; awkward positions decrease your tactile sensitivity. (2) Place your hand properly and linger there, varying the pressure of your fingers to pick up a weak pulsation. If unsuccessful, then explore the area deliberately. Avoid flitting about. (3) Do not confuse the patient's pulse with your own pulsating fingertips. If you are unsure, count your own heart rate and compare it with the patient's. The rates are usually different. Your carotid pulse is convenient for this comparison.

Using the backs of your fingers, *note the temperature of the feet and legs*, comparing one side with the other.

Coldness may suggest arterial insufficiency, especially when it is unilateral. When bilateral, however, it is more frequently due to a cold environment or anxiety.

Special Maneuvers for Suspected Arterial Insufficiency. If arterial insufficiency is suspected, elevate both legs so that the feet are above the level of venous pressure (about 30 cm or 12 inches). Ask the patient to move his feet up and down at the ankles for about 30 or 60 seconds. These maneuvers drain the feet of venous blood, unmasking the color produced by the arterial supply.

Increased pallor in arterial insufficiency.

Inspect for unusual pallor. (Mild pallor is normal.) Then have the patient sit up with his legs dangling down. Note the time required for:
   1. Return of color to the skin (usually about 10 seconds).
   2. Filling of the veins of the feet and ankles (usually about 15 seconds).

Delayed color return and venous filling in arterial insufficiency

Note any unusual rubor (redness) or cyanosis of the dependent feet and legs.

Dusky rubor in arterial insufficiency

If all pulses below the femorals are diminished or absent, listen over the femoral arteries for bruits. If the femoral pulses are also absent, listen for bruits in the abdomen

A localized systolic bruit may indicate the point of partial arterial occlusion.

Palpate for edema. Press firmly with your thumb for at least 5 seconds behind the medial malleolus, over the dorsum of the foot and over the shin. Note any pitting edema.

See Table 16-3, Some Peripheral Causes of Edema (p. 270).

Palpate the calf for signs of deep phlebitis. Squeeze the calf muscles by compressing them against the tibia. Note any tenderness. Note also any increased firmness or tension of the muscles.

Tenderness, increased firmness and tension suggest phlebitis in the calf.

If you suspect thrombophlebitis of the calf, check for Homans's sign. With the patient's leg extended at the knee, dorsiflex the foot and note any pain or soreness in the calf. Feel also for increased muscular resistance to dorsiflexion as compared to the opposite side.

Calf pain or soreness on dorsiflexion of the foot suggests thrombophlebitis, as does increased muscular resistance to this maneuver. Unfortunately, thrombophlebitis frequently exists without any physical signs at all.

Ask the patient to stand and *inspect the saphenous system for varicosities.* If present, look for redness or discoloration and palpate for tenderness or cords.

Special Maneuvers for the Evaluation of Varicose Veins. The Trendelenburg test is used to evaluate the competence of the valves in the great saphenous vein and in the communicating veins between the superficial and deep venous systems. Elevate the patient's leg to 90 degrees to empty it of venous blood. Place a tourniquet around the upper thigh tightly enough to occlude the great saphenous. Ask the patient to stand. Normally it takes about 35 seconds for the saphenous vein to fill from below. Release of the tourniquet at 60 seconds produces no sudden increment in venous filling if the saphenous valves are competent.

Redness and tender cords suggest phlebitis.

See Table 16-4, Signs of Incompetence of the Venous Valves (p. 271).

TABLE 16-1

TABLE 16-1. CHRONIC INSUFFICIENCY OF ARTERIES AND VEINS

CHRONIC ARTERIAL INSUFFICIENCY
ADVANCED

No edema

Skin shiny, atrophic

Nails thick, ridged

Ulcer of toe

CHRONIC VENOUS INSUFFICIENCY
ADVANCED

Edema

Brown pigment

Ulcer of ankle

	CHRONIC ARTERIAL INSUFFICIENCY	CHRONIC VENOUS INSUFFICIENCY
Pulses	Decreased or absent	Normal, though may be difficult to feel through edema
Color	Pale, especially on elevation; dusky red on dependency	Normal, or cyanotic on dependency
Temperature	Cool	Normal
Edema	Absent or mild	Present, often marked
Skin changes	Thin, shiny, atrophic skin; loss of hair over foot and toes; nails thickened and ridged	May show brown pigmentation around ankles, stasis dermatitis
Ulceration	If present, involves toes or points of trauma on feet	If present, develops at sides of ankles
Gangrene	May develop	Does not develop

TABLE 16-2

TABLE 16-2. COMMON ULCERS OF FEET AND ANKLES

	CHRONIC VENOUS INSUFFICIENCY	ARTERIAL INSUFFICIENCY	TROPHIC ULCER
	Pitting *Ulcer* *Pigment*	*Ulcer* *Shiny, atrophic skin* *Gangrenous toe*	*Thickened skin* *Ulcer*
Location	Inner, sometimes outer ankle	Toes, feet, areas of trauma e.g., the shin	Pressure points
Surrounding skin	Pigmented, sometimes fibrotic	No pigment or callus, may be atrophic	Calloused
Pain	Not severe	Often severe, unless neuropathy masks it	Absent
Associated gangrene	Absent	May be present	In uncomplicated trophic ulcer, absent
Associated signs	Stasis dermatitis, pigmentation, edema, cyanosis of foot on dependency	Atrophic skin, pallor of foot on elevation, rubor on dependency	Decreased sensation, ankle jerks absent

TABLE 16-3

TABLE 16-3. SOME PERIPHERAL CAUSES OF EDEMA

	ORTHOSTATIC EDEMA	LYMPHEDEMA	LIPEDEMA	CHRONIC VENOUS INSUFFICIENCY
Process	Edema from prolonged sitting or standing	Lymphatic obstruction	Fatty deposition in legs	Deep venous obstruction or valvular incompetence
Nature of edema	Soft, pits on pressure	Soft early, becomes hard and non-pitting	Minimal if any	Soft, pits on pressure, later may become brawny
Skin thickening	Absent	Marked	Absent	Occasional
Ulceration	Absent	Rare	Absent	Common
Pigmentation	Absent	Absent	Absent	Common
Foot involvement	Present	Present	Absent	Present
Bilaterality	Always	Often	Always	Occasionally

TABLE 16-4

TABLE 16-4. SIGNS OF INCOMPETENCE OF THE VENOUS VALVES

	NORMAL	SAPHENOUS VEIN INCOMPETENT BUT COMMUNICATING VEINS COMPETENT	SAPHENOUS VEIN INCOMPETENT AND COMMUNICATING VEINS INCOMPETENT
On Standing with the Tourniquet Fastened	Slow venous filling from below	Slow venous filling from below	Rapid filling through communicating veins
On Release of the Tourniquet	No additional filling from above	Sudden additional filling from above	Sudden additional filling from above

the musculoskeletal system

ANATOMY AND PHYSIOLOGY

This section will review briefly the structure and function of joints and will describe the anatomical landmarks of several clinically important joints. Identify these landmarks first on yourself or on other normal people. Range of motion at each joint varies greatly with age and health. The figures given here, taken mainly from Beetham et al.,* are intended as general guides, not absolute standards.

Structure and Function of Joints

A typical *freely movable joint* is diagrammed at the right.

Note that the bones themselves do not touch each other within a joint but are covered by articular cartilage that forms a cushion between the bony surfaces. At the margins of the articular cartilage is attached the synovial membrane. This membrane is pouched or folded to allow for joint movement. It encloses the synovial cavity and secretes into it a small amount of viscous lubricating fluid—the synovial fluid.

The synovial membrane is surrounded by a fibrous joint capsule, which in turn is strengthened by ligaments extending from bone to bone.

Some joints, for example those between the vertebral bodies, are *slightly movable joints.* Here the bones are separated not by a synovial cavity but by a fibrocartilaginous disc. At the center of each disc is the nucleus pulposus, fibrogelatinous material that forms a cushion or shock absorber between the vertebral bodies.

*Beetham, W. P., Jr., Polley, H. F., Slocumb, C. H., and Weaver, W. F.: *Physical Examination of the Joints.* Philadelphia: W. B. Saunders Co., 1965.

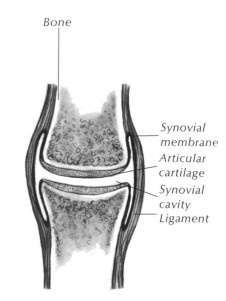

Bone

Synovial membrane

Articular cartilage

Synovial cavity

Ligament

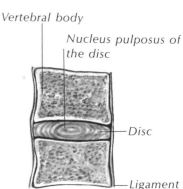

Vertebral body

Nucleus pulposus of the disc

Disc

Ligament

Bursae develop at points of friction around joints, for example between tendons and cartilage or bone or between the convex surface of a joint and the skin. A bursa is a disc-shaped, fluid-filled synovial sac that decreases friction and promotes ease of motion.

Specific Joints

Temporomandibular Joint. The temporomandibular joint forms the articulation between mandible and skull. Feel for it just in front of the tragus of each ear as the jaw is opened and closed.

Wrists and Hands. Identify the bony tips of the radius (on the lateral or thumb side) and the ulna (medially). On the dorsum of the wrist, palpate the groove of the radiocarpal or wrist joint.

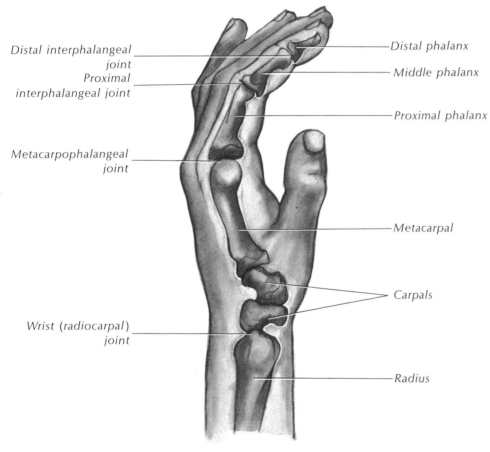
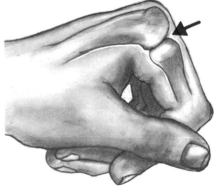

The carpal bones within the hand cannot be readily identified clinically. However, palpate each of the five metacarpals, and the proximal, middle and distal phalanges. (The thumb lacks a middle phalanx.) Flex the hand somewhat and note the groove marking the metacarpophalangeal joint. It is distal to the knuckle and can be best felt on either side of the joint.

Many tendons pass across the wrist and hand to insert on the fingers. Through much of their course these tendons travel in synovial sheaths or tunnels. Although not normally palpable, these sheaths may become swollen or inflamed.

Illustrated below and at the right is the range of motion at the wrists:

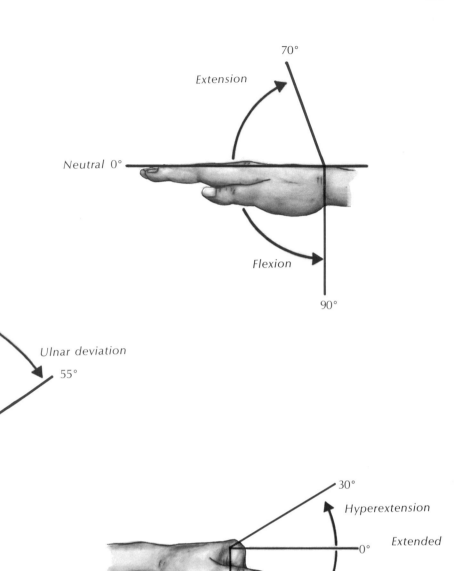

And at the joints of the fingers:

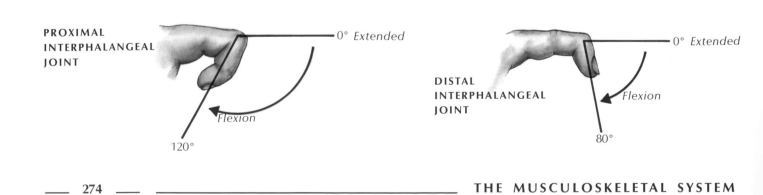

     THE MUSCULOSKELETAL SYSTEM

Elbows. Identify the medial and lateral epicondyles of the humerus and the olecranon process of the ulna. A bursa lies between the olecranon process and the skin. The synovial membrane is most accessible to examination between the olecranon and the epicondyles. Neither bursa nor synovium is normally palpable, however.

The sensitive ulnar nerve can be felt posteriorly between olecranon and medial epicondyle.

Movements at the elbow include:

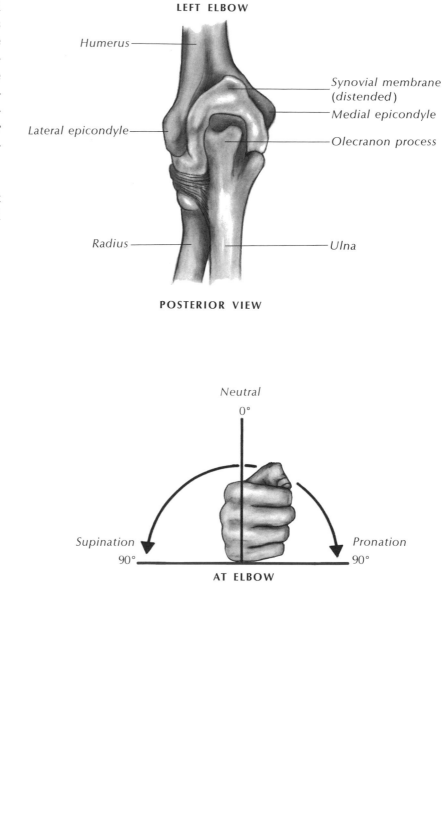

LEFT ELBOW

Humerus

Synovial membrane (distended)

Medial epicondyle

Lateral epicondyle

Olecranon process

Radius

Ulna

POSTERIOR VIEW

160°

Flexion

Extended

0°

Neutral
0°

Supination
90°

Pronation
90°

AT ELBOW

Shoulders and Environs. Identify the following landmarks: (1) the manubrium of the sternum, (2) the sternoclavicular joint, and (3) the clavicle. With your finger trace the clavicle laterally to its distal end. Now, from behind, identify the triangular scapula and follow its bony spine laterally and upward to the acromion. Place a dot of ink on its anterior tip. With your finger firmly on top of the acromion feel medially for the slightly elevated clavicle. This junction marks the acromioclavicular joint. Below and medially to this joint lies the coracoid process, a part of the scapula. Mark it with ink. Below and lateral to the joint find the greater tubercle of the humerus. Mark this also. The triangle formed by these points—the tip of the acromion, the coracoid process and the greater tubercle of the humerus—orient you to the anatomy of the shoulder.

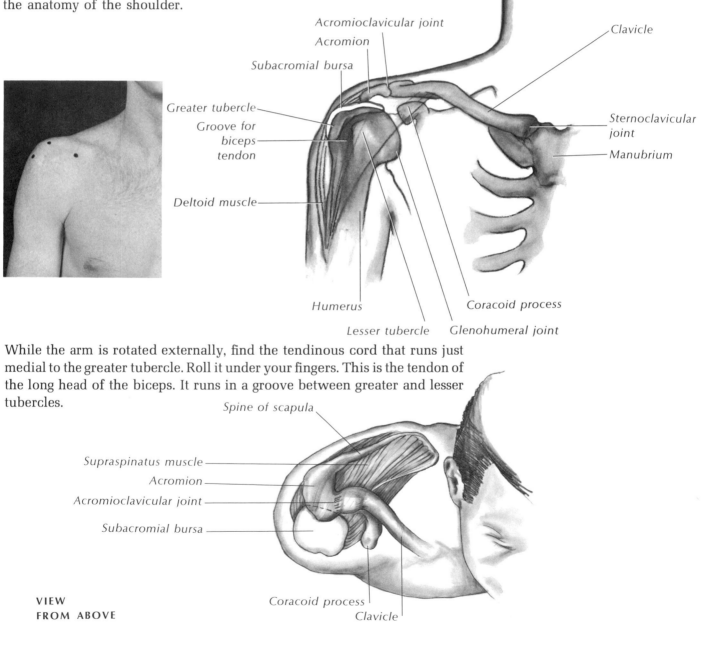

ANTERIOR VIEW

Acromioclavicular joint
Acromion
Subacromial bursa
Greater tubercle
Groove for biceps tendon
Deltoid muscle
Clavicle
Sternoclavicular joint
Manubrium
Humerus
Lesser tubercle
Coracoid process
Glenohumeral joint

While the arm is rotated externally, find the tendinous cord that runs just medial to the greater tubercle. Roll it under your fingers. This is the tendon of the long head of the biceps. It runs in a groove between greater and lesser tubercles.

Spine of scapula
Supraspinatus muscle
Acromion
Acromioclavicular joint
Subacromial bursa
Coracoid process
Clavicle

VIEW FROM ABOVE

THE MUSCULOSKELETAL SYSTEM

The arch formed by the acromion, the coracoid, and the ligament between them protects the more deeply situated glenohumeral joint, between the scapula and humerus. Although not normally palpable, the clinically important subacromial bursa lies deep to the deltoid muscle between this arch above and the humeral head below. The supraspinatus muscle, important in abducting the arm at the shoulder, inserts on the greater tubercle just deep to this bursa.

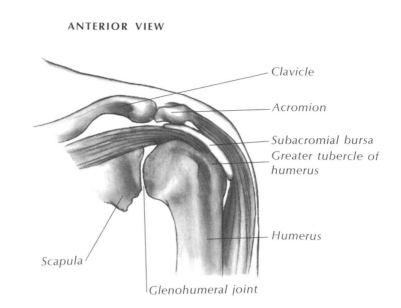

ANTERIOR VIEW

Clavicle

Acromion

Subacromial bursa

Greater tubercle of humerus

Humerus

Scapula

Glenohumeral joint

The normal range of motion at the shoulder joint is illustrated below.

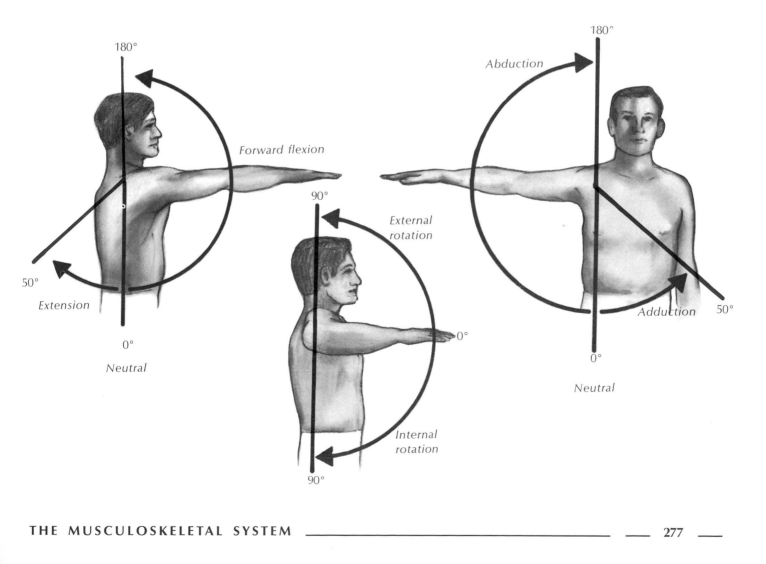

180°

Forward flexion

50°

Extension

0°

Neutral

90°

External rotation

0°

Internal rotation

90°

180°

Abduction

Adduction

50°

0°

Neutral

Ankles and Feet. The principal landmarks of the ankle are: **(1)** the medial malleolus, the bony prominence at the distal end of the tibia, and **(2)** the lateral malleolus, the distal end of the fibula. Ligaments extend from each malleolus onto the foot. The strong Achilles tendon inserts on the heel posteriorly.

Motions at the ankle joint itself (the tibiotalar joint) consist of dorsiflexion and plantar flexion.

Inversion and eversion of the foot are functions of the subtalar (talocalcaneal) and transverse tarsal joints.

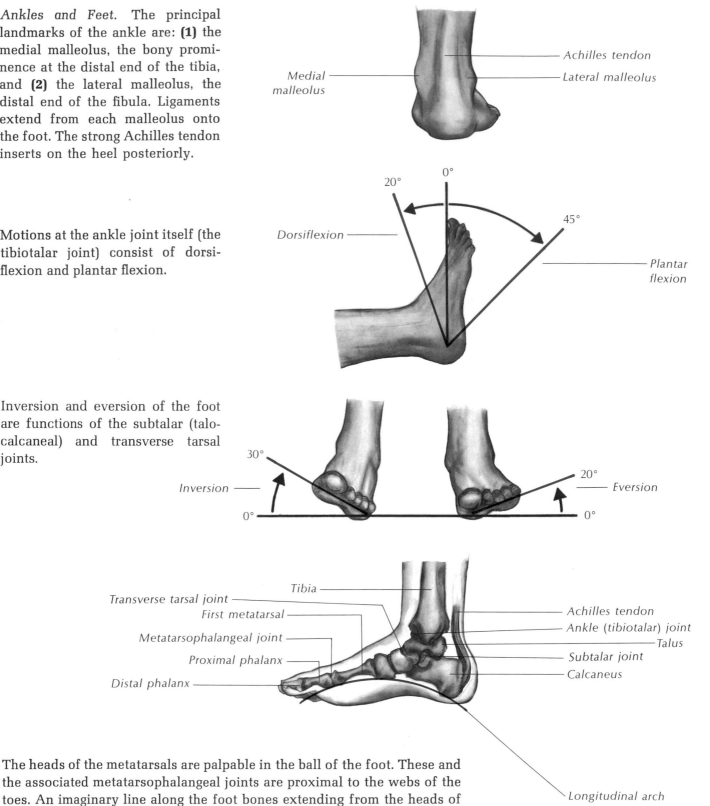

The heads of the metatarsals are palpable in the ball of the foot. These and the associated metatarsophalangeal joints are proximal to the webs of the toes. An imaginary line along the foot bones extending from the heads of the metatarsals to the calcaneus is called the longitudinal arch.

Identify the flat medial surface of the tibia—the shin. Follow its anterior border upward to the tibial tuberosity. Mark this point with a dot of ink. Now follow the medial border of the tibia upward until it merges into a bony prominence—the medial condyle of the tibia. This is somewhat higher than the tibial tuberosity. In a comparable location on the other side of the knee, find a similar prominence—the lateral condyle. Mark both condyles with ink. These three points form an isosceles triangle. On the lateral surface of the knee, somewhat below the level of the lateral tibial condyle, find the head of the fibula.

Now bring your fingertips firmly down the medial surface of the thigh along a line analogous to the inner seam of a pant leg. Your fingers will run up against an abrupt bony prominence that forms an important landmark of the knee. This is the adductor tubercle of the femur. Just below this is the medial epicondyle of the femur. The lateral epicondyle can be found comparably situated on the other side.

With the knee moderately flexed, you can now place both thumbs—one on each side of the patellar tendon—in the groove of the knee joint itself, between femur and tibia. The patella is just above this line.

Above the patella the quadriceps muscle, when contracted, can be easily identified. Observe the normal concavities on either side and above the patella. Occupying these areas is the synovial cavity of the knee joint, including an extension up behind the quadriceps called the suprapatellar pouch. Although the synovium is not normally visible or palpable, these areas may become swollen when the joint is inflamed.

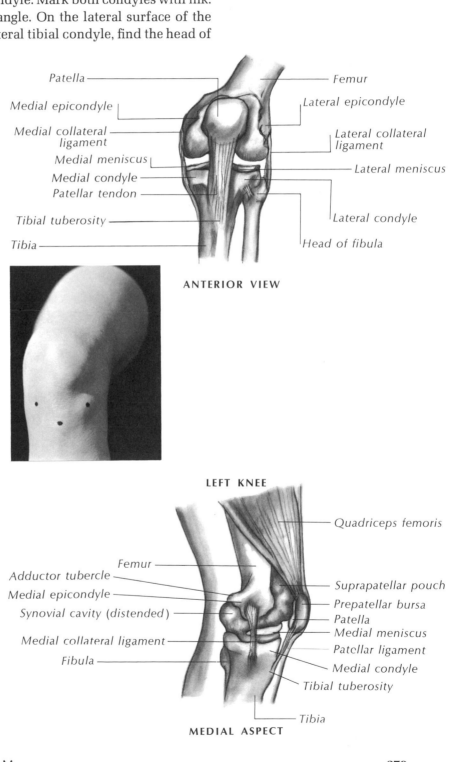

Patella — Femur
Medial epicondyle — Lateral epicondyle
Medial collateral ligament — Lateral collateral ligament
Medial meniscus — Lateral meniscus
Medial condyle —
Patellar tendon — Lateral condyle
Tibial tuberosity — Head of fibula
Tibia —

ANTERIOR VIEW

LEFT KNEE

Quadriceps femoris
Femur —
Adductor tubercle — Suprapatellar pouch
Medial epicondyle — Prepatellar bursa
Synovial cavity (distended) — Patella
Medial meniscus
Medial collateral ligament — Patellar ligament
Fibula — Medial condyle
Tibial tuberosity
Tibia

MEDIAL ASPECT

Although not normally palpable, review also the location of **(1)** the lateral and medial collateral ligaments, **(2)** the two cartilaginous menisci that form cushions between the tibia and femur and **(3)** the prepatellar bursa.

The anterior and posterior cruciate ligaments (not illustrated) cross obliquely within the knee and give it stability.

The principal movements of the knee are extension, flexion and sometimes hyperextension.

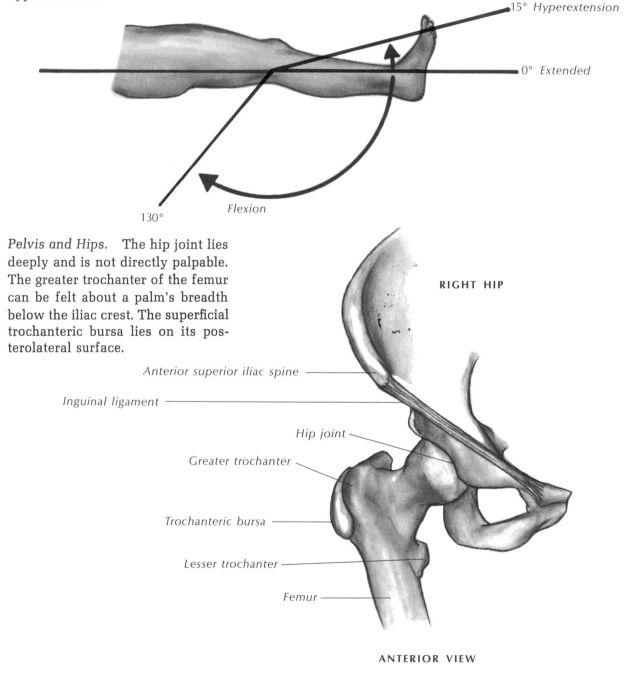

Pelvis and Hips. The hip joint lies deeply and is not directly palpable. The greater trochanter of the femur can be felt about a palm's breadth below the iliac crest. The superficial trochanteric bursa lies on its posterolateral surface.

Movements of the hip are illustrated below.

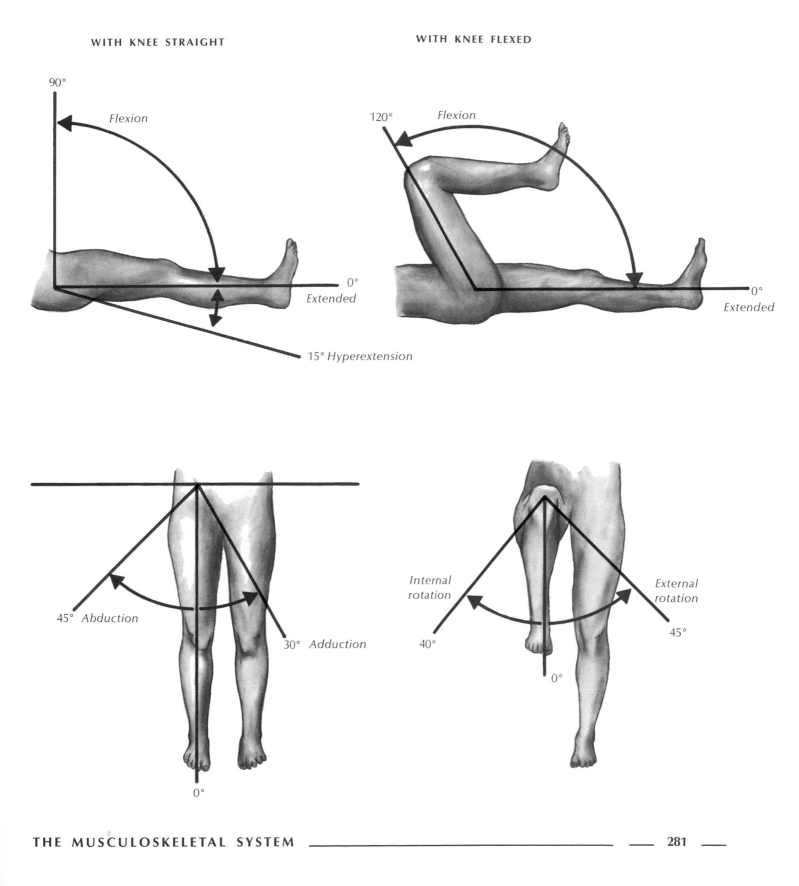

Spine. Viewing the patient from behind, identify the following landmarks: **(1)** the spinous processes, which become more evident on forward flexion, **(2)** the paravertebral muscles on either side of the midline, **(3)** the scapulae, **(4)** the iliac crests and **(5)** the posterior superior iliac spines, usually marked by skin dimples. The spinous processes of C_7 and often T_1 are unusually prominent. A line between the iliac crests crosses the spinous process of L_4.

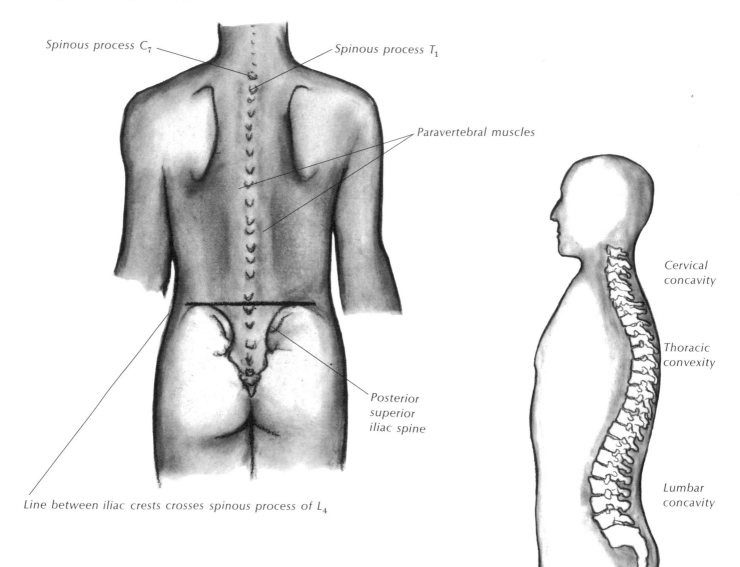

Spinous process C_7

Spinous process T_1

Paravertebral muscles

Posterior superior iliac spine

Line between iliac crests crosses spinous process of L_4

Cervical concavity

Thoracic convexity

Lumbar concavity

Viewed laterally, the spine has cervical and lumbar concavities and a thoracic convexity.

The most mobile portion of the spine is the neck, the movements of which are illustrated.

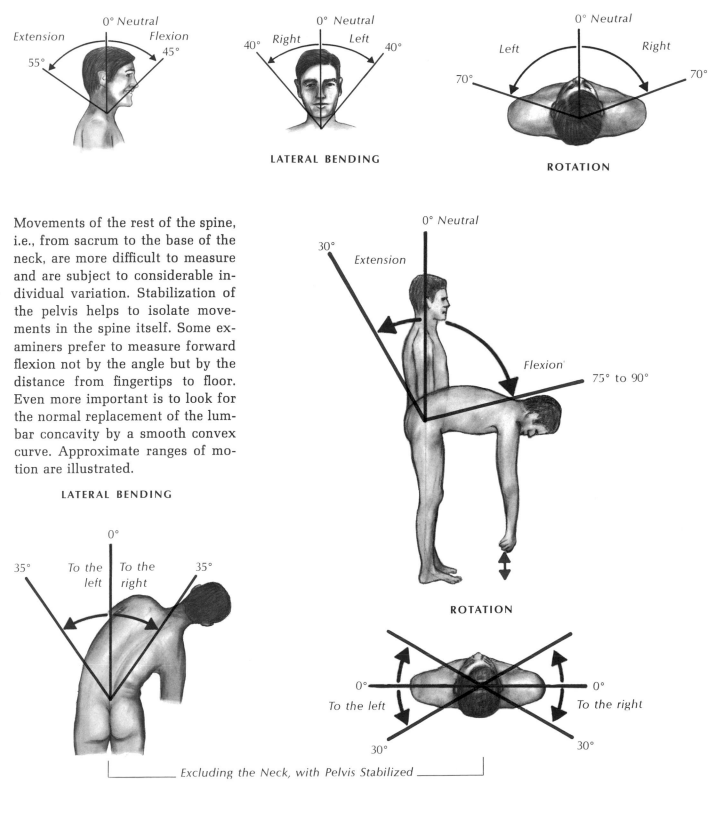

LATERAL BENDING

ROTATION

Movements of the rest of the spine, i.e., from sacrum to the base of the neck, are more difficult to measure and are subject to considerable individual variation. Stabilization of the pelvis helps to isolate movements in the spine itself. Some examiners prefer to measure forward flexion not by the angle but by the distance from fingertips to floor. Even more important is to look for the normal replacement of the lumbar concavity by a smooth convex curve. Approximate ranges of motion are illustrated.

LATERAL BENDING

ROTATION

Excluding the Neck, with Pelvis Stabilized

General Approach

Direct your assessment of the musculoskeletal system toward both function and structure. Through history and physical examination, evaluate the patient's ability to carry out the activities of daily living, for example, his ability to:

1. Walk, stand, sit, sit up, rise from a sitting position, lie down, climb, pinch, grasp, lean over.

2. Comb his hair; brush his teeth; feed, wash and dress himself; clean his perineum; turn a page.

The anatomical integrity of the system is evaluated chiefly by inspection and palpation while the body parts are at rest or going through their full range of motion. Note:

1. Deviation from or limitation in the normal range of motion, including joint instability and ankylosis (stiffness or fixation of a joint)

2. Joint swelling or deformity
   a. Thickened synovial membrane, redness, heat, tenderness
   b. Fluid in the joint capsule
   c. Bony enlargement

3. Crepitation or grating sensation as the joint moves

4. Strength

5. Condition of the surrounding tissues, including muscle atrophy, subcutaneous nodules, skin changes

Thickened synovium, warmth and tenderness suggest rheumatoid arthritis. Redness of the overlying skin suggests septic or gouty arthritis or possibly rheumatic fever.

Bony enlargement suggests degenerative joint disease.

Crepitation suggests roughening of articular cartilages, and is also felt in stenosing tenosynovitis.

Subcutaneous nodules in rheumatoid arthritis or rheumatic fever

*   *   *

Symmetrical body parts should first be compared with each other. Careful examination of each area individually can then be made.

The detail of the examination depends upon the patient's symptoms and general condition. This chapter will describe a fairly detailed examination such as you might perform on a symptomatic patient.

WITH THE PATIENT SITTING UP

Head and Neck

Palpate each temporomandibular joint just anterior to the tragus of the ear, noting any swelling or tenderness. Ask the patient to open his mouth. Feel and listen for crepitation and observe the range of motion.

Inspect the neck for deformities and abnormal posture.

Palpate for tenderness of the cervical spine and the paravertebral and trapezius muscles.

See Table 17-1, Problems in the Neck (pp. 297–298).

Test the range of motion by asking the patient to:
Touch his chin to his chest (flexion).
Touch his chin to each shoulder (rotation).
Touch each ear to the corresponding shoulder (lateral bending).
Put his head back (extension).

Hands and Wrists

Test range of motion of the fingers and wrist by asking the patient to:

1. Extend and spread the fingers of both hands.

2. Make a fist, with thumbs across the knuckles.

Dupuytren's contracture may limit full extension of the fingers.

Arthritis may limit both extension and flexion of the fingers.

3. Flex and extend his wrists, abduct and adduct them.

Inspect the hands and wrists, noting any swelling, redness, nodules, deformity, or muscular atrophy.

See Table 17-2, Swellings and Deformities of the Hands (pp. 299–301).

Palpate the medial and lateral aspects of each interphalangeal joint between your thumb and index finger, noting any swelling, bogginess, bony enlargement or tenderness.

Bony enlargement suggests degenerative joint disease. Swelling and bogginess suggest rheumatoid arthritis.

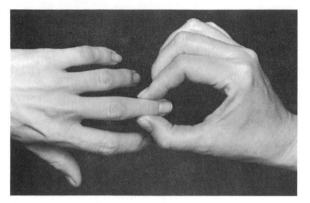

With your thumbs palpate the metacarpophalangeal joints, just distal to and on each side of the knuckle.

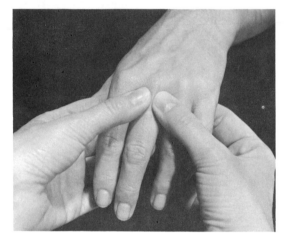

Note any swelling, bogginess or tenderness.

Palpate each wrist joint, with your thumbs on the dorsum of the wrist, your fingers beneath it. Note any swelling, bogginess or tenderness.

Swelling suggests rheumatoid arthritis if it is bilateral and lasts for several weeks.

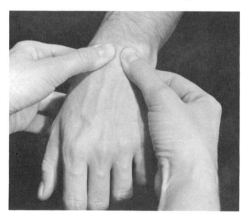

Elbows

Test the range of motion by asking the patient to bend and straighten his elbows. With his arms at his sides and elbows flexed, ask him to turn his palms up (supination) and down (pronation).

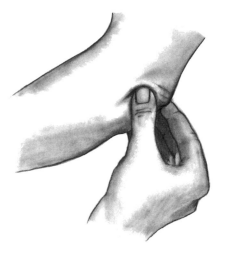

Support the patient's forearm with your opposite hand so that his elbow is flexed about 70 degrees. Inspect and palpate the elbow, including the extensor surface of the ulna and the olecranon process, noting any nodules or swelling. Palpate the groove on either side of the olecranon, noting any thickening, swelling or tenderness.

See Table 17-3, Swollen or Tender Elbows (p. 302).

Check the lateral epicondyle for tenderness.

Tender lateral epicondyle in tennis elbow

Shoulders and Environs

Test the range of motion by asking the patient to: (1) raise both arms to a vertical position at the sides of his head, **(2)** place his hands behind his neck, with elbows out to the side (external rotation) and **(3)** place his hands behind the small of his back (internal rotation). By cupping your hand over the shoulder during these movements, note any crepitation.

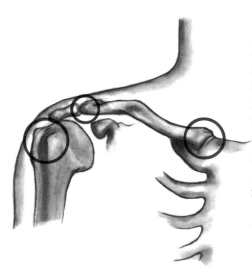

Inspect the shoulders and shoulder girdle anteriorly, noting any swelling, deformity or muscular atrophy. Inspect the scapulae and related muscles posteriorly.

Palpate for tenderness in: **(1)** the sternoclavicular joint **(2)** the acromioclavicular joint and **(3)** the shoulder itself, including the greater tubercle of the humerus and the biceps groove.

Table 17-4, Painful Shoulders (pp. 303–304).

WITH THE PATIENT LYING DOWN

Feet and Ankles

Inspect the ankles and feet, noting any deformity, nodules or swelling, any calluses or corns.

Palpate the anterior surface of the ankle joint, noting any bogginess, swelling or tenderness.

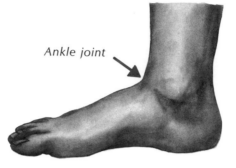

Ankle joint

See **Table 17-5,** Abnormalities of the Feet and Toes (pp. 305–306).

Arthritis of the ankle, but this may be difficult to differentiate from edema or cellulitis.

Feel along the Achilles tendon for nodules.

Rheumatoid nodules

Test for tenderness of the metatarsophalangeal joints by compressing the fore part of the foot between your thumb and fingers.

Tenderness in the small metatarsophalangeal joints is an early sign of rheumatoid arthritis. Bunion pain and acute gout affect the first metatarsophalangeal joint.

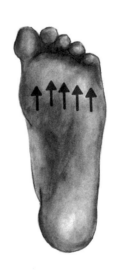

Each individual joint may be further evaluated by palpating the metatarsal heads in the sole of the foot and compressing the joints between thumb and finger.

Check the range of motion in ankles and feet:

1. Dorsiflex and plantar flex the foot at the ankle (the tibiotalar joint).

2. Stabilize the ankle with one hand, then grasp the heel with the other and invert and evert the foot at the subtalar joint.

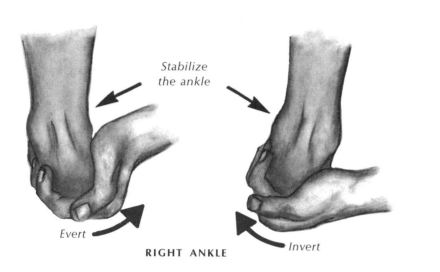

Stabilize
the ankle

Evert

Invert

RIGHT ANKLE

3. Stabilize the heel and invert and evert the forefoot, thereby testing the transverse tarsal joint.

These four maneuvers help to identify which joints of an arthritic foot are involved.

An arthritic joint is frequently painful when moved in any direction, while a ligamentous sprain produces maximal pain when the ligament is stretched. For example, in a common form of sprained ankle, inversion and plantar flexion of the foot causes pain while eversion and dorsiflexion are relatively pain free.

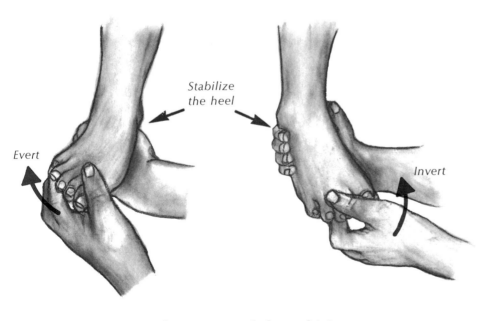

Stabilize
the heel

Evert

Invert

4. Flex the toes on the metatarsophalangeal joints.

Knees

Inspect the knees, noting their alignment and any deformity. Note any atrophy of the quadriceps muscles or loss of the normal hollows around the patella.

Bow legs (genu varum), knock knees (genu valgum) or flexion contracture (inability to extend fully)

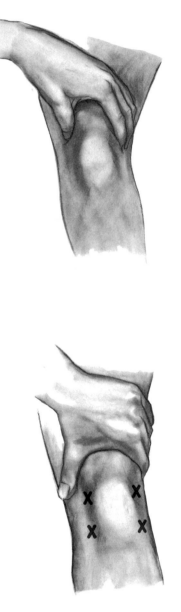

Palpate between your thumb and fingers the area of the suprapatellar pouch on each side of the quadriceps, noting any thickening, bogginess or tenderness of the synovial membrane. Feel for any bony enlargement around the knee joint.

Loss of normal hollows above and adjacent to the patella suggests synovial thickening or fluid in the knee joint.

See Table 17-6, Swellings of the Knee (p. 307).

Thickening, bogginess or tenderness suggests synovial inflammation of the knee joint.

Bony enlargement develops in advanced degenerative joint disease.

While compressing the suprapatellar pouch with one hand, palpate: **(1)** on each side of the patella and **(2)** over the tibiofemoral joint space itself. Identify any thickening, bogginess, fluid or tenderness.

Note any tenderness of the joint space or of the area near the femoral epicondyles. Palpate the popliteal space for swellings or cysts. (These are often found more easily when the patient stands with knees extended.)

See Table 17-7, Local Tenderness in the Knee (p. 308).

If a small amount of fluid in the kncc is suspected:

Look for a Bulge Sign

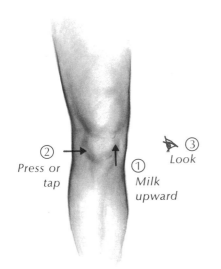

1. With the ball of your hand milk the medial aspect of the knee firmly upward two or three times to displace any fluid.

2. Then press or tap the knee just behind the lateral margin of the patella.

3. Watch for a bulge of returning fluid in the hollow medial to the patella.

A bulge indicates fluid within the knee joint. This sign can detect very small amounts of fluid but may be absent when a large amount of fluid is present under pressure.

Ballottement for a "Floating Patella."   Firmly grasp the thigh just above the knee with one hand, thus forcing fluid out of the superior portion of the joint space into the space between the patella and femur. With the fingers of your other hand, push the patella sharply back against the femur. Note a palpable tap.

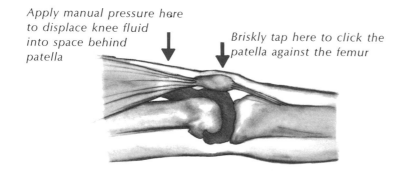

Apply manual pressure here to displace knee fluid into space behind patella

Briskly tap here to click the patella against the femur

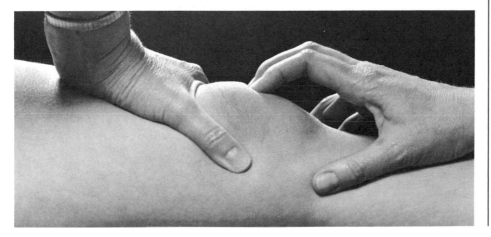

A palpable tap indicates fluid within the knee joint. Ballottement is a less sensitive test than the procedure to detect a bulge sign but it is useful when larger amounts of fluid are present.

Range of Motion at Knees and Hips.   Test rotation at the hip by rocking each of the patient's legs back and forth, in a rolling pin motion on the thigh.

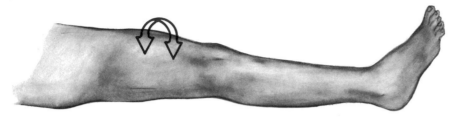

Estimate the range of motion by watching the patella and foot. Hip pain on this maneuver warrants great gentleness and caution with further tests.

Ask the patient to bend his knee up to his chest and pull it firmly against his abdomen.

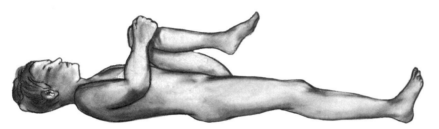

Flexion of the opposite thigh indicates a flexion deformity of that hip.

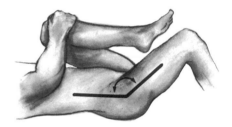

Observe the degree of flexion at the hip and knee. In addition note whether the opposite thigh remains flat on the table.

Place the patient's foot on the opposite patella. Pull the knee laterally to rotate the leg externally at the hip.

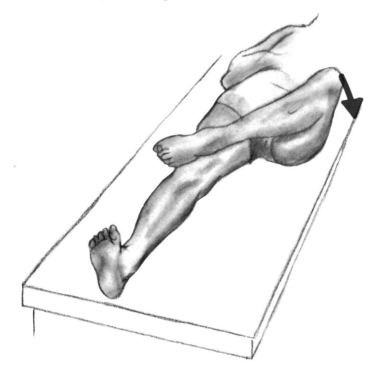

Arthritis of the hip produces pain and limitation of motion.

Then rotate the hip internally by pulling the knee medially, the foot laterally.

As you return the patient's leg to its resting position, cup your hand over the knee to detect crepitation.

WITH THE PATIENT STANDING

The Spine

The gown should allow adequate visualization of the patient's spine.

Inspect the spinal profile, noting the normal cervical, thoracic and lumbar curves.

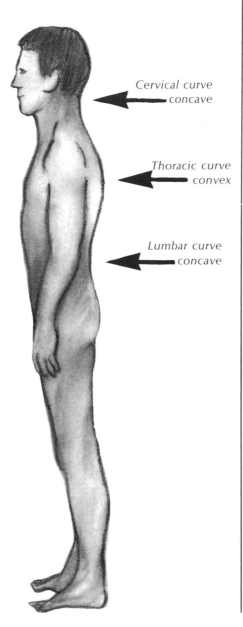

Cervical curve
concave

Thoracic curve
convex

Lumbar curve
concave

Stand behind the patient and inspect the spine for lateral curvatures. Note any difference in the height of the shoulders and of the iliac crests.

Note any knock-knee or bowleg deformity of the knees, swellings in the popliteal spaces, flat feet.

Palpate the spinous processes for tenderness and the paravertebral muscles for tenderness and spasm.

See Table 17-8, Abnormal Spinal Curvatures (pp. 309–310).

Unequal heights of the iliac crests, i.e., a pelvic tilt, suggest that the legs may be unequal in length (see p. 296). Adduction or abduction deformities of the hip may also cause a tilt.

Check the range of motion in the spine.

Ask the patient to bend forward to touch his toes (flexion). Note the symmetry of movement, the range of motion, the distance of his finger-tips from the floor, the curve in the lumbar area. As flexion proceeds, the lumbar concavity should become convex. A further way to test lumbar flexion is to place two or three fingers of the same hand on adjacent spinous processes and note their separation during flexion.

Stabilize the patient's pelvis with your hands and ask the patient to: **(1)** bend sideways (lateral bending), **(2)** bend backwards toward you (extension) and **(3)** twist his shoulders one way, then the other (rotation).

Persistence of the lumbar concavity and failure of the spinous processes to separate suggest spondylitis (arthritis of the spine).

If spondylitis is suspected, measure the patient's chest expansion in full inspiration and full expiration, using a nonelastic tape at the level of the nipple (or just above the nipples in women). Normal expansion in young adults is at least 5 or 6 cm.

Decreased chest expansion in spondylitis

Special Maneuvers

For the Carpal Tunnel Syndrome. Hold the patient's wrists in acute flexion for 60 seconds.

If numbness and tingling develop over the distribution of the median nerve, e.g., the palmar surface of the thumb, index, middle and part of the ring fingers, the sign is positive (a positive Phalen's sign). This indicates compression of the median nerve at the wrist.

For Stability of the Knee. When the patient reports giving away or buckling of the knee, test for stability. With the patient's knee extended, fix the femur in one hand, grasp the ankle with the other and attempt to adduct or abduct the leg at the knee. Normally there is almost no motion.

Mobility on abduction indicates relaxation or tear of the medial collateral ligament; on adduction, of the lateral collateral ligament.

With the patient lying down, flex the knee to 90 degrees. Stabilize the foot by gently sitting on it. Grasp the lower leg below the knee and try to push it forward and backward. Normally there is little or no movement.

Increased anterior mobility indicates anterior cruciate ligament instability; increased posterior mobility indicates posterior cruciate ligament instability.

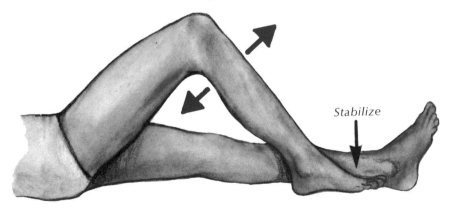

Stabilize

For a Torn Meniscus.   A torn meniscus may be suspected because of local tenderness or because of pain on abduction or adduction of the leg at the knee. (See test for mobility of the knee on the previous page.)

McMurray's test may also be helpful. Fully flex the knee of the supine patient so that the foot is close to the buttock. Place one hand on the knee so that your thumb and index finger lie on either side of the joint space. With your other hand grasp the heel and using both hand and forearm rotate the foot and lower leg laterally. Maintaining this rotation, extend the knee to a right angle. Feel and listen for a click.

See Table 17-7, Local Tenderness in the Knee (p. 308).

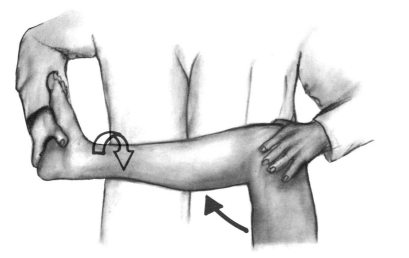

A palpable or audible click, resembling the patient's symptom, sometimes with transient pain, suggests a torn medial meniscus.

Repeat the maneuver, using medial rotation of the foot.

A click suggests a torn lateral meniscus.

For a Herniated Lumbar Disc (Sciatica).   If the patient has noted low back pain or sciatic pain, check straight leg raising. Raise the patient's relaxed leg until back pain occurs. Then dorsiflex his foot. Tight hamstrings may normally produce discomfort or pain behind the knees.

Back pain (not hamstring pain) is produced by straight leg raising and is increased by dorsiflexion of the foot when there is pressure on the lumbosacral nerve roots, as from a herniated disc.

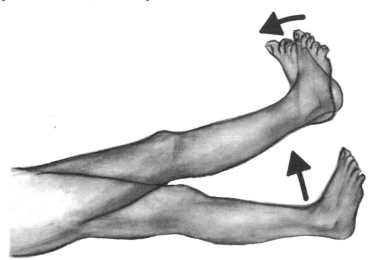

For Sacroiliac Pain.   Move the patient to one side of the examining table. While he is clasping the opposite knee firmly flexed against his abdomen, carefully lower the patient's extended leg and thigh over the edge of the examining table, thus hyperextending the leg at the hip.

In sacroiliac disease sacroiliac pain occurs on the hyperextended side.

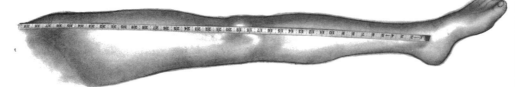

Move the patient to the other side of the table and repeat on the opposite side.

Measuring the Length of Legs.   If you suspect that the patient's legs are unequal in length, measure them. Get the patient relaxed, flat on his back, and symmetrically aligned with legs extended. With a tape, measure the distance between anterior superior iliac spine and the medial malleolus. The tape should cross the knee on its medial side.

Describing Limited Motion of a Joint.   The range of motion of a joint, when limited, should usually be described in degrees. Two examples follow. In the first the zero point of the joint cannot be reached and a flexion deformity results. The numbers in parentheses show abbreviated recordings.

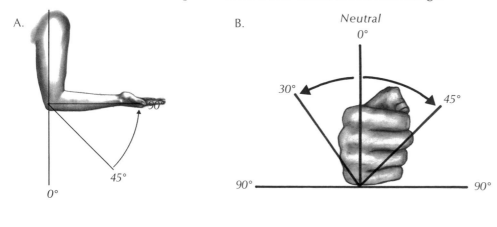

A.
The elbow flexes from 45 to 90 degrees (45° → 90°),
                    –or–
The elbow has a flexion deformity of 45 degrees and flexes further to 90 degrees (45° → 90°).

B.
Supination of elbow = 30 degrees (0° → 30°)
Pronation of elbow = 45 degrees (0° → 45°)

TABLE 17-1

TABLE 17-1. PROBLEMS IN THE NECK

MUSCLE SPASM

Acute self-limited episodes of muscle spasm and pain in the neck produce the familiar "stiff neck." Its cause is unknown. The involved muscles, usually the trapezius, are tender and cord-like to the touch. Pain is often accentuated by lateral bending away from the painful side.

More chronic areas of aching pain and tightness of the neck muscles are also common. They may be associated with chronic postural strain, tension states and depression. Look for tender muscular cords when the patient complains of chronic headache or neck pain.

HERNIATION OF A CERVICAL DISC

Acute and recurrent neck pain may be caused by herniation of an intervertebral disc that presses on a nerve root in the neck. Muscles of the neck or near the scapula on the involved side are tender and spastic. Their location varies according to the disc involved. Movements of the neck, especially extension and lateral bending toward the involved side, are limited by pain. Examine the arms for evidence of nerve root involvement: areas of diminished or absent sensation and signs of lower motor neuron damage, i.e., atrophy, fasciculations and diminished reflexes.

TABLE 17-1. (CON'T)

TABLE 17-1. (CONT'D)

CERVICAL SPONDYLOSIS

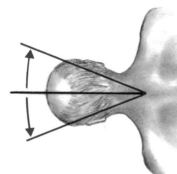

Cervical spondylosis is a chronic problem, comprising degeneration of one or more intervertebral discs in the neck, narrowing of the joint spaces and the bony spurring of degenerative arthritis. Some neck pain and limitation of neck movements are common. Two complications are important: (1) pressure on nerve roots with symptoms and signs like those of a herniated cervical disc and (2) less commonly, pressure on the spinal cord itself. The latter may produce upper motor neuron signs (weakness, spasticity and increased deep tendon reflexes) and sensory loss (especially vibration) in the legs.

ANKYLOSING SPONDYLITIS

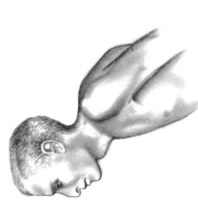

Ankylosing spondylitis usually begins in the sacroiliac joints and low back, reaching the neck only relatively late in its course. Diagnosis of the neck problem, therefore, is not usually difficult. Limitation of motion and tender spastic muscles are common early signs. The late picture of extensive disease is shown here. The head and neck are thrust forward, contrasting with the kyphotic thoracic spine. Immobility of the neck may force the patient to turn his whole body in order to look sideways.

THE MUSCULOSKELETAL SYSTEM

TABLE 17-2

TABLE 17-2. SWELLINGS AND DEFORMITIES OF THE HANDS

DEGENERATIVE JOINT DISEASE (OSTEOARTHRITIS)

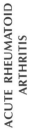

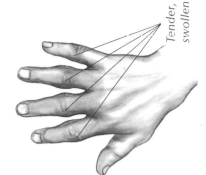

Radial deviation of distal phalanx

Heberden's node

Bouchard's node

Metacarpophalangeal joints uninvolved

Nodules on the dorsolateral aspects of the distal interphalangeal joints are the hallmark of degenerative joint disease or osteoarthritis and are called Heberden's nodes. Usually hard and painless, they affect the middle-aged or elderly and often, although not always, are associated with arthritic changes in other joints. Flexion and deviation deformities may develop. Similar nodules on the proximal interphalangeal joints, called Bouchard's nodes, are less common. The metacarpophalangeal joints are spared.

ACUTE RHEUMATOID ARTHRITIS

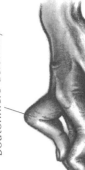

Tender, swollen

Tender, painful, stiff joints characterize rheumatoid arthritis. Symmetrical involvement on both sides of the body is typical. The proximal interphalangeal, metacarpophalangeal and wrist joints are frequently affected; the distal interphalangeal joints rarely so. Patients with acute disease often present with fusiform or spindle-shaped swelling of the proximal interphalangeal joints.

CHRONIC RHEUMATOID ARTHRITIS

As the arthritic process continues and worsens, chronic swelling and thickening of the metacarpophalangeal and proximal interphalangeal joints appear. Range of motion becomes limited and the fingers may deviate toward the ulnar side. The interosseous muscles atrophy. The fingers may show "swan-neck" deformities, i.e., hyperextension of the proximal interphalangeal joints with fixed flexion of the distal interphalangeal joints. Less common is a boutonniere deformity, i.e., persistent flexion of the proximal interphalangeal joint with hyperextension of the distal interphalangeal joint.

Rheumatoid nodules may accompany either the acute or chronic stage.

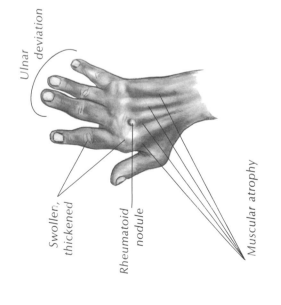

Boutonniere deformity

Swan neck deformity

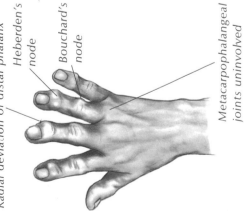

Ulnar deviation

Swollen, thickened

Rheumatoid nodule

Muscular atrophy

TABLE 17-2 (CONT'D)

TABLE 17-2. (CONT'D)

CHRONIC TOPHACEOUS GOUT

The deformities that develop in long-standing chronic tophaceous gout can sometimes mimic those of rheumatoid and osteoarthritis. Joint involvement is usually not so symmetrical as in rheumatoid arthritis. Acute inflammation may or may not be present. Knobby swellings around the joints sometimes ulcerate and discharge white chalk-like urates.

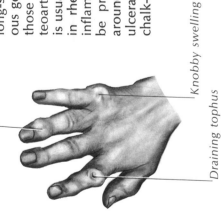

Swollen

Knobby swelling

Draining tophus

GANGLION

Ganglia are cystic, round, usually non-tender swellings located along tendon sheaths or joint capsules. The dorsum of the hand and wrist is a frequent site of involvement. Flexion of the wrist makes ganglia more prominent; extension tends to obscure them. Ganglia may also develop elsewhere on the hands, wrists, ankles and feet.

Cystic swelling

TENDON SHEATH AND PALMAR SPACE INFECTIONS

Acute Tenosynovitis

Infection of the flexor tendon sheaths (acute tenosynovitis) may follow local injury, even of apparently trivial nature. Unlike arthritis, tenderness and swelling develop not in the joint but along the course of the tendon sheath, from the distal phalanx to the level of the metacarpophalangeal joint. The finger is held in slight flexion; attempts to extend it are very painful.

Pain on extension

Swelling and tenderness along tendon sheath

Finger held in slight flexion

Acute Tenosynovitis and Thenar Space Involvement

If the infection progresses, it may escape the bounds of the tendon sheath to involve one of the adjacent fascial spaces within the palm. Infections of the index finger and thenar space are illustrated.

Early diagnosis and treatment are important.

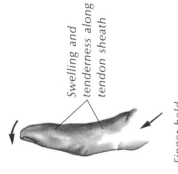

Puncture wound

Tender, swollen

TABLE 17-2 (CONT'D)

TABLE 17-2. (CONT'D)

DUPUYTREN'S CONTRACTURE

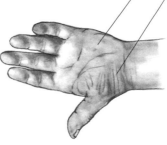

Flexion contraction

Cord

The first sign of a Dupuytren's contracture is a thickened plaque overlying the tendon of the ring finger and possibly the little finger at the level of the distal palmar crease. Subsequently the skin in this area puckers, and a thickened fibrotic cord develops between palm and finger. Flexion contracture of the fingers may gradually ensue.

FELON

Injury to the fingertip may result in infection in the enclosed fascial spaces of the finger pad. Severe pain, localized tenderness, swelling and dusky redness are characteristic. Early diagnosis and treatment are important.

Swollen, tender, dusky red

Puncture wound

THENAR ATROPHY

Muscular atrophy localized to the thenar eminence suggests a disorder of the median nerve or its components. Pressure on the nerve at the wrist is a common cause (the carpal tunnel syndrome). Hypothenar atrophy suggests an ulnar nerve disorder.

Normal hypothenar eminence

Flattened thenar eminence

TABLE 17-3

TABLE 17-3. SWOLLEN OR TENDER ELBOWS

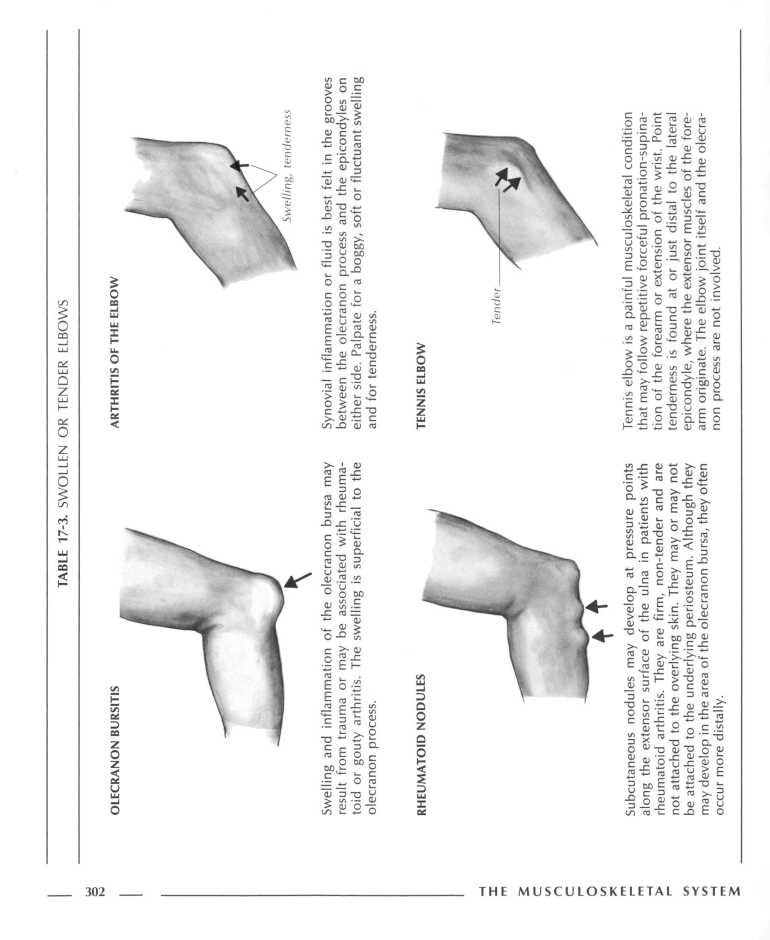

ARTHRITIS OF THE ELBOW

Swelling, tenderness

Synovial inflammation or fluid is best felt in the grooves between the olecranon process and the epicondyles on either side. Palpate for a boggy, soft or fluctuant swelling and for tenderness.

TENNIS ELBOW

Tender

Tennis elbow is a painful musculoskeletal condition that may follow repetitive forceful pronation-supination of the forearm or extension of the wrist. Point tenderness is found at or just distal to the lateral epicondyle, where the extensor muscles of the forearm originate. The elbow joint itself and the olecranon process are not involved.

OLECRANON BURSITIS

Swelling and inflammation of the olecranon bursa may result from trauma or may be associated with rheumatoid or gouty arthritis. The swelling is superficial to the olecranon process.

RHEUMATOID NODULES

Subcutaneous nodules may develop at pressure points along the extensor surface of the ulna in patients with rheumatoid arthritis. They are firm, non-tender and are not attached to the overlying skin. They may or may not be attached to the underlying periosteum. Although they may develop in the area of the olecranon bursa, they often occur more distally.

TABLE 17-4

TABLE 17-4. PAINFUL SHOULDERS*

CALCIFIED DEPOSITS IN THE SUPRASPINATUS AND RELATED TENDONS (THE ROTATOR CUFF)

Calcified deposit in the supraspinatus tendon

Extension of inflammation into the subacromial bursa

Compression with abduction

Acute inflammation associated with calcified deposits in the tendons around the shoulder (most often the supraspinatus) produces an acutely painful shoulder. The arm is held close to the side; and all motions, especially abduction and external rotation, are severely limited by pain. Tenderness is maximal below the acromion along the greater tubercle and lateral aspect of the humeral head.

Gradually the deposits work their way to the surface of the tendon, produce inflammation in the wall of the subacromial bursa or rupture into the bursa itself. The term "bursitis," which is often loosely applied to all such painful shoulder syndromes, is then appropriate.

Less severe, chronic symptoms may also be seen with calcified deposits in the rotator cuff tendons. Protruding deposits may produce characteristic twinges of pain on abduction as they are compressed between the humerus and the ligamentous arch joining acromion and coracoid. Pain begins at about 60 or 70 degrees of abduction and persists until the protrusion clears the arch at about 120 degrees.

TABLE 17-4. (CONT'D)

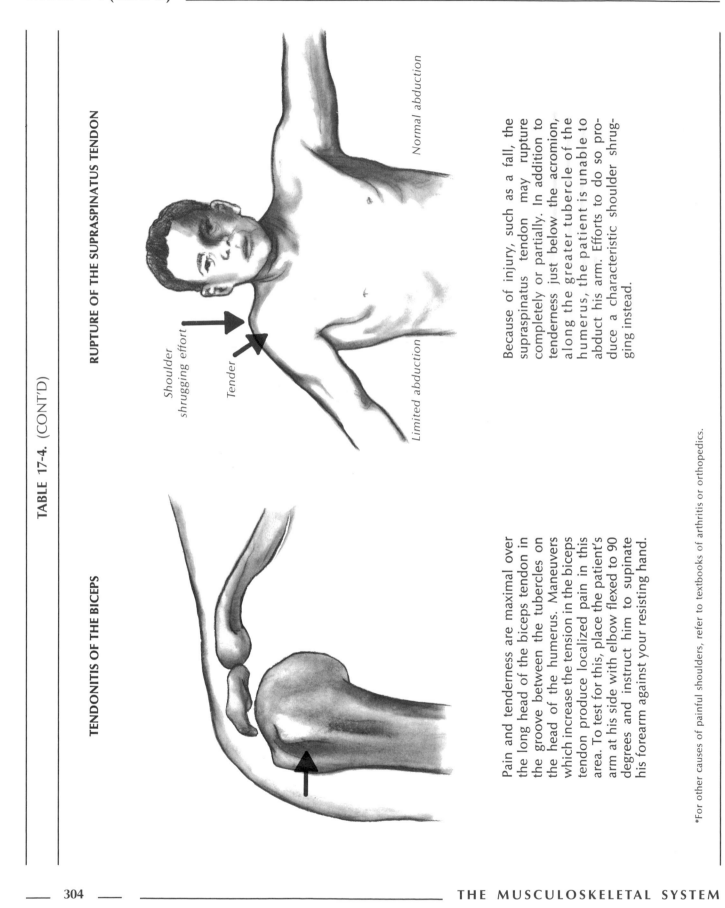

RUPTURE OF THE SUPRASPINATUS TENDON

Shoulder shrugging effort

Tender

Normal abduction

Limited abduction

Because of injury, such as a fall, the supraspinatus tendon may rupture completely or partially. In addition to tenderness just below the acromion, along the greater tubercle of the humerus, the patient is unable to abduct his arm. Efforts to do so produce a characteristic shoulder shrugging instead.

TENDONITIS OF THE BICEPS

Pain and tenderness are maximal over the long head of the biceps tendon in the groove between the tubercles on the head of the humerus. Maneuvers which increase the tension in the biceps tendon produce localized pain in this area. To test for this, place the patient's arm at his side with elbow flexed to 90 degrees and instruct him to supinate his forearm against your resisting hand.

*For other causes of painful shoulders, refer to textbooks of arthritis or orthopedics.

TABLE 17-5

TABLE 17-5. ABNORMALITIES OF THE FEET AND TOES

ACUTE GOUTY ARTHRITIS	HALLUX VALGUS	FLAT FEET

Hot, red, tender, swollen

Medial border becomes convex

Sole touches floor

The metatarsophalangeal joint of the great toe is often the first joint involved in acute gouty arthritis. It is characterized by a very painful and tender, hot, dusky red swelling which extends beyond the margin of the joint. It is easily mistaken for a cellulitis.

In hallux valgus the great toe is abnormally abducted in relationship to the first metatarsal, which itself is deviated medially. The head of the first metatarsal may enlarge on its medial side and a bursa may form at the pressure point. This bursa may become inflamed.

Signs of flat feet may be apparent only when the patient stands, or they may become permanent. The longitudinal arch flattens so that the sole approaches or touches the floor. The normal concavity on the medial side of the foot becomes convex. Tenderness may be present from the internal malleolus down along the medial-plantar surface of the foot. Swelling may develop anterior to the malleoli. Inspect the shoes for excess wear on the inner side of the soles and heels.

TABLE 17-5 (CONT'D)

TABLE 17-5. (CONT'D)

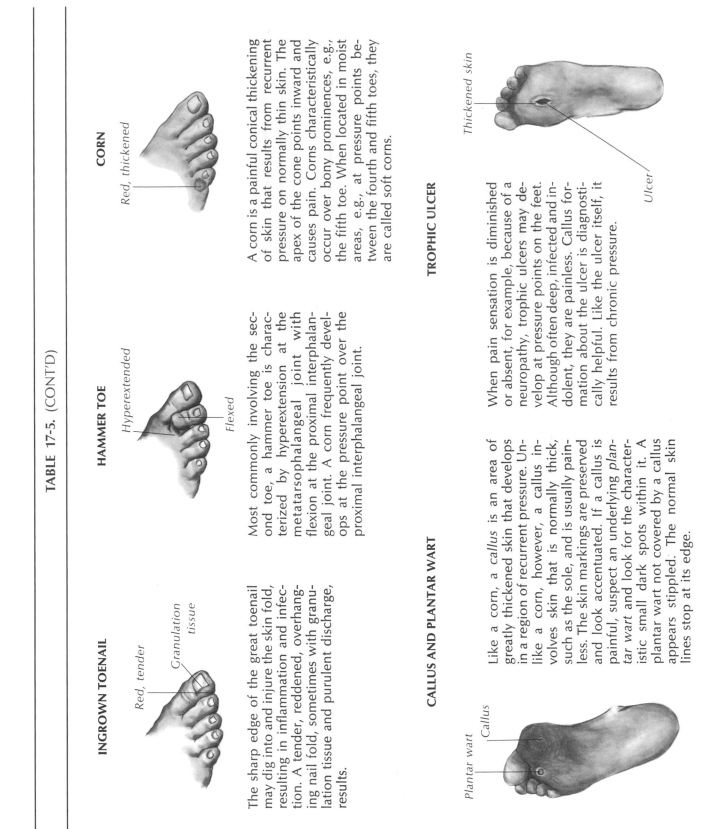

INGROWN TOENAIL

Red, tender

Granulation tissue

HAMMER TOE

Hyperextended

Flexed

CORN

Red, thickened

The sharp edge of the great toenail may dig into and injure the skin fold, resulting in inflammation and infection. A tender, reddened, overhanging nail fold, sometimes with granulation tissue and purulent discharge, results.

Most commonly involving the second toe, a hammer toe is characterized by hyperextension at the metatarsophalangeal joint with flexion at the proximal interphalangeal joint. A corn frequently develops at the pressure point over the proximal interphalangeal joint.

A corn is a painful conical thickening of skin that results from recurrent pressure on normally thin skin. The apex of the cone points inward and causes pain. Corns characteristically occur over bony prominences, e.g., the fifth toe. When located in moist areas, e.g., at pressure points between the fourth and fifth toes, they are called soft corns.

CALLUS AND PLANTAR WART

Plantar wart

Callus

TROPHIC ULCER

Thickened skin

Ulcer

Like a corn, a *callus* is an area of greatly thickened skin that develops in a region of recurrent pressure. Unlike a corn, however, a callus involves skin that is normally thick, such as the sole, and is usually painless. The skin markings are preserved and look accentuated. If a callus is painful, suspect an underlying *plantar wart* and look for the characteristic small dark spots within it. A plantar wart not covered by a callus appears stippled. The normal skin lines stop at its edge.

When pain sensation is diminished or absent, for example, because of a neuropathy, trophic ulcers may develop at pressure points on the feet. Although often deep, infected and indolent, they are painless. Callus formation about the ulcer is diagnostically helpful. Like the ulcer itself, it results from chronic pressure.

TABLE 17-6

TABLE 17-6. SWELLINGS OF THE KNEE

SWELLING IN THE KNEE JOINT

Suprapatellar Swelling

Mild to moderate

Marked

With synovial thickening or effusion the normal hollows above and on either side of the patella may be obliterated. Swelling of the suprapatellar pouch may produce fullness or even bulging. Feel for bogginess above and beside the patella and in the tibiofemoral joint space. Look for associated atrophy of the quadriceps muscle.

Bulge Sign

Remove fluid by upward compression

Press

Swelling reappears

Small amounts of fluid (4-8 ml) in the knee are demonstrable by the bulge sign. Stroke the medial aspect of the knee upward to displace the fluid, then press or tap the opposite side and watch for the fluid to return. This is a more sensitive sign of knee fluid than the patellar tap.

PREPATELLAR BURSITIS (HOUSEMAID'S KNEE)

Superficial swelling sharply limited to the prepatellar area (including the upper part of the patellar tendon) indicates fluid in the prepatellar bursa.

TABLE 17-7

TABLE 17-7. LOCAL TENDERNESS IN THE KNEE

POINTS OF MAXIMAL TENDERNESS

Medial collateral ligament

Medial meniscus

Lateral collateral ligament

Lateral meniscus

DIFFERENTIATING MANEUVERS

Ligament eased

Meniscus compressed

Meniscus eased

Ligament stretched

Tenderness maximal at the ligamentous attachment at one of the femoral epicondyles suggests a disorder of the collateral ligament. Tenderness localized below the epicondyle in the area of the joint space suggests a disorder of the meniscus.

To help distinguish further between these two, stabilize the femur and try to abduct and adduct the lower leg, using the knee as a fulcrum. Movement that stretches a diseased collateral ligament produces pain. The opposite movement compresses the meniscus which, if torn, hurts.

TABLE 17-8

TABLE 17-8. ABNORMAL SPINAL CURVATURES

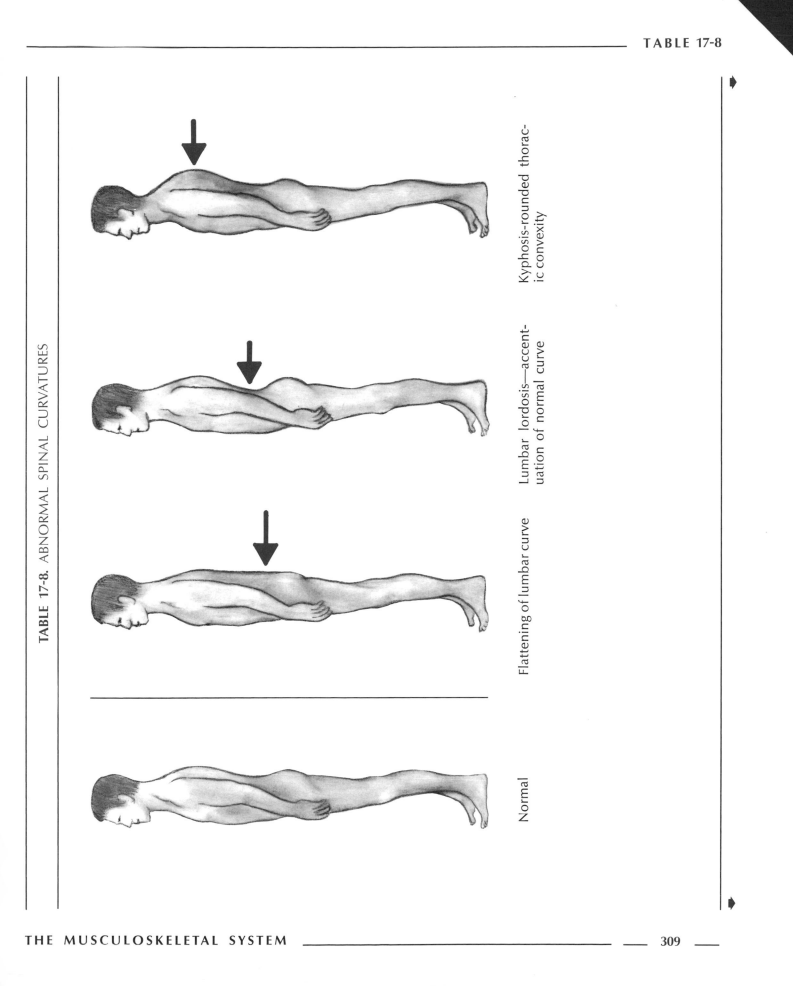

Kyphosis–rounded thoracic convexity

Lumbar lordosis—accentuation of normal curve

Flattening of lumbar curve

Normal

TABLE 17-8 (CONT'D)

TABLE 17-8. (CONT'D)

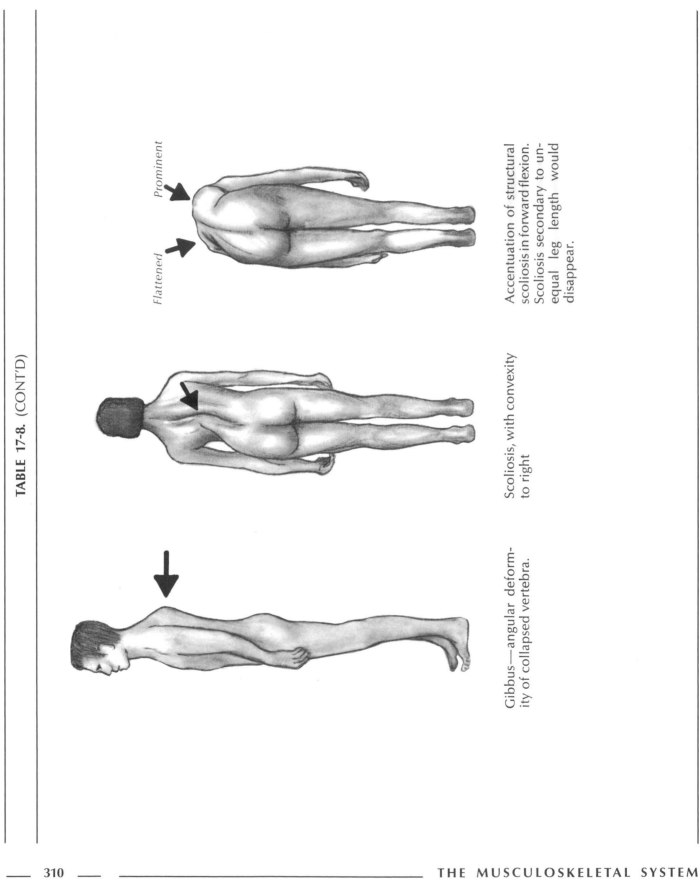

Prominent

Flattened

Accentuation of structural scoliosis in forward flexion. Scoliosis secondary to unequal leg length would disappear.

Scoliosis, with convexity to right

Gibbus—angular deformity of collapsed vertebra.

the nervous system

ANATOMY AND PHYSIOLOGY

It is impossible to review here all the anatomy and physiology relevant to the nervous system. Emphasis will be placed instead on four key topics: (1) the reflex arc and the basic organization of the motor system, (2) the organization of sensory pathways, (3) the cranial nerves and (4) the brain itself.

The Reflex Arc and Motor System

A deep tendon reflex is elicited by a brisk tap over an already partially stretched tendon. Special sensory endings in the associated muscle are stimulated and an impulse is sent up a *sensory* nerve fiber*. In its course toward the spinal cord, the sensory fiber travels together with other sensory and motor nerve fibers in a peripheral nerve.

A peripheral nerve may carry nerve fibers supplying a fairly large area of the body. Centrally, peripheral nerves are reorganized on a segmental basis into 31 pairs of *spinal nerves* (8 cervical, 12 thoracic, 5 lumbar, 5 sacral and 1 coccygeal). Within the vertebral canal, each spinal nerve separates into posterior (dorsal) and anterior (ventral) roots. The *posterior root* contains the sensory fibers. The sensory nerve impulse for the deep tendon reflex is carried on through the sensory fiber into the spinal cord where it synapses with a *motor neuron,* or *anterior horn cell.*

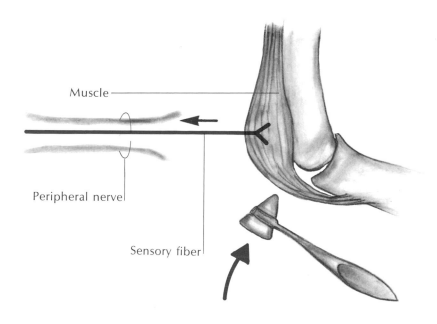

Muscle

Peripheral nerve

Sensory fiber

---

*The word "sensory," as used here, does not necessarily imply conscious sensation although many authors prefer to use the term in this restricted sense. It would be more precise to use the term "afferent," indicating the direction in which the nerve impulse travels, i.e., toward the spinal cord or brain.

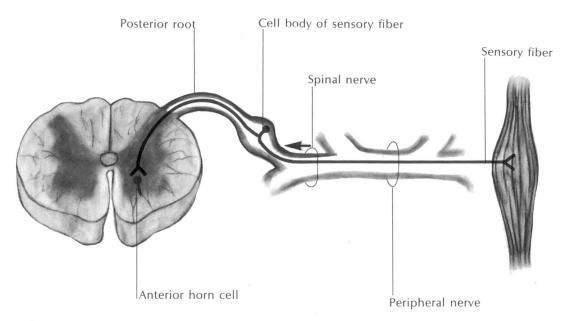

Posterior root

Cell body of sensory fiber

Spinal nerve

Sensory fiber

Anterior horn cell

Peripheral nerve

After stimulation across the synapse, an impulse is then transmitted down the motor neuron, traversing in turn the motor *anterior nerve root,* the spinal nerve and peripheral nerve. By transmitting an impulse across the neuromuscular junction, it then stimulates the muscle to a brisk contraction, completing the reflex arc.

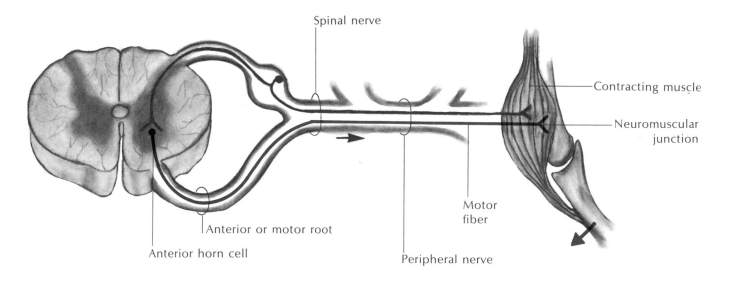

Spinal nerve

Contracting muscle

Neuromuscular junction

Anterior or motor root

Anterior horn cell

Motor fiber

Peripheral nerve

A deep tendon reflex is thus dependent upon: (1) an intact sensory nerve, (2) a functional synapse in the spinal cord, (3) an intact motor nerve fiber, (4) the neuromuscular junction and (5) a competent muscle. Such reflex activity is not dependent upon higher levels of motor function in the brain and cord. These higher motor pathways may affect reflex activity, however, and they are certainly necessary for voluntary, smooth and coordinated movements. These motor pathways include the following:

1. *The Corticospinal or Pyramidal Tract.* Nerve fibers traveling in these tracts originate in the motor cortex of the brain and travel down through the brain stem where most fibers cross over to the opposite side. They then pass on down the spinal cord where they synapse with the anterior horn cell or with intermediate neurons. Nerve fibers in the corticospinal tract mediate voluntary movement, particularly fine, discrete, conscious movement. They connect with cranial as well as spinal nerves and are often called "upper motor neurons."

2. *The Extrapyramidal Tracts.* These exceedingly complex tracts provide motor pathways between cortex, basal ganglia, brain stem and cord, but are outside the pyramidal tract system. They help to maintain muscle tone and to control body movements, especially gross automatic movements, such as walking.

3. *The Cerebellar System.* The cerebellum receives both sensory and motor input and coordinates muscular activity, maintains equilibrium and helps control posture.

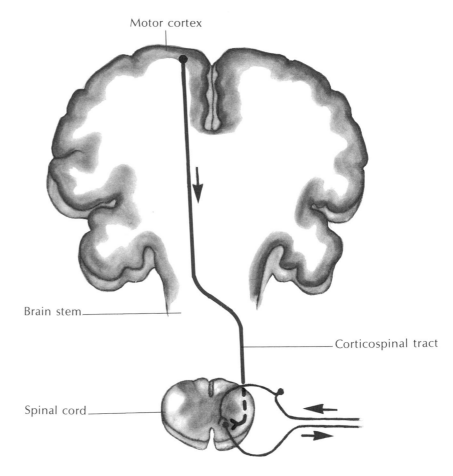

Motor cortex

Brain stem

Corticospinal tract

Spinal cord

All three of these higher motor pathways affect motor activity only through the lower motor neuron—hence its name, "final common pathway." Any movement, whether initiated voluntarily in the cortex, "automatically" in the basal ganglia or reflexly in the sensory receptor, must ultimately be translated into action via the anterior horn cell, the lower motor neuron. A lesion in any of these areas will produce effects on movement or reflex activity (see Table 18-7, pp. 354–355). The type and distribution of motor deficit produced helps the examiner to localize the lesion.

Localization is also aided by noting the *segmental levels of the reflexes* involved. The segmental levels of the common deep tendon reflexes are listed below:

Deep Tendon Reflexes	*Segmental Level*
Biceps	Cervical 5, 6
Supinator (brachioradialis)	Cervical 5, 6
Triceps	Cervical 7, 8
Knee	Lumbar 2, 3, 4
Ankle	Sacral 1, 2

Superficial reflexes require the integrity of the upper motor neuron pathways as well as the reflex arc. They are listed below. These can give information concerning both segmental and upper motor neuron disease.

Superficial Reflex	*Segmental Level*
Abdominal—Upper	Thoracic 8, 9, 10
—Lower	Thoracic 10, 11, 12
Cremasteric	Lumbar 1, 2
Plantar	Lumbar 4, 5, Sacral 1, 2

Sensory Pathways

In the preceding section, sensory impulses were discussed as part of the reflex arc. They also of course give rise to conscious sensation.

Sensation is initiated by stimulation of sensory receptors located in skin, mucous membranes, muscles, tendons and viscera. An impulse generated by one of these receptors travels along a sensory nerve fiber toward the spinal cord. In its course it usually travels with other sensory and motor nerve fibers in a peripheral nerve. The peripheral nerve is reorganized centrally on a segmental basis, divides into posterior and anterior roots and enters the spinal cord. The sensory nerve fiber follows the posterior (or dorsal) root. After entry into the spinal cord, the sensory impulse proceeds along one of two courses: (1) the spinothalamic tracts or (2) the posterior columns.

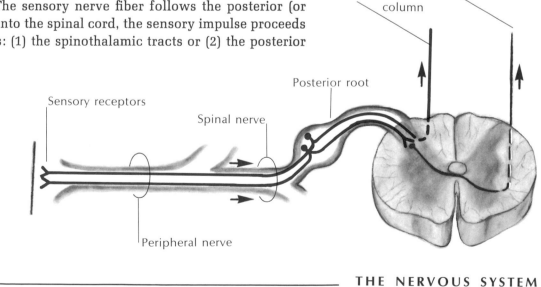

1. Within a few spinal segments from their entry into the cord, fibers conducting the sensations of pain, temperature and crude touch pass into the posterior horn of the spinal cord and synapse with a second sensory neuron. This second neuron then crosses to the opposite side just anterior to the central canal and passes upward in the *spinothalamic tracts* of the cord.

2. Fibers conducting the sensations of position, vibration and finely localized touch pass into the *posterior columns* of the cord and travel upward to the medulla where they then synapse with a second sensory neuron. This second sensory neuron also crosses over to the other side where it and the spinothalamic tracts continue on to the thalamus.

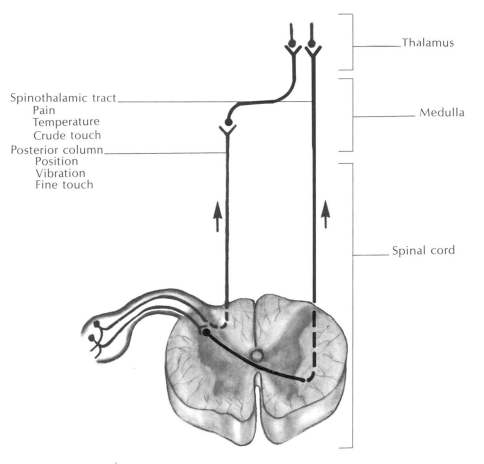

Thalamus

Spinothalamic tract
    Pain
    Temperature
    Crude touch

Posterior column
    Position
    Vibration
    Fine touch

Medulla

Spinal cord

At the thalamic level, the general quality of sensation is perceived (e.g., pain vs. cold, pleasant vs. unpleasant), but fine distinctions are not made. For full perception, a third group of sensory neurons carry impulses from synapses in the thalamus to the sensory cortex of the brain. Here stimuli are localized and discriminations made between them.

Lesions at different points in the sensory pathways produce different kinds of sensory loss. Patterns of sensory loss, together with motor findings, are therefore helpful in localizing the lesion (see Table 18-8, pp. 356–357).

Patterns of dermatomes (the skin bands innervated by the sensory or posterior nerve roots) are shown in the next two figures (pp. 316–317). Their levels are considerably more variable than the diagrams suggest and dermatomes overlap each other. Do not try to memorize their details. It is useful, however, to remember the locations of the dermatomes outlined in red on the right side of the diagrams. The distribution of a few key peripheral nerves are shown in the inserts on the left. For full charts of sensory nerve patterns, refer to texts of neurology.

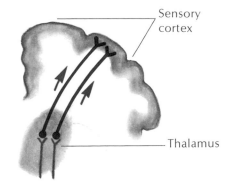

Sensory cortex

Thalamus

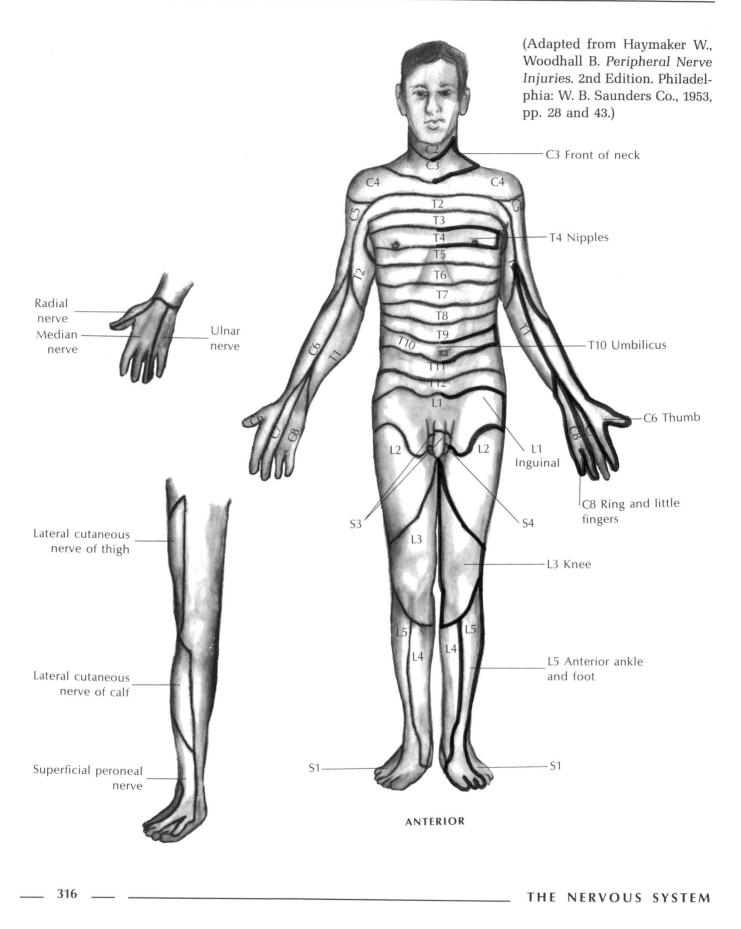

(Adapted from Haymaker W., Woodhall B. *Peripheral Nerve Injuries.* 2nd Edition. Philadelphia: W. B. Saunders Co., 1953, pp. 28 and 43.)

C3 Front of neck

T4 Nipples

T10 Umbilicus

C6 Thumb

L1 inguinal

C8 Ring and little fingers

L3 Knee

L5 Anterior ankle and foot

S1

Radial nerve

Median nerve

Ulnar nerve

Lateral cutaneous nerve of thigh

Lateral cutaneous nerve of calf

Superficial peroneal nerve

ANTERIOR

(Adapted from Haymaker W., Woodhall B. *Peripheral Nerve Injuries.* 2nd Edition. Philadelphia: W. B. Saunders Co., 1953, pp. 26 and 40.)

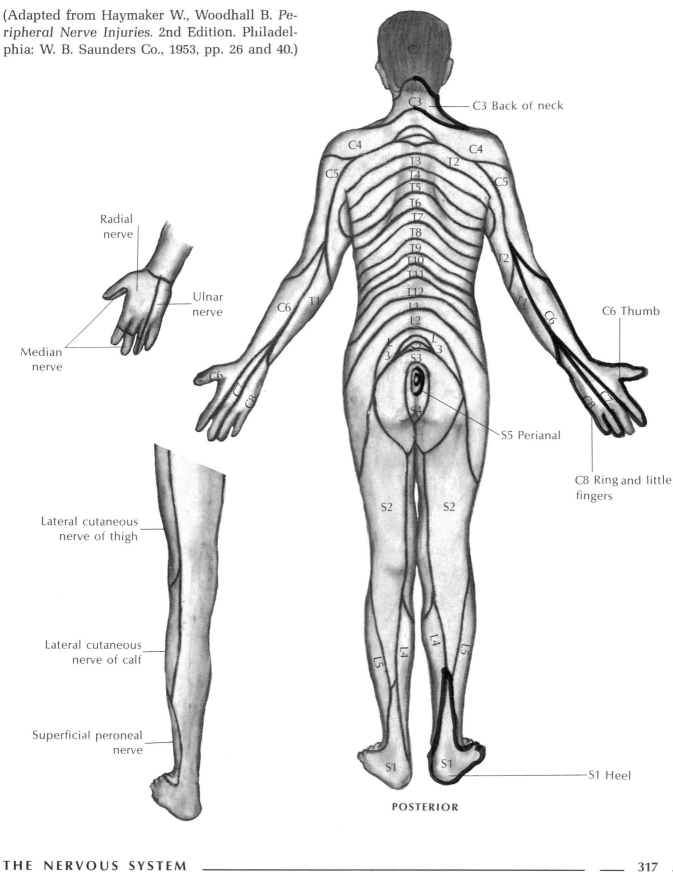

Radial nerve

Ulnar nerve

Median nerve

C3 Back of neck

C6 Thumb

C8 Ring and little fingers

S5 Perianal

S1 Heel

Lateral cutaneous nerve of thigh

Lateral cutaneous nerve of calf

Superficial peroneal nerve

POSTERIOR

The Cranial Nerves

Those functions of the cranial nerves most relevant to physical examination are summarized on these two facing pages.

No.	Nerve	Function
N1	Olfactory	Sense of smell
N2	Optic	Vision
N3	Oculomotor	Pupillary constriction, elevation of upper eyelid, most of the extraocular movements (see figure at right)
N4	Trochlear	Downward inward movement of the eye
N6	Abducens	Lateral deviation of the eye
N5	Trigeminal	*Motor*—temporal and masseter muscles (jaw clenching), also lateral movement of the jaw
		Sensory—facial. The nerve has three divisions: I. ophthalmic, II. maxillary and III. mandibular (see figure at right).
N7	Facial	*Motor*—muscles of the face, including those of the forehead, around the eyes and mouth
		Sensory—taste on anterior ⅔ of tongue

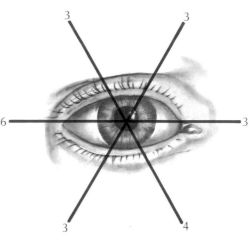

RIGHT EYE

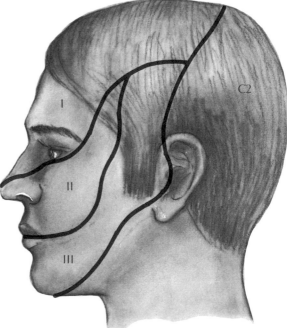

No.	Nerve	Function
N8	Acoustic	Hearing (cochlear division) and balance (vestibular division)
N9	Glosso-pharyngeal	*Sensory*—pharynx and posterior tongue, including taste
		Motor—pharynx
N10	Vagus	*Sensory*—pharynx and larynx
		Motor—palate, pharynx and larynx
N11	Spinal accessory	*Motor*—the sternomastoid and upper portion of the trapezius (see figure at right)
N12	Hypo-glossal	*Motor*—tongue

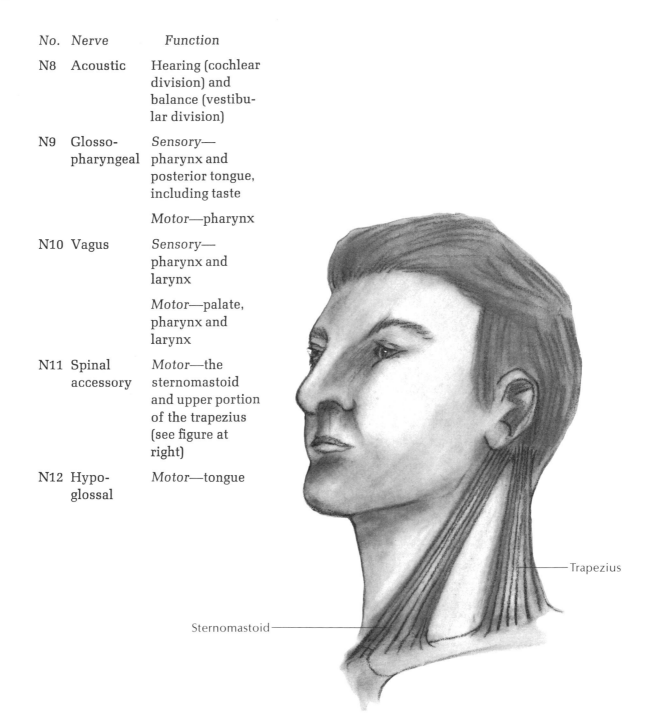

Trapezius

Sternomastoid

The Brain

The brain has three regions: the brain stem, the cerebrum and the cerebellum.

The brain stem is continuous with the spinal cord. It is traditionally divided into four sections: the diencephalon, the midbrain, the pons and the medulla.

The paired cranial nerves 2 through 12 emerge from the brain stem. Their involvement by pathological processes sometimes helps to localize neurologic lesions. The relationships of the cranial nerves to the four parts of the brain stem are summarized in the following diagram.

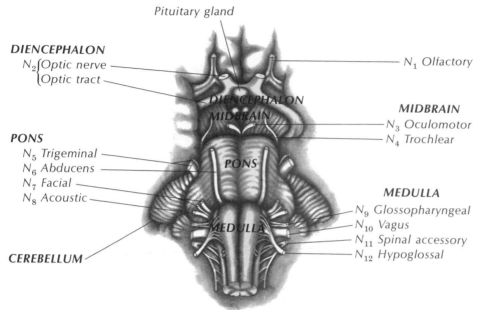

Pituitary gland

DIENCEPHALON
N_2 {*Optic nerve*
Optic tract

DIENCEPHALON

PONS
N_5 *Trigeminal*
N_6 *Abducens*
N_7 *Facial*
N_8 *Acoustic*

MIDBRAIN

PONS

MEDULLA

CEREBELLUM

N_1 *Olfactory*

MIDBRAIN
N_3 *Oculomotor*
N_4 *Trochlear*

MEDULLA
N_9 *Glossopharyngeal*
N_{10} *Vagus*
N_{11} *Spinal accessory*
N_{12} *Hypoglossal*

The cerebral hemispheres comprise the greatest mass of brain tissue. Their outer layers are formed by the cellular gray matter known as the cerebral cortex.

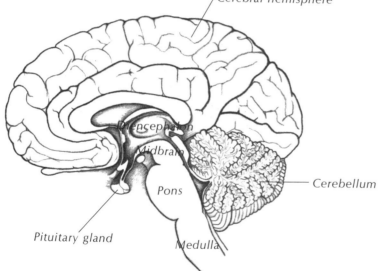

Cerebral hemisphere

Cerebellum

Diencephalon

Midbrain

Pons

Pituitary gland

Medulla

Consciousness depends upon interaction between intact cerebral hemispheres and the upper brain stem, where arousal or activating mechanisms reside. Either extensive disease of the cerebral cortex or lesions of the brain stem may impair consciousness to the point of coma.

The cerebellum is primarily concerned with coordination.

General Approach

The dilemma of how much detail to include in a "routine" examination is most apparent when testing the nervous system. The answer is determined by all the patient data you have accumulated up to this point and by further information gathered in the neurologic assessment itself. A reasonably complete but not all-inclusive examination is described in this chapter and the next. An abbreviated evaluation for the patient without apparent neurologic disease has been outlined in Chapter 3.

For efficiency, integrate certain portions of the neurologic assessment with the remainder of the examination, e.g., the survey of mental status and speech with the history and general survey, assessment of some of the cranial nerves with the head and neck, inspection of the extremities with evaluation of the peripheral vascular and musculoskeletal systems. A method of doing this has also been outlined in Chapter 3. Think about and describe your findings, however, in terms of the nervous system as a whole.

Organize your thinking into five categories: (1) mental status and speech, (2) cranial nerves, (3) the motor system, (4) the sensory system and (5) reflexes.

Survey of Mental Status and Speech

Note the patient's dress, grooming and personal hygiene; his facial expression, manner and mood; his manner of speech and his state of awareness or consciousness.

See Table 18-1, Abnormalities of Speech (p. 345).

Make inquiries within the framework of interviewing that will give you information about the patient's orientation, memory, intellectual performance and judgment.

See Table 18-2, Abnormalities of Consciousness (p. 345).

If this survey suggests an abnormality, plan a more complete mental status examination as described in Chapter 19.

The Cranial Nerves

First Cranial Nerve (Olfactory). Be sure that both nasal passages are patent. Ask the patient to close his eyes. Test each nostril separately by occluding the opposite side. Ask the patient to identify odors, e.g., tobacco, coffee, soap.

Unilateral loss of smell without nasal disease suggests a frontal lobe lesion.

Second Cranial Nerve [Optic]. (See Chapter 7.)

Test visual acuity.
Inspect the optic fundi ophthalmoscopically.
Determine the visual fields by confrontation.

Third, Fourth and Sixth Cranial Nerves (Oculomotor, Trochlear and Abducens). (See Chapter 7.)

Test the pupillary reactions and extraocular movements. Identify ptosis and also nystagmus.

See Table 18-3, Nystagmus (pp. 346–347).

Fifth Cranial Nerve (Trigeminal)

Motor. While palpating the temporal and masseter muscles in turn, ask the patient to clench his teeth. Note the strength of muscle contraction.

Weak or absent contraction of the temporal and masseter muscles on one side suggests a lesion of the fifth cranial nerve. Bilateral weakness may result from upper or lower motor neuron involvement. When the patient has no teeth, this test may be difficult to interpret.

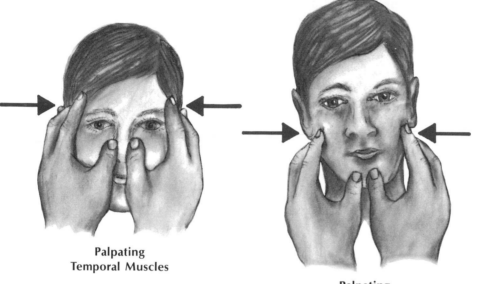

Palpating Temporal Muscles

Palpating Masseter Muscles

Sensory. With the patient's eyes closed, test the forehead, cheeks and jaw on each side for pain sensation. Suggested areas are indicated by the circles diagrammed below. Use a safety pin, occasionally substituting the blunt end for the point as a stimulus. Ask the patient to report whether it is "sharp" or "dull" and to compare sides. (Note: You have tested for pain only in areas touched with the point of the pin. The dull end is a check on the patient's reliability.)

Unilateral decrease or loss of facial sensation suggests a lesion of the fifth cranial nerve or of interconnecting higher sensory pathways. Such a sensory loss may also be associated with a conversion reaction.

If you find an abnormality, confirm it by testing *temperature* sensation. Use two test tubes filled with hot and cold water. Touch the skin and ask the patient to identify "hot" or "cold."

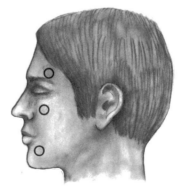

Then test for *light touch,* using a fine wisp of cotton. Ask the patient to respond whenever you touch his skin.

Test the *corneal reflex.* Ask the patient to look up. Approaching from the side and avoiding his eyelashes, touch the cornea (not the conjunctiva) lightly with a fine wisp of cotton.

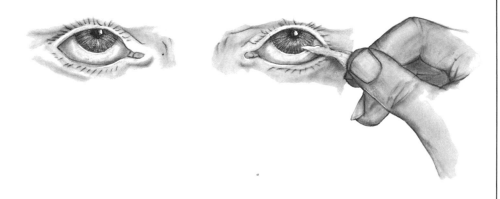

Absent blinking and tearing suggest a lesion of the fifth cranial nerve (assuming the seventh nerve is intact). Use of contact lenses may also diminish or abolish this reflex.

Note tearing and blinking, the normal reaction to this stimulus. (The sensory limb of this reflex is carried in the fifth cranial nerve, the motor response in the seventh.)

Seventh Cranial Nerve (Facial). Inspect the face, both at rest and during conversation with the patient. Note any asymmetry, e.g., of the nasolabial folds, and observe any tics or other abnormal movements. Ask the patient to:

Flattening of nasolabial fold and drooping of lower eyelid suggest facial weakness.

1. Raise his eyebrows
2. Frown
3. Close his eyes tightly so that you cannot open them

   (Test his muscle strength by trying to open them.)

4. Show his teeth
5. Smile
6. Puff out his cheeks

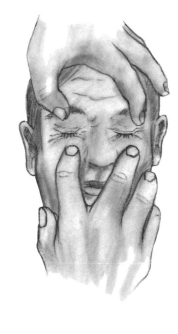

See Table 18-4, Types of Facial Paralysis (pp. 348–349).

In unilateral facial paralysis, the mouth is pulled away from the paralyzed side.

Note any weakness or asymmetry.

Eighth Cranial Nerve (Acoustic)

Assess hearing. If hearing loss is present, (1) test for lateralization and (2) compare air and bone conduction. (See Chapter 7.)

For further tests of *vestibular function* by special techniques, refer to textbooks of neurology or otolaryngology.

Ninth and Tenth Cranial Nerves (Glossopharyngeal and Vagus)

Ask the patient to say "ah" or to yawn. Observe the upward motion of the soft palate and uvula and the inward "curtain" movement of the posterior pharynx. Identify any asymmetry.
Stimulate the back of the throat and note the gag reflex.
Note any hoarseness of the voice.

Palate and uvula deviate away from the paralyzed side in a lesion of the vagus.
Hoarseness may indicate vocal cord paralysis (vagus), but, of course, has many other causes.

Eleventh Cranial Nerve (Spinal Accessory). Ask the patient to shrug his shoulders upward against your hand. Note the strength and contraction of the trapezius muscles. Ask the patient to turn his head to each side against your hand. Observe the contraction of the opposite sternomastoid and note the force of the movement against your hand.

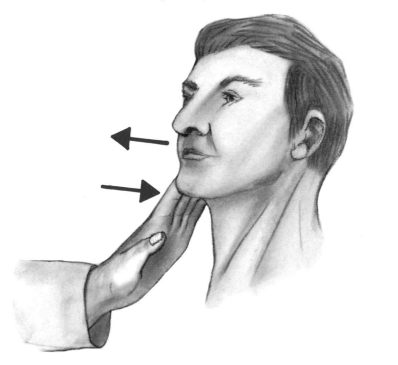

Twelfth Cranial Nerve (Hypoglossal). Inspect the patient's tongue as it lies in the floor of the mouth. Note any fasciculations (fine twitching movements of the muscle bundles, to be distinguished from the coarser restless movements often seen in a normal tongue). Ask the patient to stick out his tongue. Note any asymmetry, deviation or atrophy.

Fasciculations and atrophy suggest lower motor neuron disease. Tongue deviates toward the paralyzed side.

The Motor System

Screening Procedures, Including Gait. Ask the patient to *walk* across the room, or preferably down the hall, *turn* and come back. Observe his posture, balance, the swinging of his arms and movements of his legs. Normally, balance is easy; the arms swing at the sides; and in turning, the face and head lead the rest of the body.

See Table 18-5, Abnormalities of Gait and Posture (pp. 350–351).

Ask the patient to *walk heel-to-toe* in a straight line. If he has difficulty with this—

Done poorly in cerebellar disease.

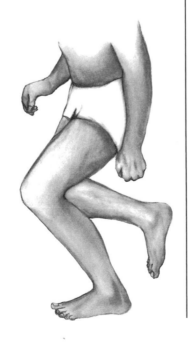

Perform a Romberg test. Ask the patient to stand with his feet together and without support from his arms. Note his ability to maintain an upright posture first with his eyes open, then with his eyes closed. (Stand close enough to protect him should he lose his balance.) Normally only minimal swaying occurs.

When examining a reasonably healthy ambulatory patient, it is convenient to survey the patient further at this point by asking him to *hop in place* on each foot in turn. The ability to do this indicates an intact motor system in the legs, normal cerebellar function and good position sense.

When a patient has ataxia from cerebellar disease, he may have difficulty standing with his feet together whether his eyes are open or closed. When a patient is ataxic because of decreased position sense, his vision can compensate for the sensory loss and he can stand fairly well with eyes open. With eyes closed, however, he loses his balance. This phenomenon constitutes a positive Romberg's sign.

Ask him to do a shallow *knee bend,* first on one leg, then on the other.

Quadriceps weakness makes a knee bend difficult or impossible.

Then ask him to *walk on his toes* and then *on his heels* — sensitive tests respectively for plantar and dorsiflexion at the ankles, as well as for balance.

Screen the motor function of the arms by testing the patient's *grip* and asking him to *hold his arms forward, palms up.* (See below for techniques.)

Further Assessment

If you detect abnormalities in screening or suspect them because of symptoms, proceed to a more detailed examination of the motor system. You may wish to alter the exact sequence of your examination to improve your efficiency or avoid tiring the patient. Keep in mind, however, the underlying organization of the assessment: inspection, assessment of muscle tone, muscle strength and coordination.

Inspection.   Inspect the muscles of limbs and trunk, noting any *atrophy, fasciculations, involuntary movements* or *abnormalities of position.*

Assessment of Muscle Tone.   Persuade the patient to relax. Take his hand with yours and while supporting his elbow, flex and extend the patient's fingers, wrist and elbow, and put his shoulder through a moderate range of motion. With practice, these actions can be combined into a single smooth movement. On each side note his muscle tone—the resistance offered to your movements.

While supporting the patient's thigh with one hand, flex and extend the patient's knee and ankle on each side. Note the resistance to your movements.

Testing Muscle Strength.   Depending upon the patient's strength, muscle power should be tested against your resistance, against gravity only or with the effects of gravity removed.

Ask the patient to close his eyes and for 20 to 30 seconds to hold his arms straight in front of him, with palms up. Watch how well he maintains this position.

Atrophy and fasciculations suggest a lower motor neuron problem.
See Table 18-6, Abnormalities of Movement (pp. 352–353).

Resistance to passive stretch is increased in upper motor neuron lesions and in Parkinsonism. Resistance to passive stretch is decreased when there is a lower motor neuron lesion. If the muscles are paralyzed, they are flaccid. Resistance to passive stretch may also be decreased when sensory neurons are destroyed or when a cerebellar lesion is present.

See Table 18-7, Differentiation of Motor Dysfunctions (pp. 354–355).

Tendency of one forearm to pronate suggests mild hemiparesis; downward drift of arm with flexion at the elbow may also occur.

On each side try to depress his outstretched arms against his resistance. Note his strength and watch the scapula on that side for winging or displacement.

Increased prominence of the scapular tip (winging) with displacement in and up suggests a weak serratus anterior muscle.

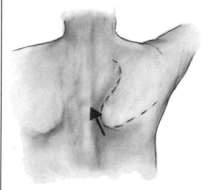

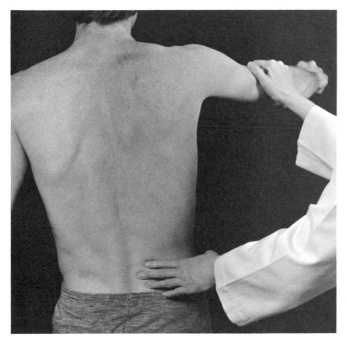

Observe,
then
press down

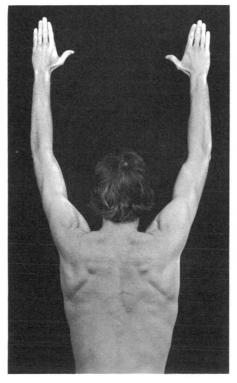

Then ask the patient to raise his arms over his head with palms forward for 20 to 30 seconds. Again observe the maintenance of this position. Try to force his arms down to his sides against his resistance. Note any weakness.

Drifting or weakness on one side suggests hemiparesis or shoulder girdle disease.

Test flexion and extension at the elbow by having the patient pull and push against your hand.

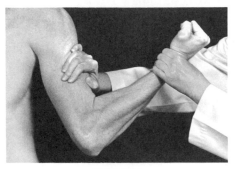

FLEXION

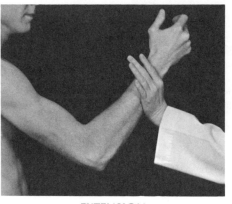

EXTENSION

Test dorsiflexion at the wrist by asking the patient to make a fist and resist your pushing it down.

Wrist drop or weakness in radial nerve disorders

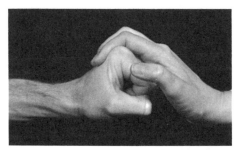

Test the grip by asking him to squeeze your fingers as hard as he can. You can avoid painfully hard gripping by offering the patient only your index and middle fingers, with the middle finger on top of the index. You should normally have difficulty removing your fingers from the patient's grip.

Grip affected by forearm muscle weakness and painful disorders of the hands

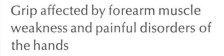

Patient

Examiner

Ask the patient to spread his fingers. Check abduction by trying to force them together.

Weak abduction in ulnar nerve disorders

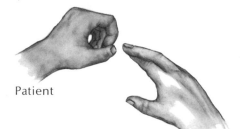

To test flexion of the fingers together with adduction and opposition of the thumb, instruct the patient to hold his thumb tightly against his fingertips. Pull your thumb between his thumb and fingers and note his strength.

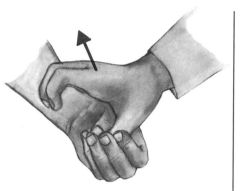

Assessment of muscle strength of the trunk may already have been made in other segments of the examination. It includes:

Flexion, extension and lateral bending of the trunk.
Excursion of the rib cage and diaphragm during respiration.

Test flexion at the hip by placing your hand on the patient's thigh and asking him to raise his leg against it.

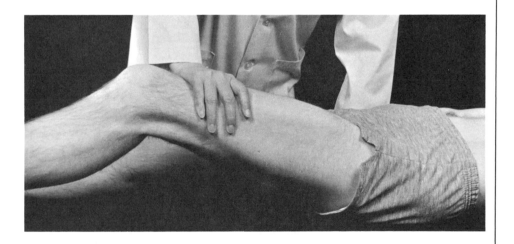

Test abduction at the hip. Place your hands firmly on the bed outside the patient's knees. Ask him to spread his legs against your hands.

Symmetrical proximal muscle weakness suggests a myopathy; symmetrical distal weakness suggests a neuropathy.

Test adduction at the hip. Place your hands firmly on the bed between the patient's knees. Ask him to bring his legs together.

Test flexion at the knee. Place the patient's leg so that the knee is flexed with his foot resting on the bed. Tell him to keep his foot down as you try to straighten his leg.

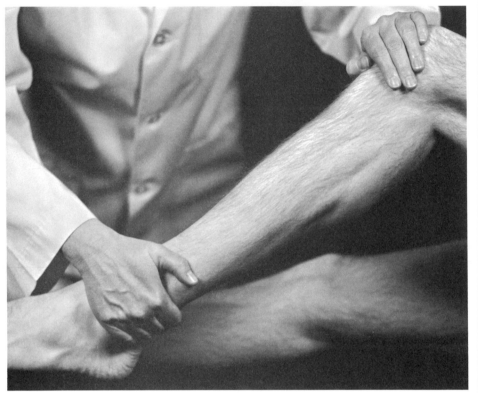

Test extension at the knee by supporting his knee and asking him to straighten his leg against your hand.

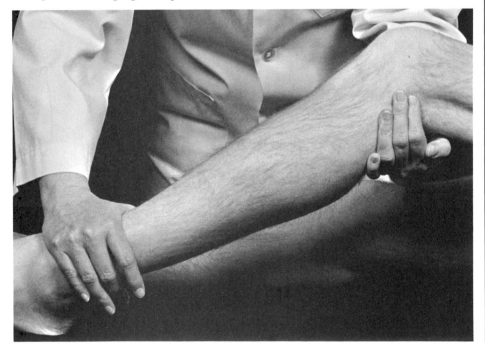

Test plantar flexion and dorsiflexion at the ankle by asking the patient to push down and pull up against your hands.

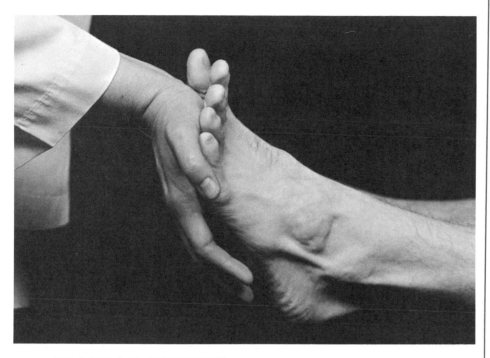

PLANTAR FLEXION

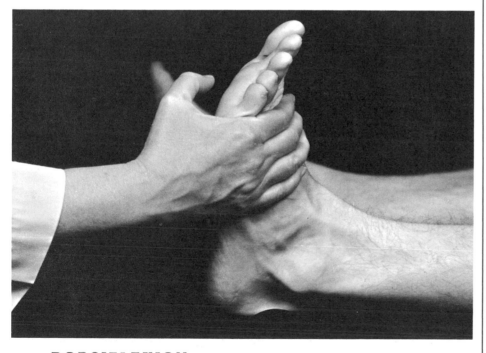

DORSIFLEXION

Assessing Coordination. Coordination in the arms and hands may be tested as follows:

1. *Rapid Rhythmic Alternating Movements.* Testing each hand separately, ask the patient to (1) pat his leg as fast as he can with his hand, (2) turn his hand over and back as rapidly as he can and (3) touch each of his fingers with his thumb in rapid sequence.

Poor coordination in cerebellar disease

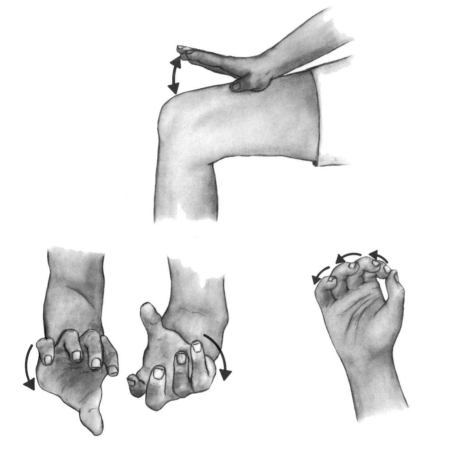

Note any slowness or awkwardness of movement. The non-dominant hand often performs slightly less well.

2. *Point-to-Point Testing.* Ask the patient to touch your index finger, then his nose alternately several times. Note any tremor or awkwardness. Repeat the maneuver with the patient's eyes closed.

Awkwardness and inaccuracy in cerebellar disease; inaccuracy only when eyes closed suggests loss of position sense.

Assess coordination in the legs with

1. *Rapid Rhythmic Alternating Movements.* Ask the patient to tap your hand as quickly as possible with the ball of each foot in turn. Note any slowness or awkwardness. The feet normally perform less well than the hands.

2. *Point-to-Point Testing.* Ask the patient to place his heel on the opposite knee, then run it down his shin to the foot. Note any tremor or awkwardness.

Awkwardness in cerebellar disease or loss of position sense

The Sensory System

Sensory testing readily fatigues the patient and then produces unreliable and inconsistent results. To avoid this problem conduct an efficient and relatively rapid survey. In a patient with no neurologic symptoms or signs, a few *screening procedures* suffice. These include: (1) assessment of pain and vibration sense in the hands and feet, (2) brief comparison of light touch over the arms and legs and (3) assessment of stereognosis, e.g., by a coin in the hands. Other patients need more complete evaluation. Examine in special detail those areas (1) where there are symptoms such as numbness or pain, (2) where there are motor or reflex abnormalities, and (3) where there are trophic changes, e.g., absent or excessive sweating, atrophic skin or cutaneous ulceration. Repeated testing at another time is often required to confirm abnormalities.

In testing a sensation:

1. Note the patient's ability to perceive the stimulus.
2. Compare sensation in symmetrical areas on the two sides of the body.
3. Compare distal and proximal areas of the extremities when testing pain, temperature and touch. Initiate the testing of vibration and position sense distally. If these are normal, omit more proximal areas.
4. Scatter the stimuli so that you cover most of the dermatomes and major peripheral nerves.
5. When you detect an area of sensory loss or hypersensitivity, map out its boundaries in detail. Stimulate first at a point of reduced sensation and move outward by progressive steps until the patient detects the change.

Symmetrical distal sensory loss suggests a peripheral polyneuropathy.

Ask the patient to close his eyes. Test sensation on the arms, trunk and legs using the following stimuli:

1. *Pain.* Use a safety pin, occasionally substituting the blunt end for the point as a stimulus. Stimulating in patterns suggested above, ask the patient to report whether it is "sharp" or "dull."
2. *Temperature.* (This may be omitted if pain sensation is normal.) Use two test tubes, filled with hot and cold water. Touch the skin and ask the patient to identify "hot" or "cold."
3. *Light touch.* Use a fine wisp of cotton. Ask the patient to respond whenever you touch his skin.
4. *Vibration.* Use a relatively low pitched tuning fork, preferably of 128 cycles per second. Tap it on the heel of your hand and place it firmly over a distal interphalangeal joint of a finger and over the interphalangeal joint of the big toe. Ask the patient what he feels. If you are uncertain whether he feels pressure or vibration, ask him to tell you

See Table 18-8, Patterns of Sensory Loss (pp. 356–357).

when the vibration stops, then touch the fork to stop it. If vibration sense is impaired, proceed to more proximal bony prominences, e.g., wrist and elbow or medial malleolus, patella, anterior superior iliac spine and spinous processes.

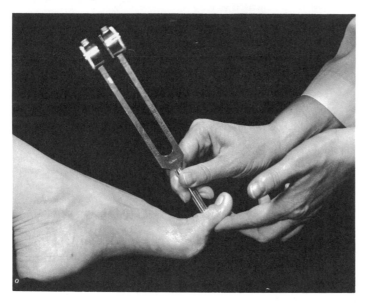

5. *Position.*   Grasp the patient's big toe, holding it by its sides between your thumb and index finger and avoiding friction against the other toes. Then move it and ask the patient to identify whether you are moving it up or down.

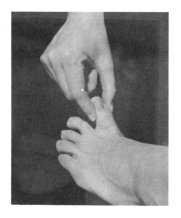

If position sense is impaired, move proximally to test it at the ankle joint. In a similar fashion test position in the fingers, moving proximally if indicated to the metacarpophalangeal joints, wrist and elbow.

6. *Discriminative Sensation.*   Testing discriminative sensation is worthwhile chiefly when other types of sensation are intact. It may also be used to evaluate posterior column function in more detail. Survey with stereognosis and proceed to the other methods if indicated.

Stereognosis.   Place a familiar small object in the patient's hand, e.g., a coin, paper clip, key, pencil, cotton ball. Ask him to identify it. Normally a patient will manipulate it skillfully and identify it correctly. Asking the patient to distinguish "heads" from "tails" on a coin is a sensitive test of stereognosis.

Discrimination may be impaired in lesions of the sensory cortex or posterior columns.

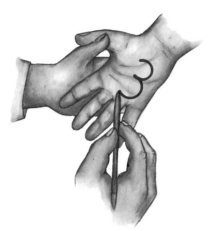

Number Identification. When motor impairment of the hand makes testing for stereognosis impractical, test the patient's ability to identify numbers. With the blunt end of a pen or pencil, draw a large number in his palm. The normal person can identify most such numbers.

Two-point Discrimination. Using the sides of two pins, touch the skin simultaneously. Alternate this stimulus irregularly with a one-point touch.

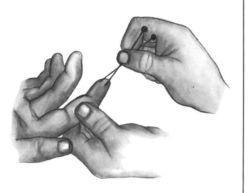

Find the minimal distance at which the patient can discriminate one from two points (normally about 2 or 3 mm on the finger pads).

Point Localization. Touch a point on the patient's skin. Ask him to open his eyes and point to the place touched. This method, together with that for extinction, is especially useful on the trunk and legs.

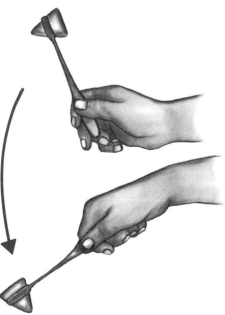

Extinction. Simultaneously stimulate corresponding areas on both sides of the body. Ask the patient where he feels it. Normally he should feel both.

Reflexes

To elicit a deep tendon reflex, (1) persuade the patient to relax, (2) position the limbs so that the muscle is mildly stretched and (3) strike the tendon briskly, producing a sudden additional tendon stretch. The patient's limbs should be symmetrically positioned and the sides compared. Hold the reflex hammer loosely between thumb and fingers so that it swings freely in an arc, yet is controlled in its direction.

With lesions of the sensory cortex, only one stimulus may be recognized.

If the patient's reflexes are symmetrically diminished or absent, use reinforcement, a technique involving isometric contraction of other muscles that may increase reflex activity. In testing arm reflexes, for example, ask the patient to clench his teeth or to squeeze his thigh with the opposite hand. If leg reflexes are diminished or absent, reinforce them by asking the patient to lock his fingers and pull one hand against the other.

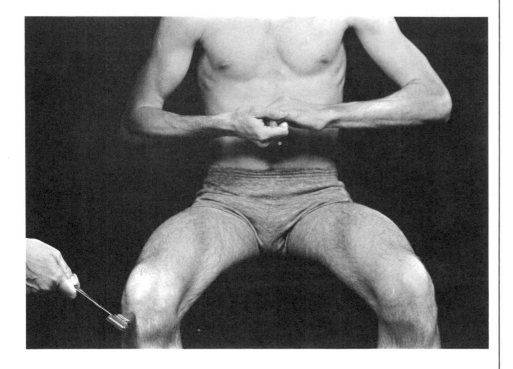

Reflexes are usually graded on a 0 to 4+ scale:

4+   very brisk, hyperactive; often indicative of disease; associated with clonus (rhythmic oscillations between flexion and extension)

3+   brisker than average and possibly but not necessarily indicative of disease

2+   average; normal

1+   somewhat diminished; low normal ⎱ If you use reinforcement,

0   no response   ⎰   indicate it.

Differences between sides are usually easier to assess than symmetrical changes.

The Biceps Reflex (C_5, C_6). The patient's arms should be partially flexed at the elbow with palms down. Place your thumb or finger firmly on the biceps tendon. Strike with the reflex hammer so that the blow is aimed directly through your digit toward the biceps tendon.

Hyperactive reflexes suggest upper motor neuron disease.

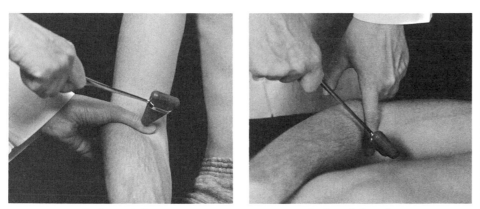

Patient sitting   **Patient lying down**

Observe flexion at the elbow and watch for and feel the contraction of the biceps muscle.

The Triceps Reflex (C₇, C₈). Flex the patient's arm at the elbow, with palm toward the body, and pull it slightly across the chest. Strike the triceps tendon above the elbow. Use a direct, not a glancing, blow. Watch for contraction of the triceps muscle and extension at the elbow.

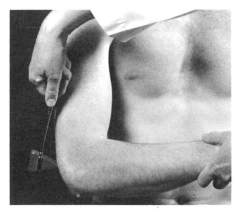

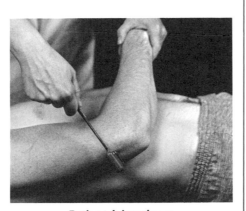

Patient sitting   **Patient lying down**

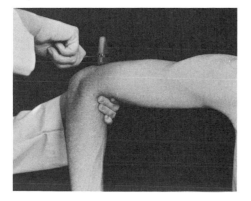

When it is difficult to get a sitting patient relaxed for a triceps reflex, an alternate method may help. Support the patient's upper arm as illustrated, and ask him to let it go limp, as if it were "hung up to dry." Then strike the triceps tendon.

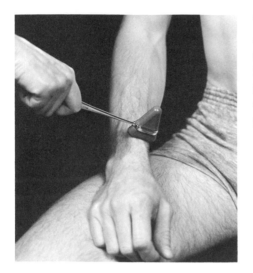

The Supinator or Brachioradialis Reflex (C₅, C₆). The patient's forearm should rest on the abdomen or in the lap, palm down. Strike the radius about 1 to 2 inches above the wrist. Observe flexion and supination of the forearm.

The Abdominal Reflexes. Test the abdominal reflexes by lightly but briskly stroking each side of the abdomen, above (T_8, T_9, T_{10}) and below (T_{10}, T_{11}, T_{12}) the umbilicus, in the directions illustrated. Use a key or tongue blade, twisted so that it is split longitudinally. Note the contraction of the abdominal muscles and deviation of the umbilicus toward the stimulus. Obesity may mask an abdominal reflex. In this situation, use your finger to retract the patient's umbilicus away from the side to be stimulated. Feel with your retracting finger for the muscular contraction.

Upper abdominal

Lower abdominal

Cremasteric

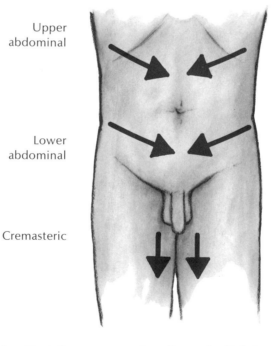

Abdominal and cremasteric reflexes may be absent in both upper and lower motor neuron disorders.

The Cremasteric Reflexes (L₁, L₂). Test the cremasteric reflexes by lightly scratching the inner aspect of the upper thigh. Note elevation of the testicle on that side.

The Knee Reflex (L₂, L₃, L₄). The patient may be either (1) sitting or (2) lying down while you support his knees in a somewhat flexed position. Briskly tap the patellar tendon just below the patella. Note contraction of the quadriceps with extension at the knee.

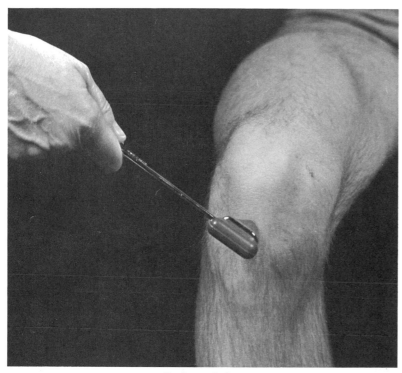

Patient sitting

Two methods are useful in examining the supine patient. Supporting both knees at once, as shown below on the left, allows you to assess small differences between knee reflexes by repeated testing of one and then the other. Sometimes, however, supporting both legs is uncomfortable for both the examiner and the patient. A comfortable alternative method by which your supporting arm is in turn supported by the patient's opposite leg is shown below on the right. Some patients are better able to relax with this method.

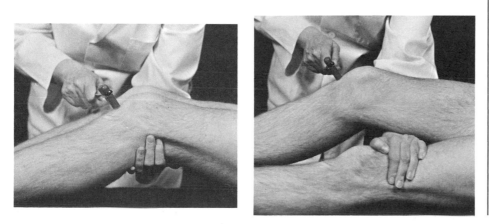

The Ankle Reflex (S_1, S_2). With the leg somewhat flexed at the knee, dorsiflex the foot at the ankle. Persuade the patient to relax. Strike the Achilles tendon. Watch for plantar flexion at the ankle. Note also the speed of relaxation after muscular contraction.

A slowed relaxation phase in the ankle reflex suggests hypothyroidism.

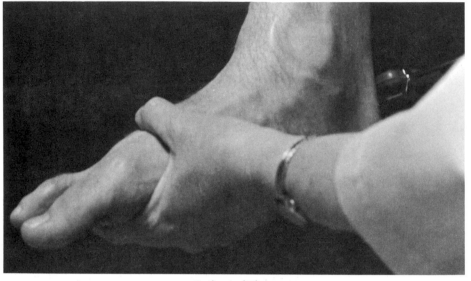

Patient sitting

When the patient is lying down, flex one leg at both hip and knee and rotate it externally so that it rests across the opposite shin. Then dorsiflex the foot at the ankle and strike the Achilles tendon.

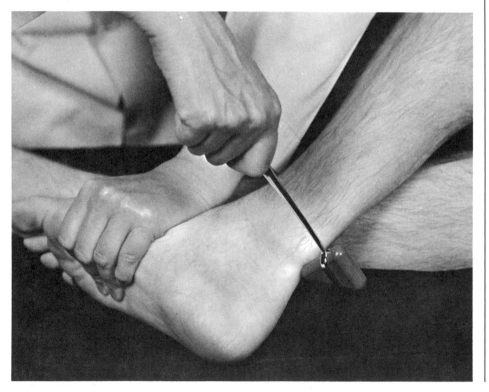

The Plantar Response (L₄, L₅, S₁, S₂).   With a moderately sharp object such as a key, stroke the lateral aspect of the sole from the heel to the ball of the foot, curving medially across the ball. Use the lightest stimulus that will provoke a response. Note movement of the toes, normally flexion.

Dorsiflexion of the great toe with fanning of the other toes indicates upper motor neuron disease (Babinski response).

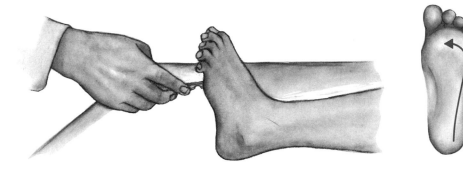

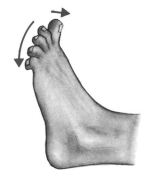

If the reflexes are hyperreactive, *test for ankle clonus.* Support the knee in a partly flexed position. With your other hand, sharply dorsiflex the foot and maintain it in dorsiflexion. Look for rhythmic oscillations between dorsiflexion and plantar flexion.

Sustained clonus indicates upper motor neuron disease.

Clonus may also be elicited at other joints, e.g., patellar clonus at the knee.

Special Maneuvers

Meningeal Signs. Testing for meningeal signs is not part of a routine examination but should be done when you suspect inflammation of the meninges, e.g., by infection (meningitis) or blood (as in subarachnoid hemorrhage). (See also pp. 388 and 417.)

With the patient recumbent, place your hands behind his head and flex his neck forward. Note resistance or pain. Watch also for flexion of the patient's hips and knees in reaction to your maneuver (Brudzinski's sign).

Pain and resistance to flexion suggest meningeal inflammation but may be due to arthritis or neck injury. Flexion of hips and knees suggests meningeal inflammation.

Flex one of the patient's legs at hip and knee, then straighten the knee. Note resistance or pain (Kernig's sign).

Pain or resistance suggests meningeal inflammation or disc disease.

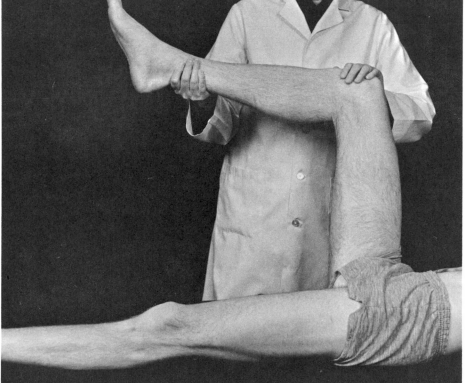

The Stuporous or Comatose Patient. Survey the patient quickly. Make sure that his airway is clear, check for evidence of bleeding and shock. (Laboratory studies and emergency management are beyond the scope of this text.)

Check his vital signs, including pulse, blood pressure and rectal temperature.

Despite the atmosphere of emergency, take several minutes and carefully observe:

His respirations

See Table 8-2, Abnormalities in Rate and Rhythm of Breathing (p. 133)

His posture and motor activity, noting especially his position in bed

The position of his head and eyes, and any spontaneous movements
Any odors
Any abnormalities of skin, including color, moisture, evidence of bleeding disorders, needlemarks or other lesions

See Table 18-9, Abnormal Postures in the Comatose Patient (p. 358)

Jaundice, cyanosis, cherry red color of carbon monoxide poisoning

As you go on with your examination, take two *important precautions:*

1. If there is any question of trauma to head or neck, do not bend the neck until x-ray examination has ruled out a fracture of the cervical spine.
2. In examining the ocular fundi do not use a mydriatic solution. It could mask important eye signs.

Proceed to a general and neurologic examination, with special attention to the following:
Examine the head carefully for signs of trauma.
Test for meningeal signs.
Examine the eyes, especially:

Bruises, lacerations, local swelling
Meningitis, subarachnoid hemorrhage

The fundi

Papilledema, hypertensive retinopathy

The pupils and their reaction to light
The extraocular movements, if possible
The corneal reflexes

See Table 7-7, Pupillary Abnormalities (pp. 92–93).

In deep coma, the presence of pupillary reflexes favors a metabolic cause; their absence favors a structural cause.

Inspect the ears and nose.

Bleeding or cerebral spinal fluid suggests a skull fracture. Otitis media

Watch for facial asymmetry.
Inspect the mouth and throat.
Examine the heart, lungs and abdomen.
Complete a neurologic examination, insofar as you are able.

Tongue injury suggests a seizure.

Three additional maneuvers are especially helpful.

1. *Assess response to stimuli,* increasing the strength of the stimulus as follows:
   a. Give a simple command.
   b. Call the patient's name.
   c. Produce pain, for example, by pressing the bony ridges above the eyes, by pinching the sides of the neck or the inner portions of upper arms and thighs.

Avoidance movements persist in stupor and light coma but are lost in deeper coma. Motor responses confined to one side suggest paralysis of the other side.

Observe how strong a stimulus is required to produce a response. Note whether motor responses are confined to one side of the body and whether stimuli from both or only one side of the body produce a response.

When a stimulus on one side of the body produces a response but a similar stimulus on the opposite side does not, suspect a sensory deficit on the latter side.

2. *Test the oculocephalic reflex (doll's eye movements).* Holding open the upper eyelids so that you can see the eyes, turn the head quickly first to one side, then to the other. Flex the neck forward, then extend it.

In a comatose patient with an intact brain stem, the patient's eyes move in the opposite direction as if still gazing ahead in their initial position (doll's eye movements).

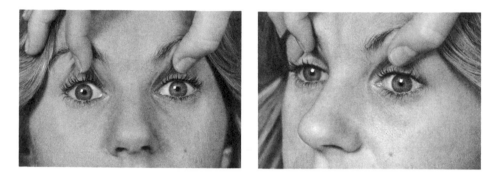

Observe the eye movements.

Unless consciously fixing their gaze, fully conscious patients move their eyes unpredictably or only slightly in the opposite direction, as shown above.

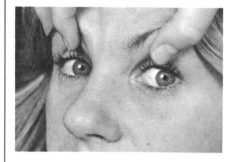

Loss of these movements suggests a lesion of midbrain or pons, or very deep coma.

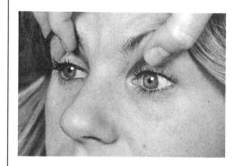

3. *Test the oculovestibular reflex with caloric stimulation.* Make sure that the eardrums are intact and the canals clear. Elevate the head to 30 degrees. With a large syringe, inject icewater through a small catheter that is lying in (but not plugging) the ear canal. Use up to 200 ml of water in order to obtain a response. Repeat on the opposite side, waiting 3 to 5 minutes if necessary for the first response to disappear.

The normal awake patient (in whom a few milliliters of icewater is often an adequate stimulus) responds with nystagmus with the quick component away from the irrigated ear.

A comatose patient with an intact brain stem responds by conjugate deviation of the eyes toward the irrigated ear.

Loss of this reflex (no response to stimulation) suggests a brain stem lesion.

TABLE 18-1. ABNORMALITIES OF SPEECH

APHASIA OR DYSPHASIA from damage to cortical speech centers.

Ranges from uncertainty or error in choice of words and syllables (dysphasia) to complete inability to speak (aphasia) despite adequate motor function of mouth and larynx

DYSARTHRIA, defective articulation due to a motor deficit involving the lips or tongue

Slurred speech, with difficulty especially in pronouncing the labial (m, b, p) and the lingual (t, d, l) consonants

CEREBELLAR DYSARTHRIA

Poorly coordinated, irregular speech with unnatural separation of syllables (scanning)

APHONIA OR DYSPHONIA due to disease of the larynx or its innervation

Ranges from a rasping hoarse voice (dysphonia) to a whisper (aphonia)

PALATAL PARALYSIS

Nasal speech

PARKINSONISM

A monotonous, weak voice

TABLE 18-2. ABNORMALITIES OF CONSCIOUSNESS*

CONFUSION

Mental slowness, inattentiveness, dulled perception of the environment, incoherence in thinking

STUPOR

Marked reduction in mental and physical activity; marked slowness and reduction in response to commands or stimuli; usually with preservation of reflexes

COMA

Unresponsiveness to stimuli; absense of most reflexes

DELIRIUM

A state of confusion with agitation and hallucinations. This state is generally considered separate from the continuum of confusion—stupor—coma.

*Because these terms are not always used with sufficient precision to ascertain changes in a patient's state of consciousness, always describe your findings in some detail. Do not simply affix the appropriate label.

TABLE 18-3

TABLE 18-3. NYSTAGMUS

Nystagmus is a rhythmic oscillation of the eyes. Analogous to a tremor in other parts of the body, it is essentially a disorder of ocular posture. Its causes are multiple, including impairment of vision in early life, disorders of the labyrinth and the cerebellar system, and drug toxicity. Nystagmus occurs normally when a person watches a rapidly moving object, e.g., a passing train. Observe the three characteristics of nystagmus listed below and on the following page. Then refer to textbooks of neurology for differential diagnosis.

DIRECTION OF THE QUICK AND SLOW COMPONENTS

Nystagmus is usually quicker in one direction than in the other and is then defined by its quicker phase. For example, if the eyes jerk quickly to the left and drift back slowly to the right, the patient is said to have nystagmus to the left.

Occasionally nystagmus consists only of coarse oscillations without quick and slow components. It is then said to be *pendular*.

NYSTAGMUS TO THE LEFT

← SLOW DRIFT TO RIGHT

QUICK JERK TO LEFT →

PLANE OF THE MOVEMENTS

The movements of nystagmus may occur in one or more planes, e.g., horizontal, vertical or rotary.

HORIZONTAL NYSTAGMUS

VERTICAL NYSTAGMUS

ROTARY NYSTAGMUS

TABLE 18-3 (CONT'D)

TABLE 18-3 (CONT'D)

FIELD OF GAZE IN WHICH NYSTAGMUS APPEARS

Example: NYSTAGMUS ON RIGHT LATERAL GAZE

Nystagmus may be present in all fields of gaze. It may appear or become accentuated on deviation of the eyes, e.g., to the side or upward. On extreme lateral gaze the normal person may show a few beats resembling nystagmus. Avoid such extreme movements and observe for nystagmus only within the field of full binocular vision.

TABLE 18-4

TABLE 18-4. TYPES OF FACIAL PARALYSIS

LOWER MOTOR NEURON PARALYSIS
Example: BELL'S PALSY

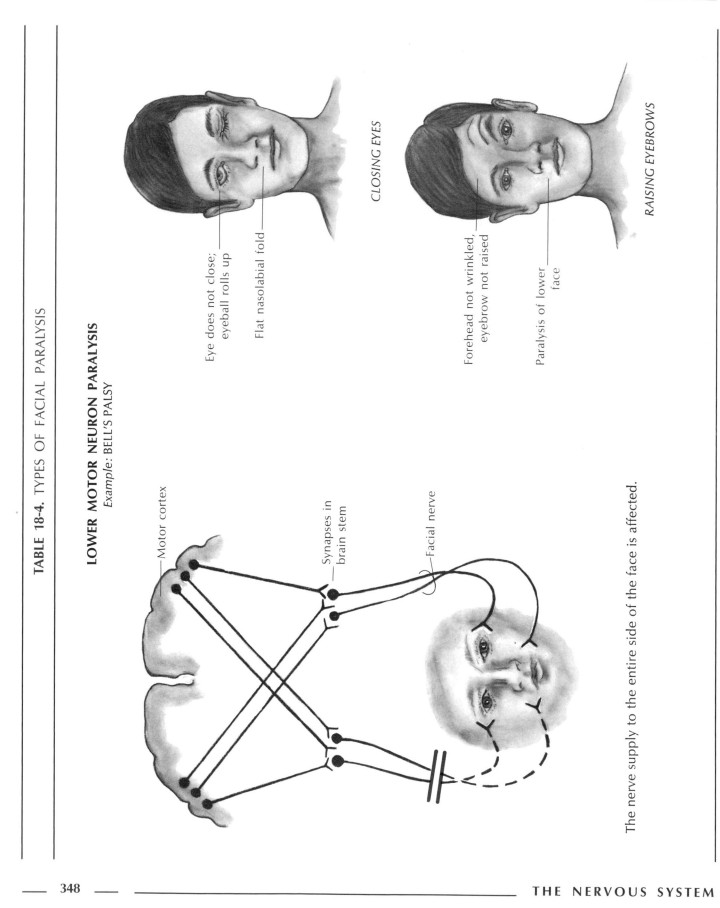

Eye does not close; eyeball rolls up

Flat nasolabial fold

CLOSING EYES

Forehead not wrinkled, eyebrow not raised

Paralysis of lower face

RAISING EYEBROWS

Motor cortex

Synapses in brain stem

Facial nerve

The nerve supply to the entire side of the face is affected.

TABLE 18-4 (CONT'D)

TABLE 18-4 (CONT'D)

UPPER MOTOR NEURON PARALYSIS
Example: HEMIPARESIS

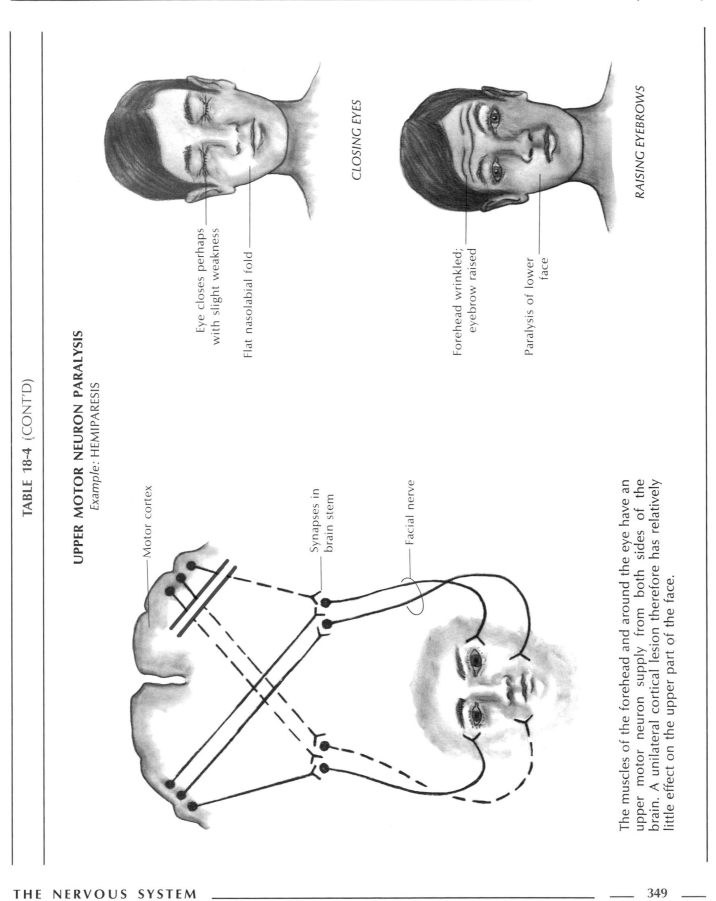

Eye closes perhaps with slight weakness

Flat nasolabial fold

CLOSING EYES

Forehead wrinkled; eyebrow raised

Paralysis of lower face

RAISING EYEBROWS

Motor cortex

Synapses in brain stem

Facial nerve

The muscles of the forehead and around the eye have an upper motor neuron supply from both sides of the brain. A unilateral cortical lesion therefore has relatively little effect on the upper part of the face.

TABLE 18-5 _____

TABLE 18-5. ABNORMALITIES OF GAIT AND POSTURE

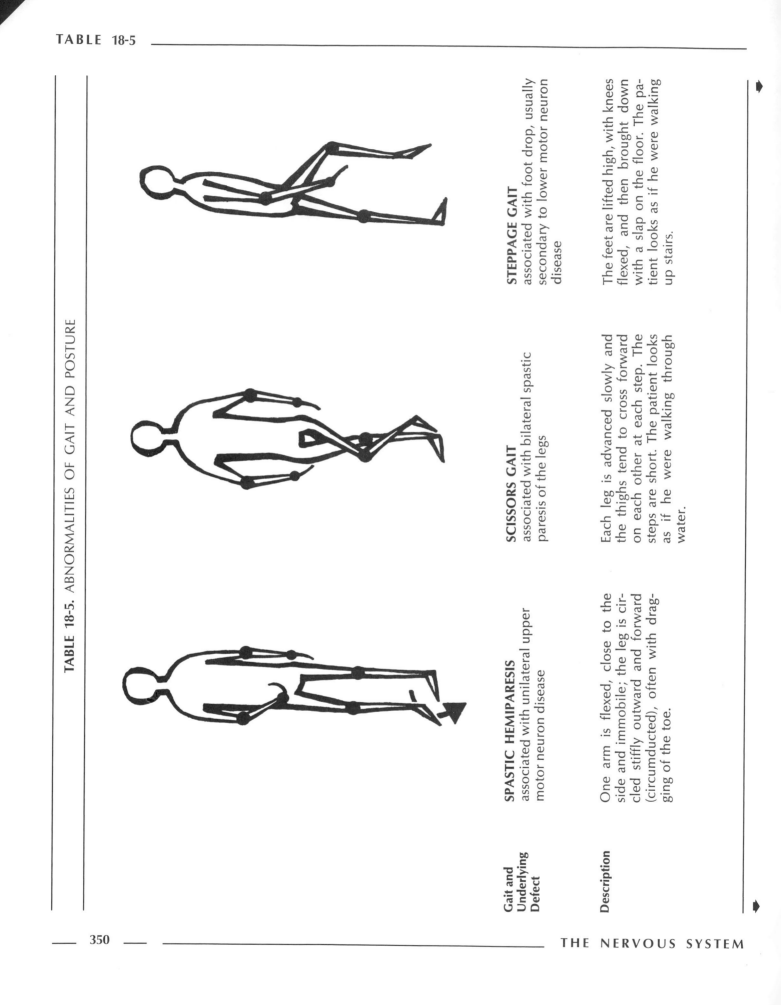

Gait and Underlying Defect	**SPASTIC HEMIPARESIS** associated with unilateral upper motor neuron disease	**SCISSORS GAIT** associated with bilateral spastic paresis of the legs	**STEPPAGE GAIT** associated with foot drop, usually secondary to lower motor neuron disease
Description	One arm is flexed, close to the side and immobile; the leg is circled stiffly outward and forward (circumducted), often with dragging of the toe.	Each leg is advanced slowly and the thighs tend to cross forward on each other at each step. The steps are short. The patient looks as if he were walking through water.	The feet are lifted high, with knees flexed, and then brought down with a slap on the floor. The patient looks as if he were walking up stairs.

TABLE 18-5 (CONT'D)

TABLE 18-5 (CONT'D)

Gait and Underlying Defect	**SENSORY ATAXIA** associated with loss of position sense in the legs	**CEREBELLAR ATAXIA** associated with disease of the cerebellum or associated tracts	**PARKINSONIAN GAIT** associated with the basal ganglia defects of Parkinson's disease
Description	The gait is unsteady and wide-based (the feet are far apart). The feet are lifted high and brought down with a slap. The patient watches the ground to guide his steps. He cannot stand steadily with feet together when his eyes are closed (positive Romberg test).	The gait is staggering, unsteady and wide-based with exaggerated difficulty on the turns. The patient cannot stand steadily with feet together, whether eyes are open or closed.	The posture is stooped, the hips and knees slightly flexed. Steps are short and often shuffling. Arm swings are decreased and the patient turns around stiffly—"all in one piece."

TABLE 18-6

TABLE 18-6. ABNORMALITIES OF MOVEMENT

Name	Description of movement	Examples
FASCICULATIONS	Visible twitching movements of muscle bundles	Together with muscle atrophy, a sign of lower motor neuron disease
TREMORS	Involuntary rhythmic tremulous movements that may be more pronounced: 1. At rest (resting tremors) 2. During a sustained posture, e.g., holding the arms forward (postural tremors) 3. During active movement (intention tremors)	1. The slow regular "pill rolling" resting tremor in Parkinsonism 2. Tremors of hyperthyroidism and anxiety 3. Cerebellar ataxia
TICS	Repetitive twitching of muscles, often in the face and upper trunk	Repetitive grimacing, winking or shoulder shrugging
CHOREA	Involuntary movements of the face, extremities or trunk that are relatively rapid, jerky, irregular and unpredictable. They may occur at rest or accompany purposeful movement.	Sydenham's chorea in rheumatic fever
ATHETOSIS	Involuntary movements of the face, extremities or trunk that are slower, more twisting and writhing than chorea. Athetoid movement may occur at rest or accompany purposeful movement.	Frequent in cerebral palsy
MYOCLONUS	Involuntary, sudden and rapid unpredictable jerks; faster than chorea	Myoclonic jerks may occur when normally falling asleep or in myoclonic seizures. A hiccup is diaphragmatic myoclonus.

TABLE 18-6 (cont'd)

TABLE 18-6. (CONT'D)

ASTERIXIS	Involuntary and brief loss of muscle tone in the out-stretched fingers and hands, resulting in nonrhythmic flapping of the fingers or entire hand. Watch one or two minutes for this sign while the patient holds his arms forward with hands cocked up and fingers spread.	Metabolic encephalopathy, e.g., severe liver disease (hence the older term, liver flap) and uremia
TARDIVE DYSKINESIA	Choreiform movements affecting primarily the tongue, lips and face, producing repetitive, involuntary grimacing, protrusion of the tongue, opening and closing of the mouth and deviations of the jaw. The hands may show lesser involvement.	A late (hence) tardive complication of psychotropic drugs, e.g., phenothiazines

TABLE 18-7

TABLE 18-7. DIFFERENTIATION OF MOTOR DYSFUNCTIONS

(1) sensory
(2) lower motor neuron
(3) corticospinal
(4) extrapyramidal
(5) cerebellar

	(1) SENSORY NEURON	(2) LOWER MOTOR NEURON	(3) CORTICOSPINAL TRACT
Process	Loss of reflex activity and tone because of interruption of the sensory limb of the reflex arc; preservation of voluntary motion	All motor functions lost when the "final common pathway" is destroyed	Paralysis and spasticity are produced with hyperactive reflexes.
Appearance	Normal	Atrophy, fasciculations	Disuse atrophy, relatively mild; no fasciculations
Muscle Tone	Decreased	Decreased	Increased (spastic)*
Voluntary Movement (Strength)	Normal	Decreased or 0	Decreased or 0
Coordination	Normal with eyes open; poor with eyes closed	(Paralyzed or weak)	(Paralyzed or weak)
Reflexes When in Affected Location:			
Deep Tendon	Absent	Decreased or 0	Increased
Plantar	Absent	(Paralyzed or weak)	Extensor
Abdominals,	Absent	Absent	Absent
Cremasterics		Absent	

*Spasticity of upper motor neuron lesion is often "clasp-knife" in character, with a gradual increase in tone followed by a sudden decrease in tone as a limb goes through its range of motion.

TABLE 18-7 (CONT'D)

TABLE 18-7 (CONT'D)

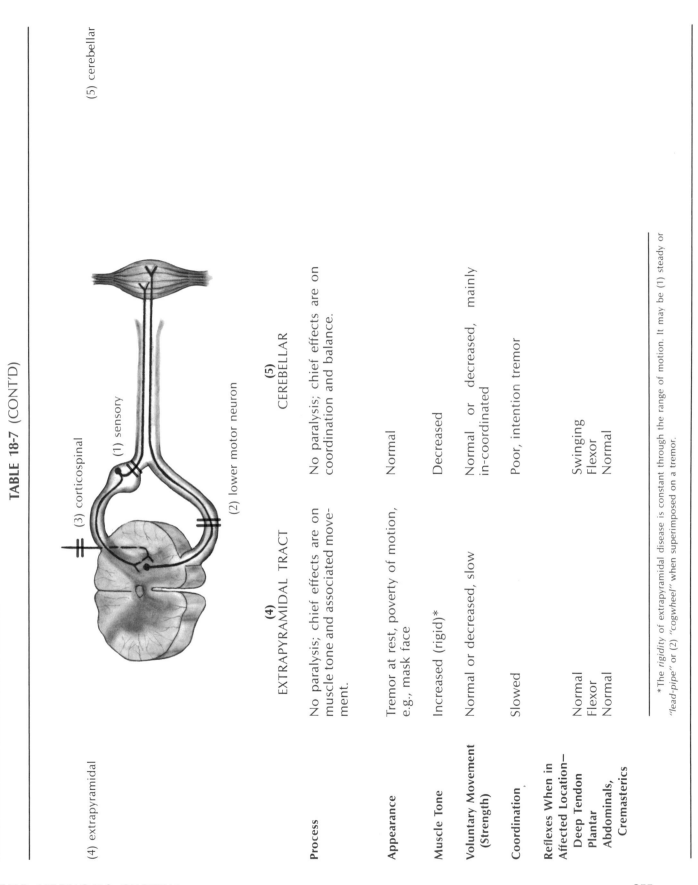

(1) sensory
(2) lower motor neuron
(3) corticospinal
(4) extrapyramidal
(5) cerebellar

	(4) EXTRAPYRAMIDAL TRACT	(5) CEREBELLAR
Process	No paralysis; chief effects are on muscle tone and associated movement.	No paralysis; chief effects are on coordination and balance.
Appearance	Tremor at rest, poverty of motion, e.g., mask face	Normal
Muscle Tone	Increased (rigid)*	Decreased
Voluntary Movement (Strength)	Normal or decreased, slow	Normal or decreased, mainly in-coordinated
Coordination	Slowed	Poor, intention tremor
Reflexes When in Affected Location— Deep Tendon Plantar Abdominals, Cremasterics	Normal Flexor Normal	Swinging Flexor Normal

*The *rigidity* of extrapyramidal disease is constant through the range of motion. It may be (1) steady or *"lead-pipe"* or (2) *"cogwheel"* when superimposed on a tremor.

TABLE 18-8

TABLE 18-8. PATTERNS OF SENSORY LOSS

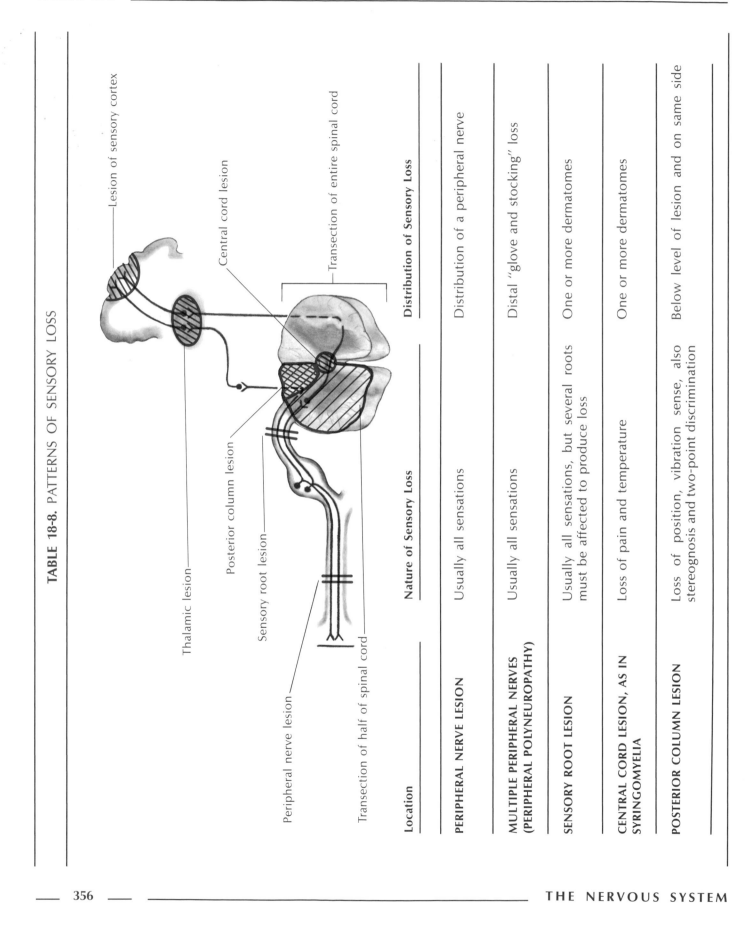

Lesion of sensory cortex

Central cord lesion

Transection of entire spinal cord

Thalamic lesion

Posterior column lesion

Sensory root lesion

Peripheral nerve lesion

Transection of half of spinal cord

Location	Nature of Sensory Loss	Distribution of Sensory Loss
PERIPHERAL NERVE LESION	Usually all sensations	Distribution of a peripheral nerve
MULTIPLE PERIPHERAL NERVES (PERIPHERAL POLYNEUROPATHY)	Usually all sensations	Distal "glove and stocking" loss
SENSORY ROOT LESION	Usually all sensations, but several roots must be affected to produce loss	One or more dermatomes
CENTRAL CORD LESION, AS IN SYRINGOMYELIA	Loss of pain and temperature	One or more dermatomes
POSTERIOR COLUMN LESION	Loss of position, vibration sense, also stereognosis and two-point discrimination	Below level of lesion and on same side

TABLE 18-8 (CONT'D)

TABLE 18-8 (CONT'D)

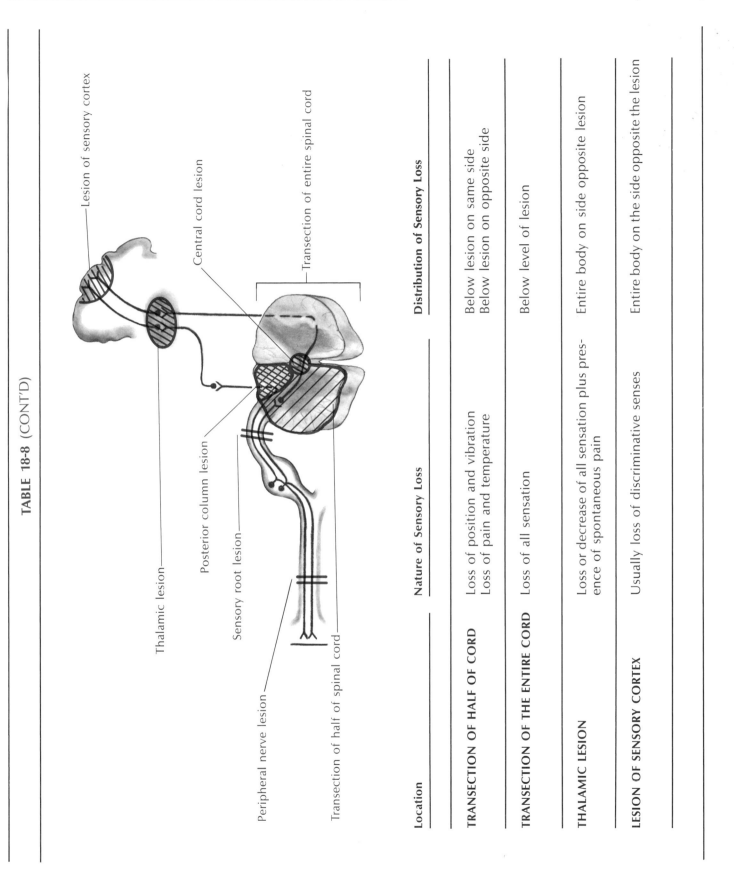

Location	Nature of Sensory Loss	Distribution of Sensory Loss
TRANSECTION OF HALF OF CORD	Loss of position and vibration Loss of pain and temperature	Below lesion on same side Below lesion on opposite side
TRANSECTION OF THE ENTIRE CORD	Loss of all sensation	Below level of lesion
THALAMIC LESION	Loss or decrease of all sensation plus presence of spontaneous pain	Entire body on side opposite lesion
LESION OF SENSORY CORTEX	Usually loss of discriminative senses	Entire body on the side opposite the lesion

TABLE 18-9

TABLE 18-9. ABNORMAL POSTURES IN THE COMATOSE PATIENT

HEMIPLEGIA (EARLY)

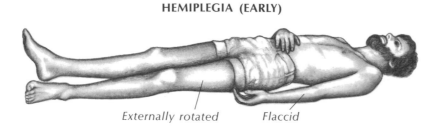

Externally rotated   *Flaccid*

Sudden unilateral brain damage involving the corticospinal tract may produce a hemiplegia or one-sided paralysis, which early in its course is flaccid. Spasticity will develop later. The paralyzed arm and leg are slack. They fall loosely and without tone when raised and dropped to the bed. Spontaneous movements or responses to noxious stimuli are limited to the opposite side. The leg may lie externally rotated. One side of the lower face may be paralyzed, and that cheek puffs out on expiration. Both eyes may be turned away from the paralyzed side.

DECORTICATE RIGIDITY

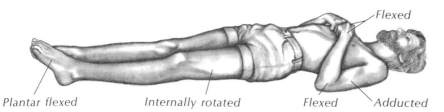
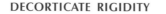

Plantar flexed   *Internally rotated*   *Flexed*   *Adducted*

In decorticate rigidity the upper arms are held tight to the sides with elbows, wrists and fingers flexed. The legs are extended and internally rotated. The feet are plantar flexed. This posture implies a destructive lesion of the corticospinal tracts within or very near the cerebral hemispheres. When unilateral, this is the posture of chronic spastic hemiplegia.

DECEREBRATE RIGIDITY

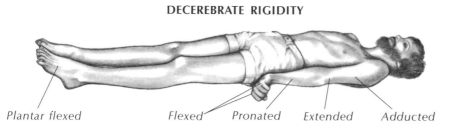

Plantar flexed   *Flexed* *Pronated*   *Extended*   *Adducted*

In decerebrate rigidity the jaws are clenched and the neck extended. The arms are adducted and stiffly extended at the elbows, with forearms pronated, wrists and fingers flexed. The legs are stiffly extended at the knees with the feet plantar flexed. This posture may occur spontaneously or only in response to external stimuli such as light, noise or pain. It is caused by a lesion in the diencephalon, midbrain or pons, although severe metabolic disorders such as hypoxia or hypoglycemia may also produce it.

mental status

TECHNIQUES OF EXAMINATION

During the course of the interview and examination, you will have made many observations relevant to the patient's mental status. This information may be sufficient for many patients; however, the presence of neurologic disease or the suspicion of emotional or intellectual dysfunction indicates further evaluation. Although the mental status examination is described separately in this chapter, much of it is best performed in the context of the medical interview. Mood and thought processes, for example, are usually best examined as the history unfolds. Assessment of memory, orientation and calculation can often be integrated into the history, thus avoiding for the patient the anxieties of a "test" situation. When further examination is necessary, simple introductory explanations should be offered.

Conduct your assessment of mental status with the same acceptance and respect for the patient that you show during other portions of the examination. At the same time, do not avoid possibly significant areas because of your own anxieties or fears of upsetting the patient.

Appearance and Behavior

Use here the observations made throughout the course of the history and examination, including:

Posture and Motor Behavior, e.g., the patient's ability to relax and his level and pattern of activity, together with their relationship to the topics under discussion or to other activities or people around him.

Dress, Grooming and Personal Hygiene. Include the style of dress and its appropriateness to the patient's age and situation.

EXAMPLES OF ABNORMALITIES

See **Table 19-1,** Manifestations of Common Mental Disorders (pp. 365–366).

Slumped posture, retarded movements of depression; restlessness, tense posture, tremors of anxiety; grimacing and mannerisms in schizophrenia

Parkinsonism and bizarre movements of head and neck in phenothiazine reactions

Unkempt appearance in depression and chronic organic brain disease; meticulous grooming of the compulsive personality

Facial Expression, including facial mobility, at rest and in interaction with others. Watch for variations with the topics under discussion.

Speech, including its:
    Quality, e.g., loudness, clarity, inflection
    Quantity, e.g., pace, volume
    Organization, e.g., coherence, relevance, circumstantiality

Manner, Mood and Relation to Persons and Things Around Him, together with variations according to the topics under discussion and to other activities or people around him. Note the patient's openness and approachability.

Mood

Assess the patient's mood, not only by observation as described above, but also by questioning. This is often best done during the interview when you can easily ask "How did (do) you feel about that?" Or more generally, "How are your spirits?" If you suspect depression, it is essential that you assess its depth and the associated risk of suicide. A series of questions like the following is useful, proceeding as far as the patient's positive answers warrant.
    Do you get pretty discouraged (or depressed or blue)?
    How low do you feel?
    What do you see for yourself in the future?
    Do you ever feel that life isn't worth living? Or that you had just as soon be dead?
    Have you ever thought of doing away with yourself?
    How did (do) you think you would do it?
    What would happen after you were dead?

Thought Processes and Perceptions

Coherency and Relevance of Thought Processes. Observation of the way in which the patient describes his history is most important here.

Thought Content. Much information about the patient's thought content has probably been revealed in the interview. Additional inquiries may be necessary, however, to ascertain specific symptoms. A stereotyped listing of questions should be avoided. Instead, if possible, put these questions in the context of the patient's history, following clues or leads provided by the patient's own words or ideas. For example:
    "What do you think about at times like these?"
    "Sometimes when people are upset like this, they can't keep certain thoughts out of their minds," or ". . . things seem unreal," etc.

Depression, anxiety, apathy, anger; facial immobility of Parkinsonism

Slow, monotonous tone of depression; pressure of speech, flight of ideas in manic conditions; incoherent circumstantial speech with neologisms (self-coined words) in schizophrenia

Uncooperativeness, evasiveness, hostility, anger, resentment, depression, tearfulness, elation, distrustfulness

Incoherent, disorganized thought in schizophrenia

In this manner, inquire about:

Compulsions—repetitive acts that the patient feels driven to do

Obsessions—recurrent, uncontrollable thoughts

Ruminations—repetitive or continuous thinking or speculations, often about abstract issues

Doubting and indecision—excessively time-consuming uncertainties about everyday decisions

Phobias—irrational fears

Free-floating anxieties—sense of ill-defined dread or impending doom

May be associated with neurotic disorders

Feelings of unreality—a sense that things in the environment are strange, unreal, remote

Feelings of depersonalization—a sense that one's self is different, changed, unreal, has lost identity

Feelings of persecution—a sense that the patient is disliked, persecuted, being plotted against

Feelings of influence—a sense that others are controlling or manipulating him

Feelings of reference—a sense that outside events, for example, radio, TV, are related to him, commenting about him, communicating with him

Delusions—false fixed beliefs

More often associated with psychotic disorders, e.g., schizophrenia

Perceptions. By a similar questioning process, inquire about:

Illusions—misinterpretations of sensory stimuli
Hallucinations—subjective sensory perceptions, independent of reality, usually auditory or visual, less commonly perceived as taste, smell or touch

Usually associated with psychotic disorders, e.g., schizophrenia, delirium

Cognitive Functions

Orientation.   By skillful questioning, the patient's orientation can often be determined in the context of the interview. For example, you can quite naturally ask the patient for specific dates or times and can inquire about the patient's address and names of his family. For some patients, more direct questions will be necessary. These can be introduced with a query such as "Do you get confused at times? For instance, what day is it to-day? . . ." In this manner determine the patient's orientation for:

1. *Time,* e.g., the time of day, the day of the week, month, date and year, duration of hospitalization

2. *Place,* e.g., of his residence, hospital, city, state

3. *Person,* e.g., his own name, the name of relatives and professional personnel

Attention and Concentration.   These include:

Digit Span.   Tell the patient that you would like to test his ability to concentrate, perhaps adding that people have trouble with that when they are in pain, or ill, or feverish, etc. Read a series of digits, starting with the shortest set and enunciating each number clearly at a rate of about 1 per second. Ask the patient to repeat them back to you. If the patient makes a mistake, give him a second try with a series of the same length. Stop after a second failure in a series of any given length. In choosing digits avoid consecutive numbers and numbers that form easily recognized dates.

5,2	5,3,8,7	3,6,7,9,5,2	9,4,7,2,5,6,1,8
9,3	2,1,7,9	4,1,5,3,7,9	3,5,8,1,4,9,7,6
6,1,7	4,7,2,9,3	7,2,4,8,3,5,9	6,1,9,8,2,5,4,3,7
8,4,1,	5,3,8,7,1	3,6,1,5,8,4,2	3,8,7,2,4,9,1,6,5

Poor performance of digit span is characteristic of organic brain disease (delirium and dementia). Performance is also limited by mental retardation.

Now, (starting again with the shortest series) ask the patient to repeat the digits to you backwards.

Normally a person should be able to repeat correctly at least five to eight digits forward and four to six backwards.

Serial 7's or Serial 3's.   Instruct the patient, "Starting from a hundred, subtract 7, and keep subtracting 7 . . ." Note the effort required and the speed and accuracy of the responses. (Writing down his answers helps you keep up with his arithmetic.) Normally, a person can complete serial 7's in 1½ minutes, with fewer than four errors. If the patient cannot do serial 7's, try serial 3's or ask him to count backward. Still easier tests are counting forward or reciting the alphabet.

Poor performance in organic brain disease, also mental retardation

Memory.   Most questions relevant to memory can be asked in the context of the interview. Include inquiries that test both:

Remote memory, e.g., birthdays, anniversaries

Recent memory, e.g., events of the day. Here it is helpful to ask questions the answers to which you can check against other sources. In addition, recent memory may conveniently be checked by giving the patient several words, for example, an object and an address. He should repeat them so that you know he heard and registered the information. Then proceed on to other parts of the examination, and after about 3 to 5 minutes ask him to repeat the words. Note the accuracy of this response, his awareness of whether he is correct and any tendency to confabulate (make up answers). Normally a person should be able to remember the words.

Poor recent memory in organic brain disease

Information.   Ask the patient questions such as the following:

1. How many days are there in a week?	**9.** Where does the sun set?
2. What must you do to water to make it boil?	**10.** Who invented the airplane?
3. How many things are there in a dozen?	**11.** Why does oil float on water?
4. Name the four seasons of the year?	**12.** What do we get turpentine from?
5. What do we celebrate on the 4th of July?	**13.** When is Labor Day?
6. How many pounds are there in a ton?	**14.** How far is it from New York to Chicago?
7. What does the stomach do?	**15.** What is an hieroglyphic?
8. What is the capital of Greece?	**16.** What is a barometer?
	17. Who wrote "Paradise Lost?"
	18. What is a prime number?
	19. What is Habeas Corpus?
	20. Who discovered the South Pole?

> Information is a good indicator of underlying intelligence. It is relatively unaffected by any but the most severe forms of psychiatric disorders.

Persons of average ability should be able to answer correctly from 8 to 13 of these questions. Take into consideration, however, the patient's cultural and educational background.

Vocabulary.   Ask the patient to give you the meaning of the following words or to use the word in a sentence.

1. Apple	**9.** Tint	**17.** Seclude
2. Donkey	**10.** Armory	**18.** Spangle
3. Diamond	**11.** Fable	**19.** Recede
4. Nuisance	**12.** Nitroglycerine	**20.** Affliction
5. Join	**13.** Microscope	**21.** Chattel
6. Fur	**14.** Stanza	**22.** Dilatory
7. Shilling	**15.** Guillotine	**23.** Flout
8. Bacon	**16.** Plural	**24.** Amanuensis

> Vocabulary is probably the best indicator of underlying intelligence. It is relatively unaffected by any but the most severe psychiatric disorders.

Persons of average intellectual ability should be able to define or use from 8 to 16 of these words. Again, keep in mind the patient's cultural and educational background.

Abstract Reasoning.   The capacity to reason abstractly is tested two ways:

Proverbs.   Ask the patient what people mean when they use some of the following proverbs.
1. A stitch in time saves nine.
2. Don't count your chickens before they're hatched.
3. The proof of the pudding is in the eating.
4. A rolling stone gathers no moss.
5. The squeaking wheel gets the grease.

> Patients with schizophrenia or organic brain disorders may often give concrete responses. Patients with low intelligence or little education may also give concrete responses or no response at all.

Note the relevance of the answers and their degree of concreteness or abstractness. (Techniques continue on p. 366).

TABLE 19-1

TABLE 19-1. MANIFESTATIONS OF COMMON MENTAL DISORDERS*

| | ORGANIC BRAIN DISORDERS | | MENTAL DEFICIENCY |
	ACUTE (DELIRIUM)	CHRONIC (DEMENTIA)	
Appearance and Behavior	Fluctuating impairment of consciousness, restlessness	May show deterioration of personal habits	
Mood	Anxiety, fear, lability	Irritability, lability	
Thought Processes and Perceptions			
Coherency and relevance	May be confused, incoherent	May become confused	
Thought content	May have delusions		
Perceptions	May have illusions, hallucinations		
Cognitive Functions			
Orientation	May be disoriented	May be disoriented	Depends on severity of deficiency
Attention and concentration	Poor	Poor	Limited
Memory: Recent **Memory: Remote**	Poor May become poor	Poor May become poor	May be poor May be poor
Information **Vocabulary**	Preserved until late Preserved until late	Preserved until late Preserved until late	Limited Limited
Abstract reasoning	Concrete	Concrete	Concrete
Judgment	Poor	Poor	May be poor
Perception and coordination	May be poor	May be poor	May be poor

*Key abnormalities in differential diagnosis are printed in red.

TABLE 19-1 (CONT'D)

TABLE 19.1. (CONT'D)

FUNCTIONAL PSYCHOSES			PSYCHONEUROTIC DISORDERS
AFFECTIVE		SCHIZOPHRENIA	
MANIC	DEPRESSIVE		
Hyperactive, elated, assertive, boistrous, with rapid emphatic speech; may become suddenly angry or argumentative	Dejected, slowed, slumped, troubled	Variable	Variable
Elation, sometimes anger and irritability	Depression, hopelessness	Blandness, impoverishment or inappropriateness of affect	Depression in neurotic depressive reaction
Rapid association of ideas which may seem illogical		Often incoherent, disorganized	
May have delusions and feelings of persecution	May have delusions, often involving guilt, self-depreciation, somatic complaints	May have feelings of unreality, depersonalization, persecution, influence and reference; delusions which are bizarre and symbolic	May have compulsions, obsessions, ruminations, indecisiveness, phobias, anxieties
May have illusions, rarely hallucinations	May have illusions, rarely hallucinations	May have hallucinations and illusions, often bizarre and symbolic	
Well-oriented	Well-oriented	Usually but not always well-oriented	
Distractable		Usually well-preserved but may be difficult to test because of inattentiveness and indifference	
		May be bizarre	

Similarities. Ask the patient to tell you how the following are alike:

1. An orange and an apple
2. A cat and a mouse
3. A child and a dwarf
4. A church and a theater
5. A piano and a violin
6. Paper and coal

Note the accuracy and relevance of the answers and their degree of concreteness or abstractness.

Patients with schizophrenia or organic brain disease often give concrete responses.

Judgment. Assess this characteristic by noting the patient's judgment with respect to his present life situation. In addition, the following questions may help evaluate his judgment and comprehension of other circumstances.

1. What should you do if you are stopped for speeding?
2. What should you do if you lose a library book?
3. What should you do if you see a train approaching a broken track?
4. Why is it better to give to an organized charity than to a street beggar?
5. Why are criminals put in prison?

Judgment may be poor in organic brain disease, mental retardation, psychotic states.

Sensory Perception and Coordination. Ask the patient to write his name on a page of blank paper. Then ask him to copy some simple figures drawn by the examiner on the page, including:

A circle   A cross   A square   A diamond   A row of dots

Poor performance suggests a problem in the perceptual, motor or intellectual processes and may be seen in organic brain disease or mental deficiency.

CHAPTER 20

the pediatric physical examination

by Robert A. Hoekelman, M.D.

INTRODUCTION

The anatomy and physiology, the techniques of examination and the normal and abnormal findings presented in the foregoing sections of this book concern themselves primarily with the adult patient. Most of what is presented is also applicable to infants and children. Children, however, in the process of development are anatomically and physiologically unique. Consequently, many of the techniques of examination, the physical findings and their significance are altered in pediatric patients.

The purpose of this section is to describe how to conduct those parts of the physical examination of infants and children that require different approaches and techniques from those used for the physical examination of adults. No attempt will be made in this section to discuss or describe findings other than the normal, variations of normal and those accompanying common pathologic conditions of infancy and childhood. Uncommon pathologic conditions will not be presented except for those few which require specific examination techniques for detection. The reader should consult the texts listed in the bibliography for complete differential diagnoses of abnormal physical findings. (Because treatment of individual organ systems here is brief, sections on techniques of examination are set off in boldface rather than presented separately as in the earlier chapters.)

In the physical assessment of a child, the examiner must consider where his patient is on the continuum of growth and development, as well as the age range that may normally exist in reaching that point. Finally, he must reflect upon the different rates of growth of the various systems of the body. For example, growth and development of the central nervous system, the lymphatic system and the reproductive system parallel neither general somatic growth nor each other. The figure at the right illustrates these differences.

Thus a physical finding such as a Babinski response is abnormal beyond the age of two years, but may be found in normal subjects prior to that age. It is essential, therefore, that the examiner of infants and children be well ac-

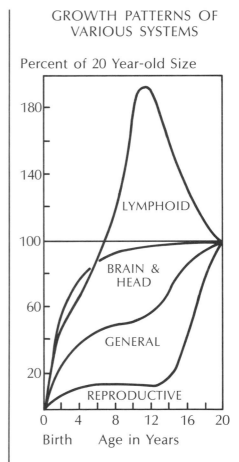

GROWTH PATTERNS OF VARIOUS SYSTEMS

Percent of 20 Year-old Size

quainted with the normal and abnormal patterns of growth and development. The scope of this text does not allow for inclusion of this information in any sequential form, nor for description of the systematic methods of testing developmental levels. Texts dealing with this information are also listed in the bibliography for the reader's use.

In this discussion of each part of the physical examination, beginning with the approach to the patient, it will be useful to consider three developmental levels: infancy (the first year); early childhood (one year through five years) and late childhood (six years and over).

APPROACH TO THE PATIENT

Infancy

The newborn should be examined briefly, immediately after birth, to determine the general condition of his cardiorespiratory, neurologic and gastrointestinal systems and to detect any gross congenital abnormalities. The infant's immediate adaptation to extrauterine life is assessed with a set of five clinical signs developed by Dr. Virginia Apgar, each scored on a 3-point scale (0, 1 or 2). The Apgar scores may range from zero to 10, using the method of scoring shown in Table 20-1. Each infant should be scored at 1 minute and 5 minutes following birth. If, at 5 minutes, the Apgar score is 8 or more a more complete examination can then be conducted.

One minute scores of 7 or less usually indicate nervous system depression. Scores of 4 or less indicate severe depression requiring immediate resuscitation.

TABLE 20-1. THE APGAR SCORING SYSTEM

Clinical Sign	Assigned Score		
	0	1	2
Heart Rate	Absent	<100	>100
Respiratory Effort	Absent	Slow and irregular	Good and crying
Muscle Tone	Flaccid	Some flexion of the arms and legs	Active movement
Reflex Irritability*	No responses	Crying	Crying vigorously
Color	Blue, pale	Pink body, blue extremities	Pink all over

*Reaction to insertion of a soft rubber catheter into the external nares

The examination should include auscultation of the anterior thorax, palpation of the abdomen, and inspection of the head, face, oral cavity, extremities and perineum. A small tube should be passed through the nose, nasopharynx and esophagus into the stomach to establish their patency. Presence of the tube in the stomach can be determined by palpation of the tip itself or by palpation or auscultation of the upper abdomen while a small amount of air is blown through the tube. Gastric contents should be aspirated in premature babies and babies born by cesarian section in order to prevent regurgitation and aspiration.

Failure to pass the tube through the nasopharynx suggests posterior nasal (choanal) atresia. Failure to pass the tube into the stomach suggests esophageal atresia usually with an associated tracheoesophageal fistula.

A more extensive examination of the newborn should be conducted within 12 hours of birth and again at approximately 72 hours of age, when the effects of anesthesia and shock of birth have subsided.

The baby should first be observed lying undisturbed in his bassinet and, then, completely undressed on an examining table.

Best results, in terms of responsiveness, are obtained 2 or 3 hours after a feeding.

The baby's cry, color, size, body proportions, nutritional status and posture should be observed as well as the respirations and movements of the head and extremities.

Normal newborns lie in a symmetrical position with the limbs semiflexed and the legs partially abducted at the hip. The head is slightly flexed and positioned in the midline or turned to one side. In normal newborns, there is spontaneous motor activity of flexion and extension alternating between the arms and legs. The forearms supinate with flexion at the elbow and pronate with extension. The fingers are usually flexed in a tight fist, but may be seen to extend in a slow athetoid posturing movement. Low amplitude, high frequency tremors of the arms, legs and body are seen with vigorous crying and even at rest during the first 48 hours of life.

In breech babies, the legs and head are extended, and the legs of a *frank* breech baby are abducted and externally rotated.

Most newborn infants are cooperative during the examination unless it is close to feeding time.

Nevertheless, auscultation of the heart and lungs and palpation of the abdomen should be accomplished when the baby is quiet, since these are more difficult to perform if the baby is crying. A sugar nipple, a bottle of formula or the tip of the examiner's finger placed in the mouth usually silences a crying baby long enough to complete these portions of the examination.

By 4 days after birth, however, tremors occurring at rest signal central nervous system disease. Asymmetrical movements of the arms or legs at any time should alert the examiner to the possibility of central or peripheral neurologic deficit, birth injuries or congenital anomalies.

Beyond this, the order of examination is of little importance except that hip abduction should be performed at the end, since this usually causes the baby to cry.

After the newborn period, throughout the rest of infancy, little difficulty should be encountered in the performance of the complete physical examination. The key to success is distraction, since infants seem to be able to attend to only one thing at a time. It is relatively easy to bring the baby's attention effectively to something other than the examination being performed.

A moving object, a light, a game of peek-a-boo, tickling or producing a variety of noises are a few of the distractions an examiner can use successfully.

Infants usually do not object to removal of their clothing. Indeed, most seem to prefer the nude state, perhaps because it allows for greater tactile stimulation. It is wise, however, to leave the diaper in place, removing it only to examine the genitalia, rectum, lower spine and hips.

Much of the examination can be performed with the infant lying or sitting in the mother's lap or held in an upright position against her breast, although this is usually not necessary except with tired, hungry or acutely ill patients.

Occasionally, almost the entire physical examination can be completed without waking a sleeping infant.

Observation of the mother-infant interaction is important. The mother's affect in talking about her infant, the manner in which she holds, moves and dresses the baby and her response to situations which may produce discomfort for her child should be noted. Breast or bottle feeding should be observed.

This may give some indication of maladaptive mothering patterns.

These observations are important in assessing malnutrition, colic, chronic regurgitation and suspected maternal deprivation.

In older infants, testing of developmental milestones such as the ability to reach for a toy, transfer a cube from one hand to the other and use of the pincer grasp in picking up a small object should be done prior to performing the general physical examination.

Early Childhood

One of the most difficult challenges facing the professional who cares for children in this age group is completing the examination without producing a physical struggle, a crying child or a distraught parent. When this is accomplished successfully, it provides a great measure of satisfaction to all involved and comes as close to "art" in practice as any other pursuit.

Gaining the child's confidence and dispersing his or her fears begins at the moment of encounter and continues throughout the entire visit. The approach may vary with the place and circumstances of the visit; however, a well-child visit will allow greater development of rapport than a visit of a child when he or she is acutely ill at home or in the hospital emergency room.

During the interview, the child should remain dressed in most instances. This may prolong the visit time, but avoids apprehension on the child's part and affords the opportunity later to observe his response to being undressed or his ability to undress himself. Children are also more apt to play quietly and interact with the mother and examiner more appropriately if fully clothed.

The child should be engaged in conversation appropriate to his age and should be asked simple questions concerning his health or illness. Making complimentary remarks about the child's appearance, dress or performance, telling a story or playing a simple trick may help to "break the ice."

This dialogue will indicate the child's level of receptive and expressive function and will give direction for approach by the examiner.

If the child responds to conversation and questions directed to him with silence, shielding of the eyes or signs of apprehension, it is wise to ignore him temporarily.

Observations during the interview should include a general assessment of degree of sickness or wellness, mood, state of nutrition, speech, cry, respiratory pattern, facial expression, apparent chronological and emotional age, posture (particularly as it may reflect discomfort) and developmental skills. In addition, parent-child interaction should be closely observed, including the amount of separation tolerated, displays of affection and response to discipline.

Abusing parents pay little or no attention to their abused child, treating him or her more like a piece of property than a person. By the same token, an abused child demonstrates no separation anxiety when physically and environmentally removed from the parents.

Specific developmental testing, such as building towers with blocks, playing ball with the examiner and performing hop, skip and jump maneuvers, is best accomplished at the end of the interview, just prior to the formal physical examination. This "fun and games" interlude more than likely will improve the child's view of the examiner and his behavior at the time of the examination.

The actual performance of the physical examination, with certain exceptions, need not take place on an examining table. In fact, some parts of the examination can best be accomplished with the child standing, sitting on the mother's lap or even sitting on the physician's lap. It is also not essential that the child be completely undressed throughout the course of the examination; often exposing only the part of the body being examined will suffice and most likely avert objection by the child. Occasionally, a child's reluctance to undress stems from the coolness of the examining room and the coldness of the examining table and instruments (including the examiner's hands) rather than from apprehension or modesty. When there are two or more siblings to be examined, it is wise to begin with the oldest, who is most likely to be cooperative and set a good example for the younger children.

Actually, only a few children resist undressing. Most will allow themselves to be stripped to their underpants and placed upon the examining table in a sitting position without objection.

During the examination, the mother should stand at the head of the examining table to the left of the examiner, who is facing the table, and to the right of the child. Again, as with the infant, distraction is the key to gaining the patient's cooperation. The child in this age group, however, is not as easily distracted as the infant; therefore, the examiner should approach the patient pleasantly and, whenever possible, explain each step of the examination prior to performing it. Demonstration of the procedure on the examiner himself or on a doll or toy animal is also very helpful to the child in gaining understanding of what is to be done. For example, the otoscope can be placed in the examiner's ear, the light flashed into his open mouth or the stethoscope placed on his chest. Allowing the child to play with the examining instruments prior to their utilization also creates an atmosphere of trust. Playing at blowing out the examining light or using the stethoscope bell as a telephone can be used as attractive diversions.

The initial "laying on of the hands" is the most crucial point of the examination, and if resistance is to be encountered, it will most likely be here. Therefore, the first contact should be in non-vulnerable areas.

Holding the patient's hand, counting his fingers and palpating his wrist and elbow while talking to him gently is most apt to meet with success.

Having both of the examiner's hands in contact with the patient's body whenever possible has a comforting effect on the patient and is less apt to produce involuntary withdrawal than will the use of one hand or a few probing fingers.

For example, when examining the heart, the left hand can be placed on the patient's right shoulder while the examiner's right hand makes contact with the chest wall in holding the stethoscope.

In a sense, the left hand acts as both a distracting and comforting force. The examiner who moves in an unhesitating, firm and graceful manner and who talks with a friendly, pleasant, reassuring voice throughout the examination is not apt to provoke apprehension.

A firm tone of voice and unequivocal instructions should be used when the child is asked to perform certain acts pertaining to the examination. He should be told what to do rather than asked to do it. For example, "Roll over on your belly" rather than "Will you roll over on your belly for me?"

Some children will cease to resist when spoken to sharply, but more than likely this will produce increased resistance. Often the child will sit or lie passively on the examining table, covering both eyes with his hands, for, to his way of thinking, if he cannot see the examiner, the examiner cannot see him. This posture can certainly be tolerated, since it does not interfere with the examination. The eyes in this instance are easily examined after the child has dressed.

The order of examination is based on performing the least distressing procedures first and the most distressing last. Thus, those parts of the examination which can be performed in the sitting position—for example, palpation, percussion and auscultation of the heart and lungs—are performed prior to placing the child in the supine position. Since lying down may make the child feel more vulnerable and provoke resistance to further examination, it should be accomplished with great care. Often supporting the head and back with the examiner's arm and moving down with the child averts apprehension. In the supine position, the abdomen should be examined first, the throat and ears next to last and the genitalia and rectum last. Examination of the genitalia and perineum, when a rectal examination is not performed, is usually less disturbing to the child than is the examination of the throat. However, to heed the mother's fastidious and perhaps modest nature, it is left to last.

The child's comfort should be paramount in conducting the examination. Immediately before an examination maneuver, he or she should be told kindly, but matter-of-factly, of the likelihood of pain or other unpleasant sensations that might result from that maneuver. In instances where the child is extremely apprehensive about one portion of the examination, i.e., the examination of the throat, it is helpful to do this first. Indeed, it may be necessary to complete the entire physical examination before obtaining the history to ensure a reasonable interview. Distasteful portions of the examination should be accomplished quickly so as to minimize the child's discomfort. However, the examiner should remember that the physical examination is designed to gather essential information, and the child's comfort may need to be sacrificed to some extent to achieve this end. A completed examination is a comfort and reassurance to the parent and examiner, while an incomplete examination is a frustration and a source of dissatisfaction to both.

On overly anxious patients

Obviously, there will be instances where resistance to the examination will be encountered. Some children will scream and yell throughout the examination, but offer no physical resistance. Most, however, will fight the examination and strive to gain an upright position and the comfort and security of mother's arms. The mother can be helpful here in verbally reassuring her child and in actually restraining the child's movements for certain portions of the examination. It is sometimes necessary to ask the mother to leave the room because she is overly sympathetic and ineffective in calming the child. Surprisingly, she may be happy to leave, but if she is asked to and refuses, the examiner should obtain the assistance of another neutral person to aid in restraining the child and make the best of it.

Rarely, for the child's sake or the mother's, it is necessary to discontinue the examination before it is completed and return to it another time.

The utilization of another person in addition to the mother to restrain the child is often helpful under ordinary circumstances; however, using mummy restraints, or other kinds of restraints has no place in the physical examination procedure.

The examiner should not convey feelings of frustration or anger, but should reassure the mother that the child's resistance is not unexpected. Her embarrassment may lead to her compounding the problem by scolding the child. Some mothers feel that when their child is uncooperative while being examined, the examiner is at fault. Others feel that such resistance is a reflection of the child's level of development of independence.

If this resistance is inappropriate for the child's age, then the examiner should consider the possibility of underlying developmental or emotional difficulties.

The neophyte examiner is apt to be less successful in examining very young children than in examining other age groups. However, with practice, perseverance and patience, he should succeed. It is difficult to teach "how to approach a reluctant child." Each examiner must learn which techniques work best for him and which approach he finds most comfortable.

Late Childhood

There is usually little difficulty in examining most children after they reach school age. Some, however, may have unpleasant memories of previous encounters with examiners and offer resistance.

The child should be questioned to determine his orientation to time and place, his factual knowledge and his language and number skills. Intelligence screening tests such as the Goodenough draw-a-man, the Durrell and the Bender may be used when there is some element of doubt concerning the child's intellectual capacity. These tests should be kept to a minimum, however, to avoid familiarity-of-content errors should formal psychological testing be necessary. Motor skills involved in writing, tying shoelaces, buttoning shirt fronts and using scissors are easily observed. Right-left discrimination for self (attained at age 6 or 7 years) and for the examiner (attained at age 8 or 9 years) is determined simply.

Modesty on the child's part may be the greatest deterrent to a successful examination. Therefore, girls, as early as age 6 or 7, should be gowned. Underpants in both boys and girls, even if the lower half of the body is draped, should be left on until their removal is required. It is usually wise for examiners who are of the opposite sex from their preadolescent and adolescent patients to leave the room while the latter disrobe. Younger children often request that siblings of the opposite sex depart and older boys frequently prefer that their mothers leave during the examination.

The order of examination in late childhood can follow that used in adults.

But it is always important at any age to withhold examination of painful areas until last.

THE GENERAL SURVEY

The rewards of careful and continuous observation have already been discussed, as well as the importance of noting general physical and behavioral signs. This section will cover the measurement of vital signs and body size, which is of particular importance in infants and children since deviations from the normal in this regard are apt to be the first and often the only indicators of the presence of disease.

For example, maternal deprivation, chronic renal disease and hyperthyroidism

Temperature

For all practical purposes, rectal temperatures should be used exclusively in pediatric patients because accurate oral temperature readings are difficult to obtain even in children over 10 years of age. In premature infants, axillary temperatures are satisfactory for close monitoring of temperature regulation.

The technique of obtaining the rectal temperature is relatively simple. In most instances, the infant or child lies prone on the examining table or his mother's lap, while the examiner separates the buttocks with the thumb and forefinger of one hand and, with the other hand, gently inserts a well-lubricated rectal thermometer, inclined approximately 20 degrees toward the table, through the anal sphincter approximately one inch into the rectum. One method for holding a child while obtaining the rectal temperature is demonstrated in the illustration on the right.

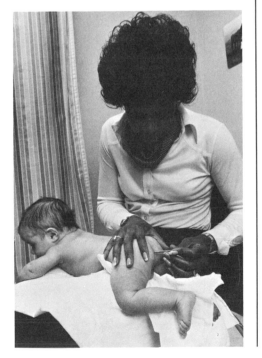

Temperature regulation in infants and children is less well controlled than in adults. The average rectal temperature is higher in infancy and early childhood, usually not falling below 99.0°F (37.2°C) until after the third year. At 18 months, 50 percent of children will have mean rectal temperatures of 100°F (37.8°C) or higher. Ranges in body temperature in individual children may be as much as 3 or more degrees Fahrenheit during the course of a single day. Rectal temperature recordings may approach 101°F, (38.3°C) in normal children, particularly in late afternoon after a full day of activity.

Pulse

The heart rate in infants and children is quite labile and more sensitive to the effects of illness, exercise and emotion than in adults. The average heart rates for pediatric patients, according to age, is shown in Table 20-2.

The heart rate may be obtained in infants by observing the pulsations of the anterior fontanelle, by palpating the carotid or the femoral arteries, or by directly auscultating the heart if the rate is very rapid. Palpation of the radial artery at the wrist may be used in older children and during early childhood with cooperative patients.

TABLE 20-2. AVERAGE HEART RATE OF INFANTS AND CHILDREN AT REST

Age	Average Rate	Two-standard Deviations
Birth	140	50
1st 6 months	130	50
6–12 months	115	40
1–2 years	110	40
2–6 years	103	35
6–10 years	95	30
10–14 years	95	30

Respiratory Rate

As with the heart rate, the respiratory rate in infants and children has a greater range and is more responsive to illness, exercise and emotion than in adults. The respiratory rate per minute ranges between 30 and 80 in the newborn, 20 and 40 during early childhood, and 15 and 25 during late childhood, reaching adult levels at age 15 years.

The respiratory rate may vary appreciably from moment to moment in premature and full-term newborn infants, with periods of rapid breathing alternating with spells of apnea. Therefore, the respiratory pattern in these circumstances should be observed for more than the usual 30 to 60 seconds to determine the true rate.

Anxiety may elevate the body temperature as witnessed by the frequency with which elevated temperatures are found on elective hospital admissions in children.

In the face of overwhelming infection, the temperature in infants may be normal or subnormal. On the other hand, during early childhood, extremely high temperature recordings (103° to 105°F, 39.5° to 40.5°C) are not uncommon, even with minor infections.

Beyond the neonatal period, a pulse greater than 180 usually indicates paroxysmal auricular tachycardia.

Respiratory rates which exceed 100 per minute are usually seen in diseases associated with lower respiratory tract obstruction, for example, bronchiolitis and bronchial asthma.

Apnea of greater than 20 seconds duration is seen in both premature infants and seemingly healthy newborns. These infants may be at risk for Sudden Infant Death Syndrome (SIDS).

In infancy and early childhood, diaphragmatic breathing is predominant and thoracic excursion is minimal; therefore, the respiratory rate is more easily ascertained by observing abdominal rather than chest excursions. Auscultation of the chest or placement of the stethoscope in front of the mouth and external nares are also useful methods of counting respirations in this age group. In older children, direct observation or palpation of thoracic movement may be used to determine the respiratory rate.

Blood Pressure

The level of systolic blood pressure climbs gradually throughout infancy and childhood. Normal systolic pressures are in the range of 50 m Hg at birth, 60 at 1 month, 70 at 6 months, 95 at 1 year, 100 at 6 years, 110 at 10 years and 120 at 16 years. The values for infants represent pressures obtained by utilizing the flush method (see description following). The diastolic pressure reaches 60 m Hg at 1 year of age and gradually increases throughout childhood to approximately 75.

Measurement of the blood pressure in infants and children is more often than not omitted from the physical examination because it has been erroneously judged to be too difficult to obtain. However, when the procedure is explained and demonstrated beforehand, most children beyond the age of 3 years are fascinated by the sphygmomanometer and are very cooperative.

Variations of blood pressure levels in normal individuals are brought on by exercise, crying and emotional upset. Because children may be anxious over the entire physical examination procedure as well as the blood pressure procedure per se, some prefer to obtain the blood pressure near the end of the pediatric examination. Others will repeat the determination at the end of the formal examination if the initial pressure was high. In anxious children with elevated blood pressure levels on repeated examinations over time, a sedative can be prescribed to allay apprehension, since most sedatives have no primary effect on the blood pressure.

Anxiety may produce elevated systolic blood pressure readings.

The use of the sphygmomanometer in determining blood pressures of children is similar to its use in adults. The width of the cuff should be one-half to two-thirds the width of the upper arm or leg, and the rubber bag should entirely encircle the extremity. A narrower cuff will elevate the pressure reading, while a wider cuff, although probably having no effect on the pressure reading, does interfere with the technique of the procedure by partially covering the brachial artery as it traverses the antecubital space. The muffling of the sound of the heart beat, used to signal the diastolic pressure in adults, is often absent in children, and the point at which the sounds disappear is recorded as the diastolic pressure. At times, especially in early childhood, the heart sounds are not audible due to a narrow or deeply placed brachial artery; in such instances, palpation of the radial artery at the wrist must be used to determine the blood pressure. The point

at which the pulse is first felt is recorded as the systolic pressure. This is approximately 10 m Hg lower than the systolic pressure determined by auscultatory means. The diastolic pressure cannot be determined by means of the radial pulse method.

In infants and very young children, smallness of the extremity and lack of cooperation preclude the use of auscultatory and palpation techniques to determine the blood pressure. However, a value lying somewhere between the systolic and diastolic pressures can be obtained by utilizing the flush technique.

With the cuff in place, an elastic bandage is wrapped around the elevated arm, proceeding from the fingers to the antecubital space and essentially emptying the capillary and venous network. The cuff is then inflated to a pressure above the expected systolic reading, the bandage is removed and the pallid arm is placed at the patient's side. The pressure is allowed to fall slowly until the sudden flush of normal color returning to the forearm, hand and fingers is observed. The endpoint is strikingly clear. This method may be used in the leg with equally good results.

For infants and young children a specific cause of hypertension can usually be determined. In older children and adolescents, however, the etiology may be obscure and in many instances observed elevated blood pressure may be a developmental phenomenon that disappears over time.

Children who demonstrate hypertension without apparent cause should be monitored on a long-term basis using percentile charts as shown below. Patients with blood pressure levels sustained above the 95th percentile should have extensive evaluations performed.

Renal disease (78 percent), renal arterial disease (12 percent), coarctation of the aorta (2 percent) and pheochromocytoma (0.5 percent) are the most common causes of hypertension in children.

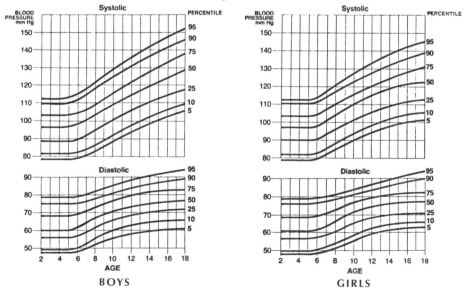

BOYS   **GIRLS**

Percentiles of blood pressure measurement in boys and girls (right arm, seated).
Reproduced with permission from the Report of the Task Force on Blood Pressure Control in Children of the National Heart, Lung and Blood Institute. *Pediatrics* 59:797–820 (Supplement) 1977.

Somatic Growth

Growth, as reflected in increases in body weight, length and girth along expected pathways and within certain limits, is probably the best indicator of health. The significance of any measure is determined by relating it to prior measurements of the same dimension, to mean values and standard deviations for that dimension as it occurs in other individuals and to measures of other dimensions in the same patient. Measures of somatic growth in infants and children, therefore, should be plotted on standard growth charts so they can be seen in these relationships.

Height. Measurement of the body length in infants is accomplished in the supine position by use of a measuring board or tray, as illustrated. If these are not available, the length should be determined by measuring the distance between marks made on the examining table paper indicating the crown and the heel of the infant. Direct measurement of the infant with a tape is inaccurate unless accomplished with an assistant holding the baby still with the legs extended. Height in older children is best measured by the child standing with his heels, back and head against the wall marked with a centimeter or inch rule. A small board held flat against the top of the child's head and at right angles to the rule is all that is required to complete the measure.

Measurements of height and weight above the ninety-seventh percentile or below the third percentile may indicate a growth disturbance and require investigation.

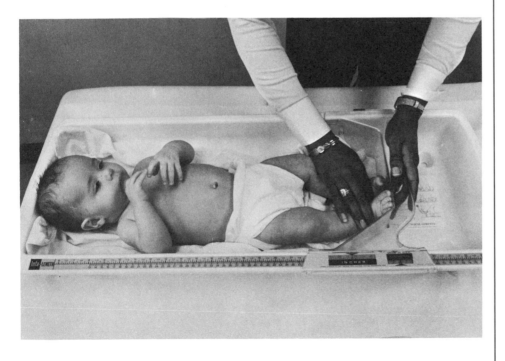

Weighing scales equipped with a height measure are not as satisfactory since children are not as likely to stand erect when not against a wall and many younger children are fearful of standing on the scale's slightly raised, unsteady base.

Weight.   Infants should be weighed directly with an infant scale, rather than indirectly by being held and weighed along with the holder. All clothing should be removed except for underpants in children beyond infancy and dressing gowns provided for girls in late childhood. Balance rather than spring scales should be used, and whenever possible the child should be weighed on the same scale at each visit.

Head Circumference.   The head circumference should be determined at every physical examination during the first 2 years of life, at least biennially thereafter, and at any initial examination at whatever age, to determine the rate of growth and absolute growth of the head.

A cloth or soft, plastic centimeter tape is preferred for this procedure, but disposable paper tapes are satisfactory.

The tape is placed over the occipital, parietal and frontal prominences so as to obtain the greatest circumference. During infancy and early childhood, this is best done with the patient supine.

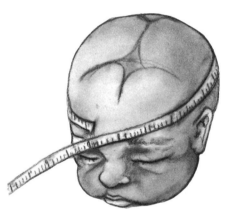

The measurement of the head circumference reflects the rate of growth of the cranium and its contents.

Chest Circumference.   This measure is obtained with the patient supine.

The tape is passed around the thorax at the level of the nipples and the measurement is taken midway between inspiration and expiration.

The chest circumference and the abdominal circumference (obtained similarly with the tape at the level of the umbilicus) are often referred to in pediatric speech, but in fact are of little value. The chest circumference, however, is sometimes used as a comparative measure for head size in that the circumference of the head is supposed to exceed that of the chest until age 2 years and be smaller than the circumference of the chest thereafter.

If growth is delayed, premature closure of the sutures or microcephaly should be considered. When growth is too rapid, hydrocephalus, subdural hematoma or brain tumor should be suspected.

THE SKIN

Infancy

The skin of the newborn infant has many unique characteristics. The texture is soft and smooth. An erythematous flush, giving the entire surface of the skin the appearance of a "boiled lobster," is present during the first 8 to 24 hours, after which the normal pale pink coloring predominates. Vasomotor changes in the subcutaneous tissue, as a response to cooling, produces a mottled appearance, particularly on the trunk, arms and legs. In normal newborns, a harlequin color change is often seen with one side of the body being red, the other pale and an abrupt line of demarcation at the midline. This phenomenon is transient and of unknown etiology. Blueness of the hands and feet (*acrocyanosis*) is present at birth and remains for several days. It may recur throughout early infancy under chilling conditions. After 4 or 5 hours, the cyanosis in the hands becomes less marked than in the feet.

This marbled, or dappled, reticular pattern is especially prominent in premature infants and cretins and in infants with Down's syndrome.

Melanotic pigmentation of the skin is not intense in most black newborns, with the exception of the nailbeds and the skin of the scrotum. Ill-defined blackish-blue areas located over the buttocks and lower lumbar regions are often seen, especially in black, American Indian and oriental babies. These areas are called *Mongolian spots* and are due to the presence of pigmented cells in the deeper layers of the skin. The spots become less noticeable as the pigment in the overlying cells becomes more prominent and eventually disappear in early childhood. There is a fine, downy growth of hair called *lanugo* over the entire body, but mostly on the shoulders and back. The amount and length vary from baby to baby, being usually prominent in prematures. Most of this hair is shed within 2 weeks. The amount of hair on the head of a newborn varies considerably, being absent entirely in some and abundant in others. All of the original hair is shed within a few months and replaced with a new crop sometimes of a different color.

If acrocyanosis does not disappear within 8 hours, cyanotic congenital heart disease should be suspected.

Generalized pallor indicates either anoxia, in which case the pulse will be slowed, or severe anemia, in which case the pulse will be very rapid.

Desquamation of the skin may be present normally at birth, varying in degree from a scattered flakiness to complete shedding of entire areas in large sheets of cornified epidermis. Also, a cheesy-white material, composed of sebum and desquamated epithelial cells and called *vernix caseosa*, is seen to cover the body in varying degrees at birth. It is always present in the vaginal labial folds and under the fingernails. A certain amount of puffiness and edema, even to the point of pitting over the hands, feet, lower legs, pubis and sacrum may be normally present, but usually disappears by the second or third day.

Normal "physiologic" jaundice which occurs in approximately 50 percent of all babies appears on the second or third day and usually disappears within a week, but may persist for as long as a month.

Natural daylight is preferred to artificial light when evaluating for the

In general, jaundice which appears within 24 hours of birth should alert one to the possible presence of hemolytic disease, and jaundice which appears or persists beyond 2 weeks of age should raise suspicions of biliary obstruction. Jaundice may indicate severe infection at any time in infancy, particularly in the newborn period.

presence of jaundice at any age. In borderline cases, pressing a glass slide against the infant's cheek will help to detect the presence of jaundice by producing a blanched background for contrast.

Older infants who are fed yellow vegetables (carrots, sweet potatoes and squash) may develop a pale yellow-orange color to the skin, which is some-times mistaken for jaundice. However, the pigmentation in this condition, called *carotenemia*, is limited to the palms, soles, nose and nasolabial folds.

Three dermatologic conditions are seen in newborns with enough frequency to deserve description. *Milia*, pinheadsized, smooth, white raised areas without surrounding erythema on the nose, chin and forehead, are caused by retention of sebum in the openings of the sebaceous glands. These areas may be present at birth, but more often appear within the first few weeks of life and disappear spontaneously over the course of several weeks. *Miliaria Rubra* consists of scattered vesicles on an erythematous base, usually on the face and trunk, caused by obstruction to the ducts of the sweat glands. *Erythema toxicum,* which usually appears on the second or third day of life, consists of erythematous macules with central urticarial wheals or vesicles scattered diffusely over the entire body, appearing much like flea bites. Eosinophiles may be seen on smear of the vesicular fluid. The cause is unknown and the lesions disappear spontaneously within a week.

Irregularly shaped reddened areas are frequently found over the occiput and on the upper eyelids, the forehead and the upper lip. The redness is due to proliferation of the capillary bed of the skin. These lesions are variously called *capillary hemangioma, nevus flammeus, nevus vasculosus and telangiectatic nevus.* They invariably disappear at about a year of age, although they may occasionally reappear, even in adulthood, when the skin is seen to flush in anger or embarrassment.

A lighted magnifying glass is useful in examining the ridges on the palms of the hands formed by the raised apertures of the sweat glands.

The patterns formed, called *dermatoglyphics,* are often helpful in diagnosing certain chromosomal defects. Finger and hand prints are usually used to study dermatoglyphic patterns at length.

Characteristic patterns may be found in patients with leukemia and schizophrenia.

The examination of the skin should go beyond observation and include palpation.

A fold of loosely adherent skin on the abdominal wall should be rolled between the examiner's thumb and forefinger to determine its consistency, the amount of subcutaneous tissue present and the degree of hydration.

The skin in well-hydrated infants and children will return to its normal position immediately upon release.

Delay in return, a phenomenon called tenting, usually occurs in dehydrated patients.

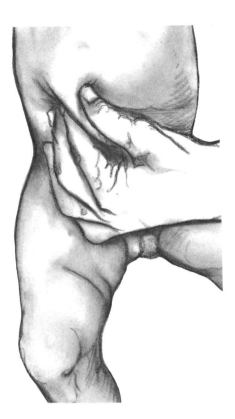

Early and Late Childhood

The skin in the normal child beyond the first year does not present any variations worthy of note. The techniques of examination and the general classification of pathologic lesions for this age are as with the adult.

THE HEAD AND NECK

Infancy

The head accounts for one-fourth of body length and one-third of body weight at birth, whereas at full maturity, it only accounts for one-eighth of body length and, for most, one-tenth of body weight. The bones of the skull are separated from one another by membranous tissue spaces called sutures. The points where the major sutures meet in the anterior and posterior portions of the skull are known as fontanelles. The sutures and fontanelles, shown in the following figure, form the basis for much of the physical assessment of the head in infancy.

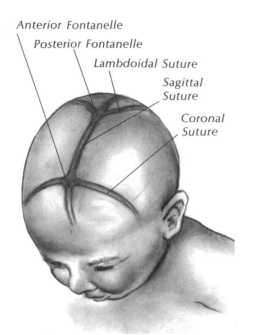

The sutures can be felt as slightly depressed ridges, and the fontanelles as soft concavities. The anterior fontanelle measures 4 to 6 cm in its largest diameter at birth and normally closes at between 4 and 26 months. Ninety percent close between 7 and 19 months of age. The posterior fontanelle measures 1 to 2 cm at birth and usually closes by 2 months of age. The intracranial pressure is reflected in the amount of tenseness and fullness seen and felt in the anterior fontanelle. Increased intracranial pressure produces a bulging, full anterior fontanelle. This is normally seen when a baby cries, coughs or is in the act of vomiting. Pulsations of the fontanelle reflect the peripheral pulse.

The anterior fontanelle is best examined for tenseness and fullness while the baby is quietly sitting or being held in an upright position.

The degree to which the anterior fontanelle is held to be an indicator of intracranial pressure and a barometer of serious central nervous system illness can be appreciated by noting that seasoned clinicians palpate the anterior fontanelle before proceeding with any other part of the physical examination.

The cranial bones of the newly born infant may overlap at the sutures to a certain degree. This phenomenon, called *molding*, results from passage of the head through the birth canal and disappears within two days. It is not seen in babies born by cesarian section.

Often newborn babies have a soft swelling with edema and bruising of the scalp over a portion of the occipitoparietal region. This is the *caput suc-cedaneum*, which is caused by drawing that presenting portion of the scalp

Increased intracranial pressure is found in infectious and neoplastic diseases of the central nervous system and with obstruction to the ventricular circulation. Decreased intracranial pressure, reflected in a depressed fontanelle, is seen as a sign of dehydration in infants.

Dilated scalp veins are indicative of long-standing increased intracranial pressure.

into the cervical os at the time the amniotic sac ruptures. The negative pressure or vacuum effect created by the loss of amniotic fluid produces distention of capillaries with extravasation of blood and fluid locally. These findings subside within the first 24 hours of life.

Examination of the infant's head should include ascertaining the shape and symmetry of the skull and face.

Asymmetry of the cranial vault (*plagiocephaly*) will occur should an infant sleep constantly on one side when in the supine position. Such positioning results in a flattening of the occiput on the dependent side and a prominence of the frontal region on the opposite side. It disappears as the baby becomes more active and spends less time in one position. In almost all instances, symmetry is restored when the position of the head becomes less constant. In utero positioning may result in transient facial asymmetries. If the head is flexed on the sternum it may produce a shortened chin (*micrognathia*), and if the shoulder is pressed on the jaw it may create a temporary lateral displacement of the mandible. The head of the premature infant at birth is relatively long in the occipitofrontal diameter and narrow in the bitemporal diameter. This relationship continues for most of the first year of life. An abnormally large head (*hydrocephaly or negacephaly*) and an abnormally small head (*microcephaly*) should be easily recognized in classical presentation, but either condition initially will require frequent observations, including measurements, for early diagnosis and institution of treatment.

If in palpating the skull of the newborn, the thumb or forefinger is pressed firmly over the temperoparietal or parietooccipital areas, the underlying bone may be felt to give momentarily, much as a Ping Pong ball would respond to similar pressure.

This condition, known as *craniotabes*, is due to osteoporosis of the outer table of the involved membraneous bone. It may result from prolonged increased intracranial pressure, from metabolic disturbances, from infection or it may be found in some normal infants on a physiologic basis.

The head may be percussed by tapping the index or middle finger directly against its surface. Percussion over the parietal bone in this manner will produce a cracked-pot sound prior to closure of the sutures. In the normal newborn similar direct percussion at the top of the cheek just below the zygoma will produce contraction of the facial muscle in the immediate area (Chvostek's sign).

This sign may persist through infancy and early childhood in some.

Transillumination of the skull is a useful procedure and should be part of every initial examination of an infant.

A second type of localized swelling involving the scalp is seen with reasonable frequency in the newborn child. The *cephalohematoma*, although not present at birth, appears within the first 24 hours and is due to subperiosteal hemorrhage involving the outer table of one of the cranial bones. The swelling, unlike the *caput succedaneum* and hematomas associated with skull fractures, does not extend across a suture. It may be small and well localized or may involve the entire bone. Occasionally bilateral, symmetrical swellings occur after difficult deliveries. Although initially soft, the swellings develop into a raised bony margin within two to three days due to the rapid deposition of calcium at the edges of the elevated periosteum. The entire process usually disappears within a few weeks, but may remain as a residual osteoma which is not resorbed for a year or two.

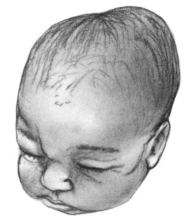

Chvostek's sign is often positive in hypocalcemic and hyperventilation tetany and in tetanus. It is obviously of no use in the diagnosis of neonatal tetany.

In a completely darkened room a standard flashlight with a soft rubber collar attached to the lighted end is placed flush against the skull at various points.

Routine auscultation of the skull to detect the presence of a bruit is of little use until a child reaches late childhood, since a systolic or continuous bruit may be heard over the temporal areas in normal children until the age of 5. Similar findings may be found in older children who have a significant anemia.

The neck of the newborn is relatively short.

It is best examined with the thumb and first two fingers while the infant is in the supine position.

Cysts are rarely found at birth, but may appear in early infancy. They are usually small, rounded and firm and can be differentiated from midline subcutaneous lesions in that they move with swallowing.

Injury to the sternomastoid muscle with bleeding into the muscle belly as it is stretched during the birth process results in wry neck (*Torticollis*). The head is tilted toward the injured side and in two or three weeks a firm fibrous mass may be felt within the muscle.

Early and Late Childhood

The examination of the head and neck beyond infancy, except as previously mentioned, should follow the procedure used in examining the adult. There are diagnostic facies in childhood that reflect chromosomal abnormalities, endocrine defects, social disease, chronic illness and other categories of disease entities. Down's syndrome, cretinism, battered child syndrome, and perennial allergic rhinitis are examples.

Parotid gland swelling in *mumps* may be difficult to detect, especially in early stages. If swelling is present above the angle of the jaw and in front of the ear, mumps, should be strongly suspected.

Palpation with the index finger along a line beginning at the outer canthus of the eye to the lower tip of the homolateral ear should produce tenderness in mumps. Swelling and tenderness above a line drawn from the

Plagiocephaly is apt to be more prominent in infants with torticollis secondary to injury to the sternomastoid muscle at birth, in the mentally and physically handicapped and in understimulated infants secondary to maternal neglect.

In hydrocephaly the eyes are deviated downward, revealing the upper sclerae and creating the "setting sun" sign as shown in the figure below.

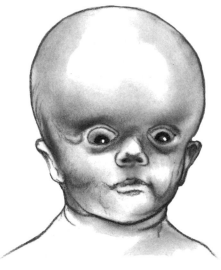

The shape of the head may be altered by premature closure of one or more of the cranial sutures (*craniosynostosis*). The resultant deformity of the skull is dependent on the sutures involved. Although palpation of affected sutures may reveal a raised bony ridge in the final stages, early diagnosis is made by roentgenographic means.

Craniotabes is found in hydrocephaly, rickets and congenital syphilis

angle of the jaw to the mastoid process are present in mumps while swelling and tenderness below this line are found in cervical adcnitis.

Neck mobility is an important determinant in considering central nervous system disease, especially meningitis.

Suppleness or rigidity may be determined by cradling the head in the examiner's hands with the child in the supine position. By supporting the child's head, literally in the examiner's hands, it can be moved easily in all directions and any resistance, especially to flexion, readily detected.

A cracked pot sound when elicited in older infants and children whose sutures should be closed is suggestive of separation of sutures secondary to increased intracranial pressure.

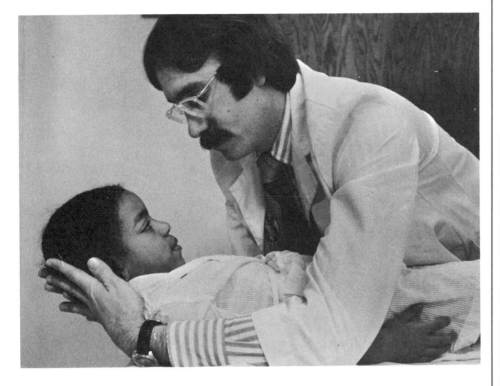

In infancy and early childhood, this is a more reliable test for nuchal rigidity and meningeal irritation than Brudzinski's sign or Kernig's sign (see p. 343).

Nuchal rigidity may be detected in early and late childhood by asking the child to sit up with his legs extended on the examining table. Normally he should be able to sit upright and voluntarily touch his chin to his chest. Younger children may be persuaded to flex their necks forward by getting them to look at a small toy or a light beam placed on their upper sternum.

Transillumination occurs when the cerebral cortex is partially absent; thinned; or displaced by accumulation of extra cortical fluid.

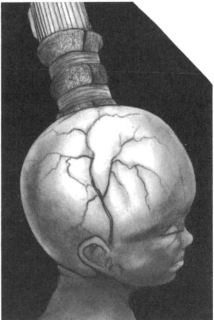

Bruits heard in non-anemic older children suggest increased intracranial pressure or an intracranial arteriovenous shunt or aneurysm.

When meningeal irritation is present, the child assumes the *tripod position* and is unable to assume a full upright position or perform the chin-to-chest maneuver (see figure on right).

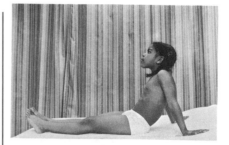

A *thyroglossal duct fistula* or *cyst* may be seen or felt in the midline immediately superior to the thyroid cartilage.

Remnants of the three lower branchial clefts may be seen as skin tags, cysts or fistulae along the anterior border of the sternomastoid muscle.

THE EYE

Infancy

It is somewhat difficult to examine the eyes of the newborn because the lids are ordinarily held tightly closed. Attempts at separating the lids usually increases the contraction of the orbicularis oculi muscles. Since bright light causes the infant to blink his eyes, the newborn's eyes should be examined under subdued lighting conditions.

The examiner can gain a clear view of the sclerae, pupils, irides and extraocular movements by holding the baby upright in the extended arms and turning slowly in one direction. When the baby is rotated with his head held in the midline, his eyes look in the direction toward which he is being turned.

When the rotation stops, they look in the opposite direction following a few quick unsustained nystagmoid movements. Conjugate eye movements develop rapidly after birth, but definitive following movements are not seen for a few weeks. Searching nystagmus is not uncommon immediately after birth. During the first 10 days of life, the eyes do not move when the head is turned, but remain in their original position as the head is slowly moved through its full range of motion. This so-called *doll's eye test* will detect paresis of the

If nystagmus is present after a few days it may be indicative of blindness.

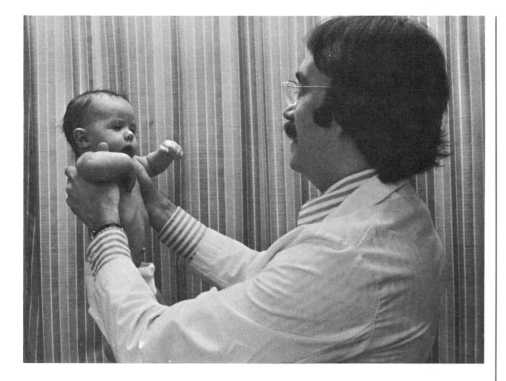

abducens nerve and weakness of the lateral rectus muscle. Intermittent alternating convergent strabismus is frequently seen or reported by parents during the first 6 months of life. Should it persist beyond that time or become unilateral sooner, or if divergent strabismus is observed at any time, the baby should be referred to an ophthalmologist.

Small subconjunctival, scleral and retinal hemorrhages are common in newborns. As the pupillary reactivity to light is poor during the first 4 to 5 months, reactions are best observed by first shading one eye and then uncovering it. The *optical blink reflex,* wherein the infant blinks his eyes and dorsiflexes his head in response to a bright light, is normally present in all newborns and may be used to test light perception. Inequality of the size of the pupils in both bright and subdued light is not uncommon but should be considered significant if it is constant over time and associated with other ocular or central nervous system findings. In all babies, the corneal reflex is present at birth.

The irides should be inspected for the presence of a cleft (*coloboma*) and for *Brushfield's spots.* The latter appear as white specks scattered in a linear fashion usually around the entire circumference of the iris and, although present in some normal infants, strongly suggest *Down's syndrome.* The presence of prominent inner epicanthal folds along with an upward outer slant to the eyelids is also suggestive of this malady. Chemical conjunctivitis, due to instillation of silver nitrate into the eyes at birth, occurs frequently in normal infants and is characterized by edema of the lids and inflammation of the conjunctivas with a purulent discharge.

The *setting sun sign,* in which the eyes are constantly gazing downward, occurs in hydrocephalus, but is also seen briefly in some normal newborns.

If retinal hemorrhages are extensive, severe anoxia or subdural hematoma should be suspected.

Dacryocystitis and *nasolacrimal duct obstruction* with ocular discharge and tearing may follow chemical conjunctivitis.

Opacities of the cornea, the anterior chamber or the lens or retinal anomalies will interrupt the light pathway and give a partial red reflex or a white reflex. In infants, *cataracts, a*

Demonstration of the red reflex is accomplished by setting the ophthalmoscope at "0" diopter and viewing the pupil at a distance of approximately 10 inches. Normally a red or orange color is reflected from the fundus through the pupil.

A funduscopic examination should be performed on all infants. Normally, the examination can be postponed until between 2 and 6 months of age, when the infant is most cooperative, unless the ocular or neurologic examination dictates that it be done immediately.

A mydriatic (10 percent phenylephrine with 1 percent mydriacyl—2 drops in each eye every 15 minutes over a 45-minute period) is essential for proper visualization. The baby can be placed in a supine position on the examining table or on the mother's lap or be held upright over her shoulder. Should the baby need calming, a sugar nipple can be used. Lid retraction can be accomplished, if necessary, with the examiner's thumb and first finger or by using an opened paper clip should the examiner's free hand be needed to hold the infant's head in midline. The method of funduscopic examination is otherwise the same as with adults. The cornea can ordinarily be seen at +20 diopters, the lens at +15 diopters, and the fundus at "0" diopters.

The optic disc is paler in infants, the peripheral vessels are not well developed and the foveal light reflection is absent. Papilledema is rarely seen, even with markedly increased intracranial pressure, since the fontanelles and open sutures absorb the increased pressure. Until age 3, the sutures will separate sufficiently to prevent papilledema. If vascular or optic disc anomalies are found, the parents' fundi should be examined to determine a possible genetic origin and prognosis for the findings.

The development of central vision progresses from birth, when only light perception is thought to be present, to adult visual levels attained at approximately 6 years of age.

The assessment of vision in the newborn is based on the presence of visual reflexes: direct and consensual pupillary constriction in response to light; blinking in response to bright light and to an object moved quickly toward the eyes; and opticokinetic nystagmus produced by the rapid movement of vertical black lines across the visual fields.

Those visual reflexes imply that both light perception and some degree of visual acuity are present shortly after birth. Opticokinetic testing on one group of newborns, $1\frac{1}{2}$ to 5 days after birth, demonstrated a visual acuity of at least 20/670 in 93 percent. That this acuity improves is evident, even without refractive measurement references. At 2 to 4 weeks, fixation on objects occurs; at 5 to 6 weeks, coordinated movements in following an object are seen; at 3 months the eyes converge and the baby begins to reach for

---

persistent posterior lenticular fibrovascular sheath and *retrolental fibroplasia* may cause an abnormal light reflex. Beyond infancy, *retinal detachment, chorioretinitis* and *retinoblastoma* should be suspected when an abnormal retinal reflex is encountered.

Retinal hemorrhages associated with intracranial bleeding are accompanied by dilated, congested, tortuous, retinal veins.

various sized objects at various distances, and finally, eye-hand coordination and the ability to focus are accomplished. At the age of 1 year, normal visual acuity is in the range of 20/200.

Failure to progress along these lines may indicate mental deficiency as well as diminished or absent vision.

Early Childhood

When examining a child in this age group, the most important condition the examiner must detect is *amblyopia exanopsia*. This is not the most serious ophthalmologic disease, but, in comparison to others of significance, it is the most prevalent and offers, with early intervention, the best prognosis. Improvement in this condition is unlikely if treatment is instituted after the sixth year of life. Amblyopia means reduced vision in an otherwise normal eye, and the reduced vision in this situation is due to disuse. Essentially, because of disconjugate fixation, two images are received by the optic cortex, one of which is suppressed to avoid diplopia or images of unequal clarity. One eye then becomes "lazy" and stops functioning to its full capacity and visual acuity in that eye is reduced markedly by suppression of central (foveal) vision. Since the two most common causes of amblyopia exanopsia are *strabismus and anisometrophia* (an eye with a refractive error 1.5 diopters greater than its pair), it is important to be able to test for muscle weakness and for visual acuity accurately.

Obstructive amblyopia is secondary to a cataract, corneal opacity or severe ptosis.

Muscle weakness causing deviation of one eye inwardly (*esotropia*) or outwardly (*exotropia*) may be detected by the *Hirschberg test,* the *prism test* or the *cover test.*

The Hirschberg test requires the reflection of a light on the cornea of each eye. The patient's attention is attracted to a light held at the examiner's

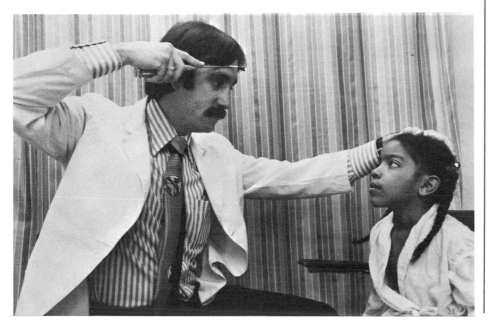

midforehead. While the eyes are fixed upon the light, its reflection on each cornea is noted. The patient's head is first held fixed in the midline and then is turned to the left and right, while fixation is maintained, to determine change in the corneal reflection pattern on lateral gaze. The reflections on each cornea should be symmetrically placed; thus, the type and degree of tropia can be determined by noting the pattern of asymmetrical placement of the reflections. The normal pattern and those with esotropia and exotropia are shown to the right.

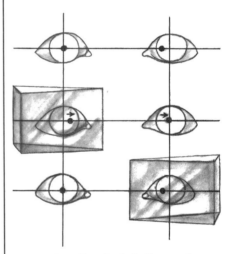

NORMAL PATTERN

RIGHT ESOTROPIA

RIGHT EXOTROPIA

The prism test is conducted in much the same way as the Hirschberg test.

Again the patient's attention is attracted to a light held at the examiner's midforehead. While the eyes are fixed upon the light, a 4-diopter prism is held, base out, in front of one eye while the other eye is observed by the examiner. If the observed eye moves inward or outward and remains in whichever position it has moved, strabismus is present. The opposite eye is tested in the same way.

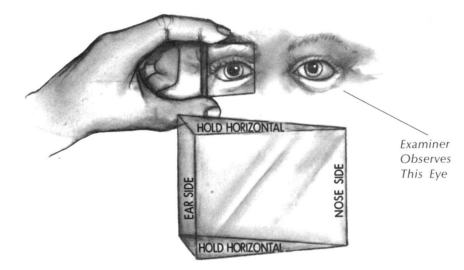

HOLD HORIZONTAL

EAR SIDE

NOSE SIDE

HOLD HORIZONTAL

Examiner Observes This Eye

Prism Test in Left Esotropia

The cover test is the most sophisticated of the three tests for strabismus, as it detects frank strabismus, differentiates the type of deviation and determines the characteristics of any latent deviation.

The patient's attention is again attracted to the midforehead light. The examiner's hand is placed on the top of the child's head and his thumb is placed in front on one eye while the other is observed for movement. The thumb is then removed and both eyes are observed for movement. If either

or both eyes move, a strabismus is present. The test is then repeated with the thumb covering and uncovering the other eye.

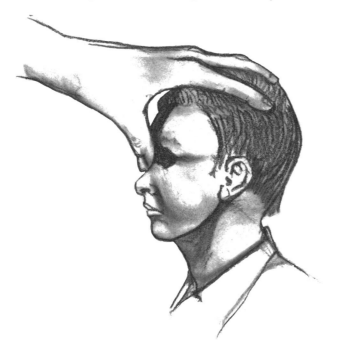

The combination of movements observed allows for differential diagnosis of the strabismus in question. The results of using the cover test, or what is more properly called the cover-uncover test, in monocular right esotropia are shown at the right.

Testing visual acuity in early childhood is not a simple matter. The variables of the child, the examiner, the testing environment and the test itself all contribute significantly to the outcome and should be given careful attention if valid results are to be obtained. Unfortunately, there is no testing method which accurately measures visual acuity in children under the age of 3 years. Since each eye must be tested separately to detect amblyopia, one eye must be covered by an elastoplast bandage to ensure complete occlusion. Resistance to placement of the patch may be overcome by calling it a "pirate's patch." A child with amblyopia might accept the patch on the amblyopic eye, but not on the good eye.

For accurate measures of visual acuity in this age group, some form of opticokinetic testing would seem to hold the most promise. However, two other types of tests used will be mentioned here as illustrations, without any enthusiasm as to their worth.

The miniature toy test utilizes identical sets of small toys representing familiar objects. The child is given one set and the examiner, keeping the other, asks the child to match each toy as it is shown to him at a distance of 10 feet. Worth's test uses five balls ranging from $\frac{1}{2}$ to $1\frac{1}{2}$ inches in diame-

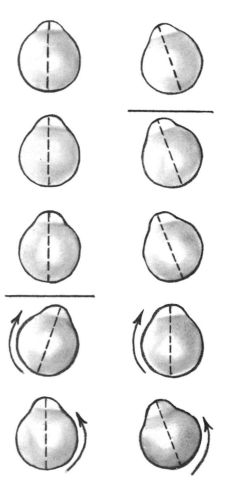

ter. Beginning with the largest, each is individually thrown on the floor by the examiner and retrieved by the child.

In children over the age of 3, the *Snellen E chart* (a form of direct visual testing) is very adequate. Most youngsters will cooperate in indicating, either verbally or by positioning of the fingers, in which direction the E is pointing. For those who initially have difficulty with this test, a single E card can be sent home with the child for practice purposes. Charts with pictures instead of Es are often used, but have no special advantage, nor do any other testing methods generally available. The visual acuity at age 3 years is ± 20/40, at age 4 to 5 years, ± 20/30 and at 6 to 7 years, 20/20.

Visual field examination in infants and in early childhood can be done with the child sitting on the mother's lap.

The head is held in the midline while an object such as a dangling measuring tape case or a small toy is brought into the child's field of vision from several points behind, above and below him. Deviation of the eyes in its direction indicates that the child has seen the object.

Late Childhood

The eye problems and methods of examining the eye for this age group have been covered in the adult section. In general, vision testing machines used for mass screening in schools tend to underrate visual acuity and produce over-referrals.

Simple refractive error can be distinguished from organic causes of diminished vision by asking the child to take his vision test looking through a pinhole punched in a card. Visual acuity improves using the pinhole card when refractive errors are present, but not when organic ocular disease exists.

THE EAR

Infancy

Normally the ear joins the scalp on or above the extension of a line drawn across the inner and outer canthus of the eye.

Small, deformed or low-set auricles may give indication of associated congenital defects, especially renal agenesis or anomalies.

Examination of the ear in the immediate neonatal period establishes the patency of the external auditory canal only, since the tympanic membranes are obscured by accumulated vernix caseosa for the first 2 or 3 days of life. In

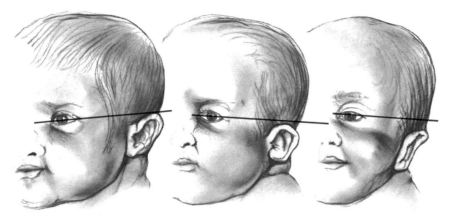

NORMAL EARS   PSEUDO LOW-SET EARS   TRUE LOW-SET EARS

infancy, the external auditory canal is directed upward from the inside; therefore, the pinna should be pulled gently downward for best visualization of the ear drum. The light reflex on the tympanic membrane is diffuse and does not assume the cone shape for several months.

A small skin tab, cleft or pit is frequently found just forward of the tragus and represents a remnant of the first branchial cleft.

Hearing in infancy can be tested by observing a blinking of the eyes in response to a sudden sharp sound, which should be produced at a distance of 12 inches from the ear by snapping the fingers, clapping the hands or utilizing a bell or other kinds of mechanical noise-making devices. Care should be taken that the sound production does not produce an airstream that could evoke the blink reflex.

The acoustic blink reflex is difficult to elicit during the first 2 or 3 days of life and may disappear temporarily after it is elicited a few times. This is a crude test at best, and the absence of blinking in response to sound is not diagnostic of deafness nor does its presence give complete assurance of normal hearing. At 2 weeks, the infant may jump in response to a sudden noise and at 10 weeks may respond by momentary cessation of body movements. Between 3 and 4 months of age, the eyes and head will turn toward the source of sound. Even before this, an increase in respiratory rate may occur when familiar sounds are heard.

Because the parents' impression of the baby's auditory acuity is usually correct, when a mother is concerned that her baby cannot hear, it should be assumed that he cannot hear until proven otherwise.

Early Childhood

The examination of the ear becomes more difficult as the child grows older. Greater resistance is encountered since the ear canals are sensitive and the child cannot observe the procedure.

Often it is helpful simply to place the otoscopic speculum gently into the external auditory canal of one ear, removing it instantly and repeating the procedure on the other. Then the examiner can begin again, taking the necessary time in the actual examination with a child whose apprehensions have been allayed.

The ears can be successfully examined even in a struggling child if care is taken in restraining him and in manipulating both ear and otoscope gently.

The patient should be placed in the supine position, by the mother or an assistant, with his arms held extended close to the sides of his head, limiting its movement from side to side. The examiner approaches the child from the right side and leans across his lower chest and upper abdomen, restricting movements of the trunk. A third person may be required to hold the feet and legs if the child struggles unduly; however, this is rarely necessary.

This same restraining procedure may be used for examination of the eyes, nose and throat, as illustrated below.

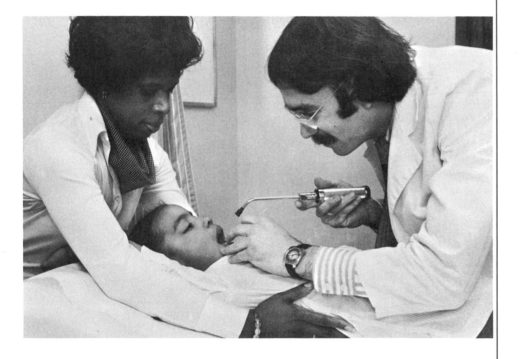

When the right ear is being examined, the child's head is turned to the left and held firmly in this position by the lateral aspect of the examiner's right hand. The examiner holds the otoscope in his right hand in an inverted position and manipulates the auricle with his left hand. In this age group, the external auditory canal is directed downward and forward from the inside, and the pinna must be pulled upwards and backwards to afford the best visualization. The thumb and forefinger of the right hand which hold the otoscope are buffered from sudden movements of the child's head by the restraining right hand and the forearm which rests firmly on the examining table. See the illustration on page 397.

When the left ear is examined, the patient's head is turned to the right and held firmly in this position by the lateral aspect of the examiner's left hand

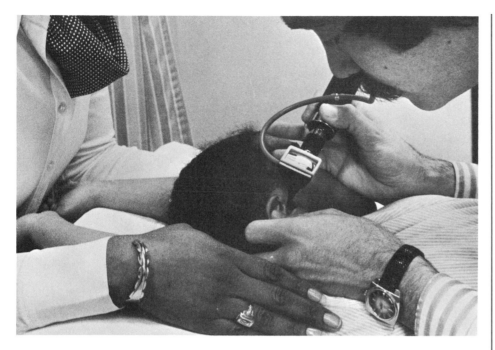

and wrist. The thumb and forefinger of the left hand manipulate the auricle and the right hand holds the otoscope in an inverted position. The lateral aspect of the fifth finger of the right hand is held against the patient's head to provide a buffer against sudden movement by the patient. This procedure is demonstrated in the following figure.

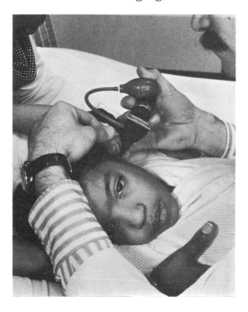

The speculum of the otoscope should be as large in diameter as will allow for comfortable ¼ to ½ inch penetration. This provides maximum visualization of the canal and drum and a reasonable seal to observe the effects of pneumatic otoscopy. Some examiners attach a rubber tip to the end of the speculum to gain a tighter, more comfortable seal.

Pneumatic otoscopy is accomplished by observing the tympanic membrane as the pressure in the external auditory canal is increased or decreased. This is done by introducing and removing air from the canal in applying positive and negative pressures with a rubber squeeze bulb (as shown in the figure below) or by blowing and sucking on a rubber tube attached to the otoscope.

When air is introduced into the normal ear canal, the tympanic membrane and its light reflex are seen to move inward. When air is removed, the tympanic membrane moves outward, toward the examiner. This to and fro movement of the tympanic membrane has been likened to the luffing of a sail.

This movement is absent in chronic middle ear infection (*serous otitis media*) and diminished in some cases of acute otitis media.

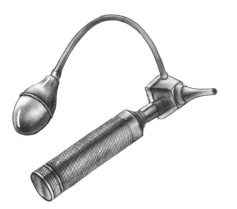

Cerumen accumulation within the ear canal, obscuring a view of the tympanic membrane is commonly found in children. Very often this is unilateral. There are several instruments and ear washing techniques that may be used to remove ear wax comfortably, but they will not be described here. Accumulation of purulent material and debris in the ear canal is found in *otitis externa* and in *otitis media* with a ruptured tympanic membrane. In either event, nothing is to be gained in washing out the ear canal.

Otitis media and otitis externa may be differentiated clinically by gentle movement of the pinna, which will cause exquisite pain in otitis externa, but no discomfort in purulent otitis media.

Simple auditory screening in this age group can be accomplished by whispering at a distance of 8 feet.

The child should be asked questions or given commands and care should be taken that lip reading is not allowable. In addition, tuning forks can be used to screen for hearing with the examiner using his own auditory acuity as the control.

If these screening methods reveal any diminution of hearing, a full audiometric testing should be performed. Furthermore, all children should be given a full-scale acoustic screening test with an audiometer prior to beginning school, as should any child at whatever age with delayed speech development or with non-motor speech defects. Because of their complexity, audiometric screening devices used for older children are often unsatisfactory for use in early childhood and direct referral to a hearing and speech center may be more appropriate when delayed or defective speech is present.

Significant, temporary hearing loss may follow an episode of otitis media for as long as 4 months.

Late Childhood

As the child grows older, the ease and technique of examining the ears and testing the hearing approaches the levels and methods for adults. There are no unique abnormalities or variations from the normal concerning the ear and its function in this age group, as compared with other age groups, including the "selective deafness" some children and adolescents demonstrate in hearing only what they choose when spoken to in either soft or loud voices by their parents and teachers.

THE NOSE, AND THROAT

Infancy

Obstruction to the nasal passages in newborn infants occurs with *choanal atresia* and with displacement of the cartilage of the vomer during delivery.

Passage of a number 14 French catheter through each nostril into the posterior nasopharynx will detect these anomalies. Patency of the nasal passages may also be determined by holding the infant's mouth closed and occluding each nostril alternately.

This will not stress a normal baby, since most newborns are nasal breathers. On the other hand, occluding both nares simultaneously and allowing the mouth to open will cause considerable distress. Indeed, some infants are unable to breath through their mouths at all (*obligate nasal breathers*).

The mouth of the newborn is edentulous. The gums are smooth with a raised 1-mm serrated fringe of tissue on the buccal margins. Occasional white pearl-like retention cysts are seen along the ridges and are often mistaken for teeth—they disappear spontaneously within a month or two.

Rarely, supernumary teeth are found. These are soft, without enamel, and are shed within a few days.

Petechiae are commonly found on the soft palate after birth.

The frenulum of the upper lip may be quite thick and extend from the superior aspect of the inner lip to the posterior portion of the upper gum, creating a deep notch in its midline. The frenulum of the tongue varies in consistency from a thin filamentous membrane to a thick, fibrous cord. Its length varies so that it may attach midway on the undersurface of the tongue or at its very lip. A heavy fibrous frenulum that extends to the tip of the

Epstein's pearls, pinhead-sized, white or yellow, rounded elevations which are located along the midline of the hard palate near its posterior border, are due to retained secretions and disappear within a few weeks or months.

tongue may interfere with its protrusion (*tongue tie*). However, there will be no difficulties encountered with nursing or speech if the tongue can be extended as far as the alveolar ridge.

Visualization of the pharynx is best accomplished while a baby cries. This is true throughout infancy and early childhood. A tongue blade produces strong reflex elevation of the base of the tongue and obstructs the view of the infant's pharynx. Tonsillar tissue is not seen in the newborn.

There is little saliva produced during the first 3 months of life. As the infant beings to produce saliva, drooling occurs, since there are no lower teeth to provide a dam for retention.

Early and Late Childhood

The anterior portion of the nose can be easily visualized by pushing up the tip of the nose. A large-bored speculum attached to the otoscope is sufficient for seeing deeper into the nostrils.

Examination of the mouth may present difficulties in early childhood and restraints are usually needed (see figure on p. 396). The young child may be more comfortable sitting in the mother's lap as shown here.

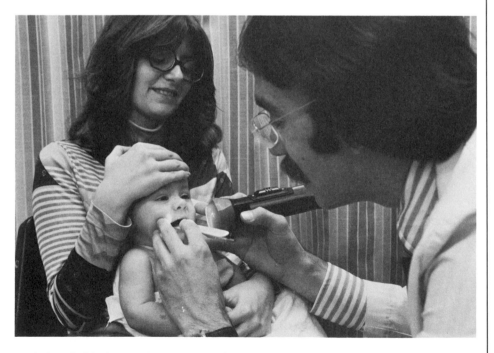

If the child clamps his teeth and purses his lips, the tongue blade can be easily pushed through the lips, along the buccal mucosa and introduced between the alveolar ridges behind the molars. This produces a gag reflex and, with it, complete visualization of the pharynx.

Oral moniliasis (*thrush*) is a common malady in infants, usually contracted from mothers with vaginal moniliasis. In thrush, a lacy white material with an erythematous base is seen on the surface of the oral mucous membranes. It is difficult to remove, distinguishing it from milk curds which wipe away easily.

The presence of large amounts of saliva in the newborn suggests a *tracheoesophageal fistula.* A shrill or high pitched cry in infancy may be indicative of increased intracranial pressure. A hoarse cry should make one suspect hypocalcemic tetany or cretinism, while absence of any cry suggests severe illness or mental retardation. A continuous inspiratory and expiratory stridor may be due to a relatively small larynx (*infantile laryngeal stridor*) or delay in the development of the cartilage in the tracheal rings (*tracheomalacia*).

A direct assault on the front teeth will only meet with failure and a splintered tongue blade. Most children, however, are not that resistant and can be easily enticed to open their mouths, especially if they do not see a throat stick in the examiner's hand. A child who can stick out his tongue and say "aahh!" does not require further manipulation for complete visualization of his pharynx. A good examiner can determine all that needs to be known with one quick look. Older children will permit placement of the tongue blade on one side of the base of the tongue and then the other. A transilluminator attachment to the oto-ophthalmoscopic handle is more useful than the standard penlight or flashlight in that its giraffe-like configuration allows for delivery of concentrated light in the recesses of the oral cavity and the pharynx.

Of course, the transilluminator may be used to transilluminate the sinuses when sinusitis is suspected. This requires a completely dark room and a cooperative child.

The frontal sinuses are transilluminated by firmly placing the tip of the light above each eye against the inner aspect of the supraorbital ridge of the frontal bone.

Normally one sees a faint glow of light transmitted through the bone outlining the sinus on the same side.

The maxillary sinuses are transilluminated by placing the neck and head of the light in the patient's mouth with the tip pressed against first one side and then the other of the hard palate. The patient is instructed to seal his lips around the shaft of the transilluminator attachment while the examiner looks for the maxillary sinus glow on the corresponding side of the face.

The appearance of the tongue may indicate disease. The *coated* tongue is nonspecific, the *smooth* tongue is found in avitaminosis, the *geographic* tongue in many allergic conditions, and the *strawberry* and *raspberry* tongues at specific stages of scarlet fever. The *scrotal* and *fissured* tongues have no significance. (See Table 7-21, p. 109.)

The teeth should be examined for timing and sequence of eruption, number, character, condition and position. Abnormalities of the enamel may reflect past or present, general or localized disease. Malocclusion should be looked for in late childhood. Most malocclusion and misalignment of teeth due to thumb sucking in early childhood is reversible if the habit is substantially arrested by age 6 or 7 years. When examining for maxillary protrusion (*overbite*) or mandibular protrusion (*underbite*), one should be careful not to fall into the trap of asking the child to "show his teeth," as the upper and lower teeth are aligned reflexly when they are presented for inspection.

Rather, the child should be asked to bite down as hard as possible. The examiner then, upon parting the lips, will observe the true bite.

Transillumination is absent or diminished when sinusitis is present.

Green coloration of the teeth is seen following severe erythroblastosis fetalis, grayish mottling of the enamel may result from administration of tetracycline in infancy and early childhood, caries reflect poor nutrition and oral hygiene, and black lines along the gingival margins signal the ingestion of heavy metals.

Malocclusion is most often due to hereditary predisposition, but may be due to chronic mouth breathing secondary to obstruction to the nasal airway. Maxillary overgrowth is associated with chronic hemolytic anemia while mandibular overgrowth occurs rarely in juvenile rheumatoid arthritis affecting the temporomandibular joint.

The primary teeth erupt in a more predictable fashion in contrast to when they are shed or when the secondary teeth arrive. At age 7 months, most infants have two upper and two lower central incisors. From that point on, four teeth are added every four months, so there are eight at 11 months, 12 at 15 months, 16 at 19 months and a full complement of 20 at 23 months. Normally, the shedding of primary teeth coincides with the eruption of corresponding secondary teeth and begins at the end of early childhood between 6 and 7 years of age, ending in early adulthood at age 17 to 22 years.

When the throat is examined, the size and appearance of the tonsils should be noted. In both early and late childhood, the tonsils are relatively large, in view of the abundance of lymphoid tissue at this time of life (see figure on p. 367). They appear even larger as they move out of their fossae toward the midline and forward when the gag reflex is elicited or the tongue is voluntarily protruded and the traditional "aahh!" is sounded. The tonsils usually have deep crypts on their surface which often have white concretions or food particles protruding from their depths. This is no indication of disease current or past.

The adenoids are not ordinarily visible unless extremely enlarged or unless the soft palate is elevated with the tongue blade to expose them in the nasopharynx. Adenoidal size can be determined indirectly by noting the degree of posterior nasal obstruction present when the patient sniffs through each nostril and by the nasal quality they produce in the voice. Their size may also be determined directly by palpation. In most instances, where adenoidal palpation is carried out, the history is one of recurrent fever, headaches and cough and the diagnoses of *chronic adenoiditis* and *adenoidal abscess* are entertained.

> **During examination, the child is positioned and restrained as for examination of the throat (see figure on p. 396). Three tongue blades taped together are placed, with the examiner's left hand, between the molars and are then turned on edge to ensure wide exposure. The examiner's plastic-gloved right index finger is placed into the nasopharynx through the mouth behind the soft palate, and very rapidly the adenoidal and surrounding lymphoid tissue is palpated and thoroughly massaged. The procedure is accomplished with three or four quick strokes of the finger.**

The child and parents should be warned that this procedure is uncomfortable and is likely to be followed by vomiting of copious amounts of bloody mucus.

> **The same method may be used to palpate a peritonsillar abscess to determine the presence or absence of fluctuation and the posterior pharyngeal wall to determine the presence and state of a retropharyngeal abscess.**

Koplik's spots, although a diagnostic sign in their dénouement, deserve description. Their appearance on the buccal mucosa opposite the first and second molars in a child with fever, coryza and cough is proof positive of prodromal measles (*rubeola*), and the appearance of a generalized maculopapular rash within 24 hours can be predicted with certainty. Koplik's spots appear as grains of salt on individual erythematous bases. Their number varies dependent upon when in the course of the illness they are observed. When three or more appear in a particular spot, they should be easily recognized.

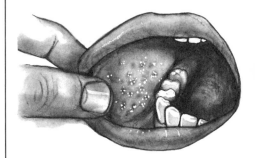

A white exudate over the surface of the tonsils is suggestive of *streptococcal tonsillitis;* a thick gray adherent exudate suggests *diphtheritic tonsillitis;* and necrosis of the tonsilar tissue without exudate suggests *infectious mononucleosis.* All three conditions produce a fetid odor, but none distinguishable from the others. When one tonsil appears inflamed and unilaterally protrudes toward the midline and forward, *peritonsillar abscess* is an almost certain diagnosis.

Absence or asymmetry of movement of the soft palate in response to gagging and phonation, which is indicative of paralysis or weakness, should be noted. Asymmetry and corresponding voice change are often seen for varying periods following tonsillectomy.

THE THORAX AND LUNGS

Infancy

The configuration of the infant's thorax is rounded with the anteroposterior diameter being equal to the transverse diameter. The *thoracic index*, which is the ratio of the transverse diameter to the anteroposterior diameter, is 1 at birth. At 1 year of age it is 1.25, and it reaches 1.35 at 6 years without much change thereafter.

The chest wall in infancy is thin with little musculature, and the bony and cartilaginous rib cage is very soft and pliant. The tip of the xiphoid process is often seen protruding anteriorly immediately beneath the skin at the apex of the costal angle.

The breasts of the newborn in both male and female are often enlarged and engorged with secretion of a white liquid called witch's milk. This is due to maternal estrogen effect and lasts only a week or two.

The respiratory rate and patterns of infancy and early childhood are discussed on p. 376. Expirations are more prolonged than inspirations at this age. The predominantly diaphragmatic breathing produces a simultaneous drawing in of the lower thorax and protrusion of the abdomen on inspiration and the reverse on expiration—termed *paradoxical breathing*.

Tactile fremitus can be utilized in infancy by palpation of the chest when the baby cries. The whole hand, palm and finger tips, placed over the anterior, lateral or posterior thorax will detect gross changes in transmission of sound through the parenchyma of the lung, the pleura and chest wall of the infant. Percussion of the infant's chest may be done directly by tapping the thoracic wall with one finger or indirectly by using the finger-on-finger method.

The percussion note is normally hyperresonant throughout. Any decrease in hyperresonance detected over the lung fields has the same significance as dullness or flatness in the adult.

The bell or small diaphragm stethoscope should be used when auscultating the infant's chest to allow for maximum localization of findings.

The child who has a croupy cough, hoarseness, difficulty swallowing and signs of upper respiratory tract obstruction is suspect of having acute *epiglottitis*. In such a case, the epiglottis is markedly swollen and cherry red. Invoking the gag reflex in this instance could produce complete laryngeal obstruction and a fatal outcome. Therefore, great care must be taken in examining the throat. It should be done, if at all, only once and then deftly and gently with the child in the upright position, with a tracheostomy set at hand for use in the event that complete upper airway obstruction should result from the examination procedure. The danger of such obstruction is sufficiently great that many examiners prefer to omit direct examination of the throat in suspected cases of acute epiglottitis and rely upon lateral x-rays of the neck to establish the diagnosis.

Pectus excavatum may be manifest in early infancy by marked midline substernal retractions with normal respirations, but it and other asymmetric thoracic deformities such as *pectus carinatum* do not ordinarily become evident until early childhood (see p. 93).

When paradoxical breathing alters to predominant thoracic breathing, intra-abdominal or intrathoracic pathology which precludes the use of the diaphragm should be suspected.

The breath sounds will be louder and harsher than in adults because the stethoscope is closer to the origin of the sounds. Normally, infant breath sounds are bronchovesicular in character. Breathing in newborns is usually intermittently slow and shallow, then rapid and deep, so the examiner must be both patient and opportunistic. Often breath sounds will be diminished on the side of the chest opposite the direction in which the head is turned. There may be fine crepitant rales at the end of deep inspiration in normal newborns and older infants. Crying fortunately will produce all of the deep breaths one could want and actually enhances auscultation, except in the unusual baby who cries on inspiration as well as expiration. Because of the smallness of the thoracic cage and the ease of sound transmission within, breath sounds are rarely entirely absent. Even with atelectasis, effusion, empyema and pneumothorax, breath sounds are diminished rather than absent. In infants, pure bronchial breathing is rarely heard, even when consolidation is present. Wheezes, which are palpable, and audible vibrations caused by air rushing through a narrow lumen, occur more frequently in infancy and early childhood than in older children and adults because the small lumen of the tracheobronchial tree is easily narrowed by slight swelling of the mucous membrane or by small amounts of mucus. Rhonchi and rales are often heard together and may be confused one with the other. However, distinction between the two is necessary and can be made by listening with the bell at the mouth and comparing what is heard there with what is heard through the chest wall. Rhonchi can be heard transorally, rales cannot.

Extension or other movement of the head with inspiration indicates use of accessory muscles of respiration and usually accompanies severe respiratory disease.

Both dullness and flatness may be elicited in infants when consolidation of the lung, an intrathoracic mass or pleural fluid are present.

An inspiratory wheeze is indicative of narrowing high in the tracheobronchial tree while an expiratory wheeze indicates narrowing lower down.

Early and Late Childhood

Breast development for girls may begin normally as early as the eighth year. Asymmetrical growth with resulting differences in size of the breasts during preadolescence is the rule; symmetrical anlages are the exception. Completion of growth through adolescence corrects these inequalities in most instances. Parents and the young lady herself must be reassured, even if no mention of the subject is made by them. The preadolescent and adolescent female should be given the benefit of complete examination of the breasts periodically as part of the total physical examination.

Physical findings on examination of the lungs in early and late childhood reveal many of the characteristics of those found in infancy, due to the continued relative lack of musculature and subcutaneous tissue overlying the thorax. Respiratory patterns are more regular and increasing cooperation is obtained with age.

The stethoscope may be a threatening instrument to the very young child; therefore, success in placing it upon the chest will be enhanced if the child is told what it is and is allowed to manipulate it or even to listen through it.

Tactile and vocal fremitus is usually easily generated through small talk with the child. A surprising number will go the "99" and "1, 2, 3" routes.

Gaining the child's cooperation in deep breathing and breath holding is not that difficult either and demonstration by the examiner will usually suffice. Having the child attempt to blow out a match held too far away for immediate success seldom fails to produce full inspiration.

THE HEART

The examination of the heart in infants and children is, with few exceptions, conducted in the same manner as with the adult. The femoral pulses assume greater importance since their diminution, as compared to the radial pulse, or their absence may be the only findings to raise suspicion of *coaractation of the aorta* in infancy and early childhood.

They are easily felt by palpating along the inguinal ligament midway between the iliac crest and the symphysis pubis.

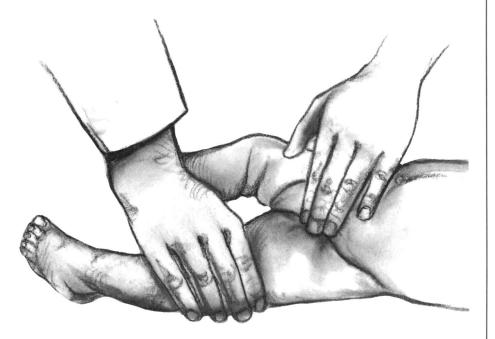

The physical indications of severe heart disease include those not found with the stethoscope. Poor weight gain, delayed development, tachypnea, tachycardia, a prominent, active, heaving or thrusting precordium, cyanosis and clubbing of the fingers and toes all signal cardiac disease. Heart failure is marked by venous engorgement, pulsus alternans, gallop rhythm and hepatic enlargement. Pulmonary and peripheral edema appear late. Peripheral edema is more likely to be due to renal rather than cardiac failure.

Since the respiratory rate may approximate the heart rate in infancy, breath sounds may be thought to be murmurs.

Occlusion of the nares momentarily will interrupt the respirations long enough to clarify this issue.

There are some distinct characteristics of the cardiac findings in normal infants and children which are not found in adults. The apical impulse (PMI), which is often visible, is at the level of the fourth interspace until age 7 years when it drops to the fifth interspace. It is to the left of the midclavicular line until age 4 years, at the midclavicular line between 4 and 6 and moves to the right of it at 7. The heart percusses relatively larger because of its more horizontal position and the overlying thymus gland at its base. *Sinus arrhythmia* is almost always present and *premature ventricular contractions* are quite common. The heart sounds are louder because the chest wall is thinner and they are of higher pitch and shorter duration. S_1 is louder than S_2 at the apex. Splitting of S_2 at the apex, producing an extra heart sound, is found in 25 to 33 percent of children. S_2 is louder than S_1 in the pulmonic area.

In the pediatric cardiac examination, the murmur assumes great significance in differential diagnosis, because more than half of all children (indeed, some say all) develop an innocent murmur at some time during childhood and because significant heart disease in the pediatric age group is infrequent in the absence of a murmur. Therefore, the examiner must distinguish between the innocent and the organic murmur. It has been customary to grade the intensity of murmurs on a scale of 1 to 6 as shown on p. 154.

The *innocent murmur* has received over 120 labels indicative of its benign or functional nature, its origin or its auscultatory characteristics. It is systolic in timing, usually of short duration and of grade 3 or less in intensity and has an empty, low pitched, vibratory, musical groaning quality to its sound. It is usually loudest along the left sternal border, either in the second or third intercostal spaces or in the fourth or fifth intercostal spaces medial to the apex. It is poorly transmitted, is heard best in the supine position and may vary in its intensity and its presence with changes in position, with the phase of respiration, after exercise and from day to day. The most important characteristic of the innocent murmur is that it is heard in the absence of any other demonstrable evidence of cardiovascular disease.

The non-innocent or organic murmurs are due to congenital or acquired heart disease. Almost all acquired heart disease productive of murmurs in childhood is due to acute rheumatic fever. An organic murmur first appearing before 3 years of age is almost always due to a congenital cardiac defect, and one first appearing after that age is usually due to rheumatic valvulitis.

The murmurs of congenital cardiac defects are due to abnormal communications between the arterial and venous circuits of the heart and great vessels and to valvular deformities. For the most part, they are rough, coarse and harsh in character, systolic in timing and usually heard best at the base of the heart. The murmurs of *ventricular septal defect* and of *patent ductus arteriosus* have been described on pp. 166 and 172. Those of *aortic stenosis* and *pulmonic stenosis* are described on p. 167.

The presence or absence of cyanosis may be helpful to the examiner in differentiating the various types of congenital heart disease that present with similar murmurs (see Table 20-3 on the next page).

When S_2 is equal to or greater than S_1 at the apex, prolongation of the P-R interval should be suspected. Splitting of S_2 in the pulmonic area may be found normally, but is frequently present in *mitral stenosis* and *bundle branch block.*

Murmurs of grade 3 or higher usually indicate the presence of heart disease.

In *atrial septal defect,* a grade 1 to 3 rough, coarse systolic murmur is heard at the second and third left interspaces. It is less harsh than the murmur of a ventricular septal defect, is rarely accompanied by a thrill and is not widely distributed. The murmur of *coarctation of the aorta* (adult type) is heard in the same area, is louder, is transmitted to the back medial of the scapula and may be accompanied by a visible pulsation and palpable thrill at the suprasternal notch. It is also associated with decreased to absent femoral pulses and elevated blood pressure in the upper extremities. The murmurs associated with *tetralogy of Fallot, pure pulmonic stenosis, tricuspid atresia, transposition of the great vessels* and *Eisenmenger's complex* are grades 1 to 3 in intensity, are systolic in timing, may be heard best at the left second and third

More often than not, the final diagnostic impression must await the results of electrocardiograms, chest x-rays, fluoroscopic examinations, cardiac catheterization and more sophisticated studies.

Of the murmurs associated with acquired rheumatic heart disease, three of the four are heard at the apex and two of these three—the murmurs of mitral and aortic valvular stenosis and insufficiency—are diastolic in timing and are described on p. 17. The tricuspid and pulmonic valves are rarely involved sufficiently in the rheumatic process to produce murmurs.

The examiner of a child's heart should be able to differentiate normal from abnormal findings. Final decisions regarding specific abnormalities must often be left to the pediatric cardiologist whose experience and access to special diagnostic tools will more likely bring accurate diagnoses and appropriate management. Therefore, early referral of the infant or child found to have evidence of congenital or acquired heart disease should be made to a pediatric cardiologist.

THE ABDOMEN

Infancy

The abdomen in infants is protuberant due to poorly developed musculature.

The umbilical cord should be checked routinely at birth for the number of vessels present. Normally two umbilical arteries and one umbilical vein are present.

The umbilicus in the newborn may have a relatively long cutaneous portion (*umbilicus cutis*) or a relatively long amniotic portion (*umbilicus amnioticus*). In either event, the amniotic portion dries up within a week and falls off within two. The skin retracts to become flush with the abdominal wall during the same time period.

Infants are prone to umbilical hernias, ventral hernias and diastasis recti. However, these are not usually discernible until 2 or 3 weeks of age. All are easily detected with crying.

The presence of diastasis recti may reflect a congenital weakness of the abdominal musculature (rare) or be the result of a chronically distended abdomen. Most, however, are normal variants and disappear in early childhood.

interspaces, are not well transmitted, may or may not be accompanied by a thrill and have no individual distinguishing characteristics. These murmurs may be absent in infancy. In addition, palpable liver pulsations may be present with tricuspid atresia and pure pulmonic stenosis.

TABLE 20.3 CYANOSIS AND CONGENITAL HEART DISEASE

No Cyanosis	Septal defects—small
	Patent ductus arteriosis
	Pure pulmonic stenosis—mild
	Coarctation of the aorta
	*Right coronary artery
	*Subendocardial fibroelastosis
	*Glycogen storage disease
Early Cyanosis	Tetralogy of Fallot—severe
	Tricuspid atresia
	Transposition of the great vessels
	Isolated dextro or levulocardia
	Two- and three-chambered hearts
	Severe pulmonic stenosis with intact ventricular septum
Late Cyanosis	Eisenmenger complex
	Pure pulmonic stenosis—mild
	Tetralogy of Fallot
	Septal defects—large

*Present with cardiac enlargement, tachycardia and tachypnea, but without a heart murmur.

A newborn with a concave abdomen should be immediately investigated for diaphragmatic hernia with displacement of some of the abdominal organs into the thoracic cavity.

A high correlation between a single umbilical artery and a variety of congenital anomalies exists.

Failure of the navel to heal with granulomatous tissue forming at its base occurs frequently.

A superficial abdominal venous pattern is observable until puberty. Abdominal reflexes are usually absent until after the first year of life.

Palpation of the infant's abdomen is relatively easy.

Relaxation is obtained by holding the legs flexed at the knees and hips with the left hand and palpating with the right.

The liver edge and spleen tip are more often palpable than not, and frequently both kidneys can be felt by using the technique described for adults. The bladder is often felt and normally percussed to the level of the umbilicus. The descending colon is easily felt and may present as a sausage-like mass in the left lower quadrant. Any abdominal masses of other origin are easily outlined.

Cysts, which occur rarely, may be differentiated from solid tumors by transillumination.

The spasm and rigidity encountered in a crying infant will usually be avoided with a bottle feeding or a sugar nipple administered during palpation of the abdomen.

Percussion of the infant's abdomen is accomplished as in the adult, but the examiner must make allowance for a greater amount of air within the stomach and the intestinal lumen since infants frequently swallow air when feeding and crying.

Auscultation of the abdomen should be accomplished before palpation. During auscultation, metallic tinkling every 10 to 30 seconds is heard normally.

The abdominal examination technique is altered when *pyloric stenosis* is suspected.

The infant should be placed unclothed in the supine position with the examiner standing at the foot of the table. A bright light is directed, at table height, across the abdomen from the patient's right side. A bottle of sugar water or milk is then fed to the infant and the abdomen is observed closely. When pyloric stenosis is present, peristaltic waves are seen to go across the upper abdomen from left to right. These become increasingly large and frequent as the feeding progresses as shown in the figure on the next page.

Inevitably, the baby will vomit with projectile force. At this point, deep palpation in the right upper quadrant will most likely reveal the presence of an olive-sized pyloric mass. Similar palpation with the baby in the prone position may prove more successful.

The defect in the abdominal wall at the umbilicus may be as large as 1½ inches in diameter and the hernia itself may protrude 3 to 4 inches out from the abdominal wall when intra-abdominal pressure is increased. Most umbilical hernias disappear by 1 year of age.

Dilated veins may indicate portal vein obstruction. The direction of venous flow in portal hypertension in veins below the umbilicus is downward.

Since the infant is essentially an abdominal breather, diminished abdominal excursions signal intra-abdominal or intrathoracic pathology. On the other hand, an *increase* in abdominal breathing suggests pulmonary disease.

In *Hirschsprung's disease* (congenital megacolon), a midline suprapubic mass representing a feces-filled rectosigmoid is often found.

An increase in pitch or frequency of bowel sounds or marked diminution is indicative of intestinal obstruction and ileus, respectively. A venous hum is a sign of portal hypertension.

Early and Late Childhood

Protuberance of the abdomen, apparent when the child is is an upright position and disappearing when the child lies down, is noted in most children until adolescence.

Ticklishness is almost universal when the hand first touches the abdominal wall. This disappears in most cases, particularly if the child is distracted by conversation and by the examiner placing the whole hand flush on the surface for a few moments without making initial probing movements with the fingers. With those children who persist in their sensitivity, placement of the child's hand under the examiner's, as shown in the illustrations on this page, will reduce apprehension and increase relaxation of the abdominal musculature. Light superficial palpation of all quadrants should precede deep palpation. The last area to be examined is that which the history suggests as the site of pathology.

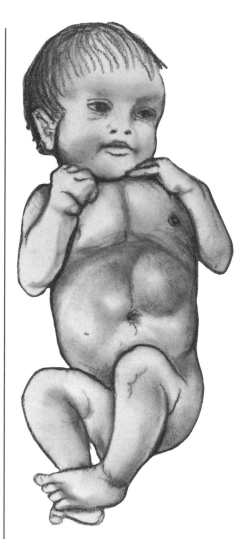

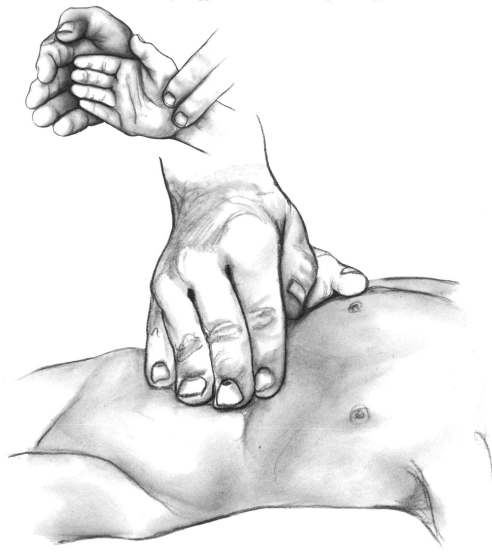

Tenderness may be determined by direct response of the child or may be detected by a change in the facial expression or the pitch of the child's cry.

The liver and spleen are easily palpated in most children. The edge of the liver is normally felt 1 to 2 cm below the right costal margin. It is sharp, soft and moves easily when pushed from below upward during deep inspiration. The size of the liver is better determined by percussion than palpation.

A pathologically enlarged liver is usually palpable at more than 2 cm below the costal margin and has a rounded, firm edge.

The spleen is also, as a rule, felt easily in most children. It is likewise soft with a sharp edge and presents as a downward tongue-like projection along the lateral aspect of the left upper quadrant.

It often can be palpated between the thumb and forefinger of the right hand by following the technique used in palpating the aorta as shown on pp. 211–212, and is found to be freely moveable.

Epigastric pulsations are seen normally, but also may be due to enlargement of the right ventricle with its pulsations transmitted through the diaphragm.

The aorta and its pulsations are easily felt on deep palpation of the abdomen to the left of the midline.

Because the omentum is poorly developed in early childhood, localization of intra-abdominal infection or other inflammatory reaction is less apt to occur than in late childhood and adolescence. Whenever serious pathology occurs within the abdomen, tenderness and spasm are usually diffuse, indicating generalized peritonitis.

In acute appendicitis in this age group, localization of the inflammation may be demonstrated by eliciting pain in the right lower quadrant. This is accomplished in the case of an anterior lying appendix by having the patient attempt to raise his head while the examiner's hand pushes down on the forehead. When the appendix lies retrocecally over the psoas and obturator muscles, positive psoas and obturator signs are present (see p. 212).

The examination for inguinal hernia in this age group is similar to that performed on the adult and should be done with the patient standing.

As the child's cough may be of insufficient strength to demonstrate a reduced hernia, the hernia can be sometimes demonstrated if the child attempts to lift a heavy object such as the end of the examining table or a chair which seats the examiner.

THE GENITALIA AND RECTUM

Infancy

Examining the genitalia in the male infant presents no difficulties. The foreskin is adherent to the glans penis, covers it completely and has a tiny orifice at its distal end. It does not retract over the glans until the infant is several months old and only then if it has been stretched on a regular basis.

Hypospadias is present when the urethral orifice presents at some point along the ventral surface of the glans or the shaft of the penis. The foreskin in these instances is incompletely formed ventrally.

Most male infants in our society are circumcised in the immediate neonatal period so that the glans is exposed to its base.

The testes are normally found in the scrotum, or in the inguinal canal, from which they can easily be milked down into the scrotum.

Hydroceles of the testes and the spermatic cord are common in infancy and often associated with actual or potential inguinal hernias. Hydroceles may be differentiated easily from hernias in that the former transilluminate and are not reducible.

In the newborn female the labia minora are prominent. They quickly atrophy and become almost non-existent until puberty. More often than not, there is a bloody mucoid vaginal discharge during the first week of life due to the maternal estrogen influence on the vaginal mucosa. A serosanguinous vaginal discharge may supplant this for a week or two more.

The perineal structures, the urethral orifice, the hymen and the vaginal mucosa are easily visualized by separating the labia with the thumb and forefinger of one hand, pressing them posteriorly and laterally while pressing anteriorly and ventrally with the tip of one finger of the other hand placed within the rectum.

The genitalia of both male and female breech babies may be markedly edematous and bruised for several days following delivery.

The rectal examination of infants (and of patients in early and late childhood) should be accomplished with the patient in the supine position.

The feet are held together in the midline and the knees and hips flexed upon the abdomen with one hand while the index finger of the other hand is introduced into the rectum. Once this is done, the first hand is placed upon the abdomen to conduct a bimanual examination. The index finger is preferred for the rectal examination, even in infancy, because of its greater tactile sensitivity. Slight bleeding and protrusion of the rectal mucosa is not uncommon upon removal of the examining finger, regardless of its size.

Early and Late Childhood

Penile size in early childhood and prepubescence is of no significance. Indeed, in obese boys, the fatpad over the symphysis pubis may envelop the penis, obscuring it completely. Hyperactive cremasteric reflexes may cause apparent undescended testes.

The cremasteric reflex can be abolished by having the child sit in a crosslegged squatting position on the examining table as illustrated. A diagnosis of undescended testicle should not be made until the inguinal canal and scrotum have been palpated with the patient in this position.

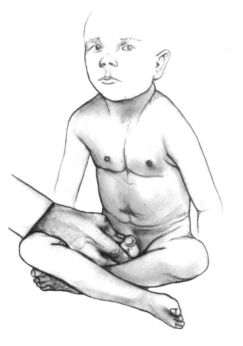

Examination of the female genitalia in this age group may be enhanced by using the child's own hands to distract and reassure her, as shown.

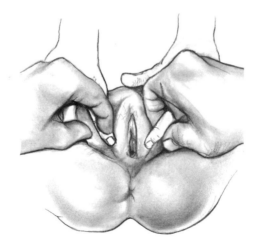

The hymenal orifice and the vaginal mucous membranes may be visualized better if the child coughs or takes a deep breath while the labia are separated.

Greater relaxation and cooperation may be obtained on the rectal examination if the child is asked to breathe in and out rapidly "like a puppy dog" as demonstrated by the examiner.

Perianal skin tabs are common and have no significance. Bimanual rectoabdominal palpation in females will reveal a small midline mass which is the cervix. Any other mass that is palpable on this examination should be considered abnormal, since none of the other anatomical structures are normally palpable until adolescence. Vaginoabdominal palpation as a method of examining the pelvic structures and direct visualization of the vagina and cervix are not considered as part of the ordinary physical examination in childhood. When these procedures are indicated on the basis of the history of abdominal or perineal findings, they are best accomplished with an otoscope equipped with a vaginal speculum.

Fusion of the labia minora is commonly seen. It may be partial, with only the posterior portion of the labia fused, or it may be complete as shown in the illustration. A thin membrane which joins the labial edges is easily lysed with a cotton swab or a probe.

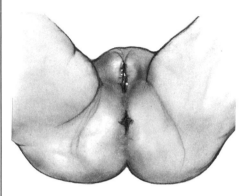

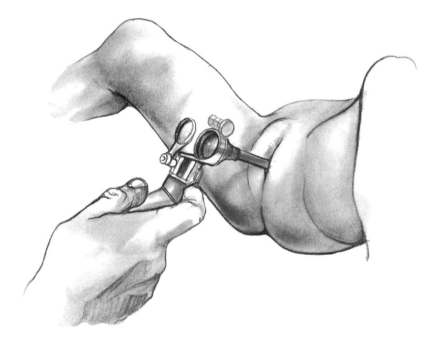

Secondary sexual hair growth parallels the development of other secondary sexual characteristics. Pubic hair may appear sparsely as early as the eighth year. Axillary, facial, body, arm and leg hair proliferate in that order as puberty is approached and undergone.

THE MUSCULOSKELETAL SYSTEM

Infancy

The range of motion at all joints is greatest in infancy and gradually lessens throughout childhood to adult levels.

At birth, the feet may appear deformed if they retain their intrauterine positioning. Such positional deformities can be distinguished by the ease with which the affected foot can be manipulated to neutral and over-correction positions. Scratching or stroking the positionally deformed foot will cause it to assume a normal position. Adduction of the forefoot distal to the metatarsal-tarsal line (*metatarsus adductus deformity*) is commonly found. Correction occurs spontaneously within the first 2 years of life.

During infancy there is a distinct bowlegged growth pattern. This begins to disappear at 18 months of age when a transition from bowlegs to knock-knees occurs. The knock-knee pattern usually persists from 2 until 6 to 10 years of age when a balancing takes place and, for most, the legs straighten. Some babies exhibit a twisting or torsion of the tibia inwardly or outwardly in the coronal plane. This invariably corrects itself during the second year of life.

When the infant stands, his legs are set wide apart and the weight is borne on the inside of the feet. When walking is accomplished, a wide-based gait is used for the first year or two. This causes a certain degree of pronation of the feet and incurving of the Achilles tendons when they are viewed from behind.

The longitudinal arch in infancy is obscured by adipose tissue, giving the foot the appearance of being flat. This is accentuated by pronation of the foot so that the infant is often misdiagnosed as being flatfooted.

The hips of all infants should be examined for signs of dislocation.

The baby is placed in the supine position with the legs pointing toward the examiner. The legs are flexed to right angles at the hips and knees and abducted until the lateral aspect of each knee touches the examining table. When a congenitally dislocated hip is present, the femoral head, which, in this condition lies posterior to the acetabulum, will be seen, felt and sometimes heard to "click" as it enters the acetabulum at some point in the 90 degree abduction arc. This maneuver and finding are known as Ortolani's test and sign. The test is more sensitive if the examiner's middle fingers are placed over the greater trochanter of the femur and the thumbs over the lesser trochanter, as shown in the accompanying three figures.

True deformities do not allow manipulation to even the neutral position.
When the forefoot is twisted inward on its longitudinal axis (inverted) in addition to being adducted, *metatarsus varus* exists (see figure). *Talipes varus* is present when the forefoot is adducted and the entire foot is inverted. Both of these foot deformities require orthopedic correction.

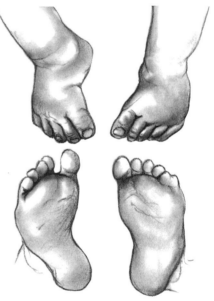

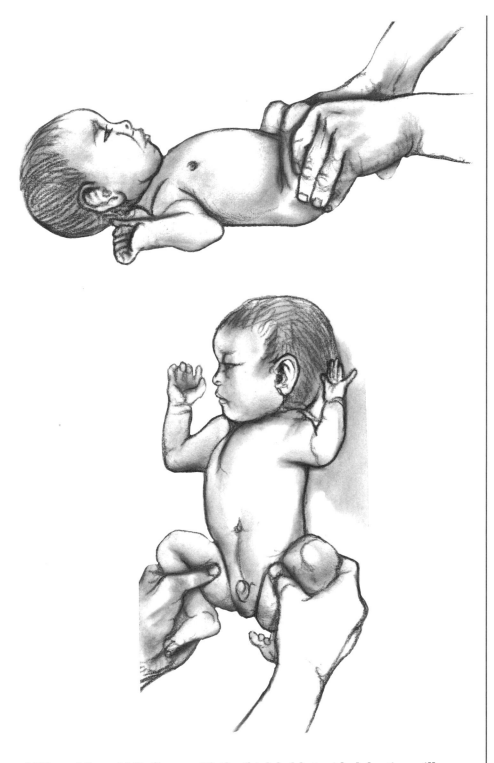

Lifting of the middle finger with the thigh held at mid-abduction will cause reduction of the dislocated hip. The test is more sensitive if the pelvis is steadied with one hand applying pressure from above downward while the other hand performs the maneuver shown.

Unstable (non-dislocated but potentially dislocatable) hips may be detected by exerting backward and outward pressure with the examiner's thumb placed medially over the lesser trochanter. The femoral head can be felt slipping onto the posterior lip of the acetabulum and, when the pressure is released, back into the hip socket (Barlow's sign).

Beyond the newborn period, as the muscles surrounding the hip increase in strength, the "click" of the Ortolani sign is less obtainable, and decreased abduction of the legs, at the hip, on one or both sides, becomes the significant finding in detecting unilateral or bilateral congenital dislocation of the hip.

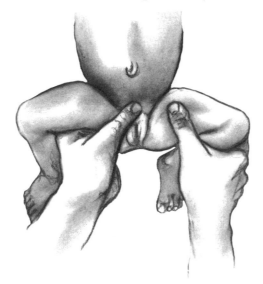

Early and Late Childhood

The presence of musculoskeletal difficulties in this age group can often be detected by closely observing the child in various postures, such as, from the front and rear standing upright with the feet together; walking; stooping to obtain an object from the floor; rising from the supine position; and touching the toes or shins while standing.

In childhood the thoracic convexity is decreased and the lumbar concavity is increased.

Severe hip disease may be detected by observing the child from behind as he shifts his weight from one leg to the other. The pelvis is seen to tilt toward the diseased hip when weight is borne on the affected side and to remain level when the weight is borne on the unaffected side (Trendelenburg's sign). Shortening of the leg in hip disease may be determined by comparing the distance from the anterior superior spine of the ilium to the medial malleolus on each side.

If the spinous processes are marked with a felt-tip pen when the child is bent forward, early scoliosis is more easily detected with the spine then observed in the upright position.

THE NERVOUS SYSTEM

Infancy

The findings on the neurologic examination in infancy, especially in the newborn period, differ markedly from those present in children and adults.

The central nervous system at birth is underdeveloped and functions at subcortical levels. Cortical function develops slowly after birth and cannot be tested in its entirety until early childhood. Thus in the newborn period and early infancy, findings of normal brainstem and spinal functioning do not ensure an intact cortical system, and abnormalities of the brainstem and spinal cord may exist without concomitant cortical difficulties. There are a number of specific reflex activities (*infantile automatisms*) found in the normal newborn which disappear in early infancy.

The neurologic examination in infancy, for the most part, will enable the examiner to detect extensive disease of the central nervous system, but will be of little use in pinpointing minute lesions and specific functional deficits.

The general appearance, positioning, activity, cry and alertness of the newborn baby should be noted as these observations are an important part of the neurologic assessment for this age group.

Motor function should be tested by putting each major joint through its range of motion to determine whether normal muscle tone, spasticity or flaccidity are present.

Beyond the newborn period, throughout infancy, specific gross and fine motor coordination testing can be accomplished by utilizing an age appropriate protocol such as the *Denver Developmental Screening Test*. This test also assesses social and language development. Discrepancies in achievement in the motor and communication areas may suggest whether the deficit is in the motor, sensory or intellectual spheres. Knowledge of when developmental landmarks are normally achieved is essential in assessing the function of the infant's nervous system.

The sensory examination in infants is rather limited in terms of defining neurologic disease. Thresholds to touch, pain and temperature are higher than in older children and reactions to these stimuli are relatively slow.

Gentle stroking of various parts of the body will usually produce movement or withdrawal of a stimulated extremity or change in the facial expression. If a pin is used vigorously enough, crying will result.

The cranial nerves are tested in infancy as in the adult. The difficulties encountered in assessing the function of the first, second, and eighth nerves have already been mentioned.

The twelfth nerve is easily tested by pinching the nostrils of the infant. This produces a reflex opening of the mouth and raising of the tip of the tongue.

The absence of infantile automatisms in the neonate or the persistence of some beyond their expected time of disappearance may indicate severe central nervous system dysfunction.

Postural indicators of severe intracranial disease include persistent asymmetries, predominant extension of the extremities and constant turning of the head to one side. Marked retroflexion of the head, stiffness of the neck and extension of the arms and legs (*opisthotonus*) is an indicator of severe meningeal irritation seen in intracranial infection or hemorrhage and in brainstem irritation (see Figure below).

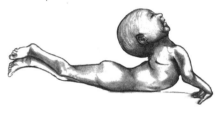

Absence of withdrawal when a painful stimulus is applied to an extremity indicates anesthesia or paralysis. However, if a change in facial expression or a cry is elicited in the absence of withdrawal, paralysis is indicated rather than anesthesia. With spinal cord lesions, the extremity will withdraw in response to pain, but there will be no concomitant change in the baby's facial expression or cry.

If twelfth nerve paresis is present, the tongue tip will deviate toward the affected side.

Because the corticospinal pathways are not fully developed in infants, the spinal reflex mechanisms (deep tendon reflexes and plantar response) are variable in infancy. Their presence in exaggerated form or their absence have very little diagnostic significance unless there is asymmetry of response or change in response from a previous testing.

The technique for eliciting these reflexes is similar to that used with adults, except that the examiner's semiflexed index finger can substitute for the neurologic hammer, its tip acting as the striking point. The thumbnail is an adequate stimulus for eliciting the plantar response.

The Babinski response to plantar stimulation can usually be elicited in most normal infants and until 2 years of age in many children. The triceps reflex is usually not present until after 6 months of age. Rapid, rhythmic plantar flexion of the foot in response to eliciting the ankle reflex (*ankle clonus*) is a common finding in newborns. As many as eight to ten such contractions in response to one stimulus may occur normally (*unsustained ankle clonus*).

When the contractions are continuous (*sustained ankle clonus*), severe central nervous system disease should be suspected.

Ankle clonus may also be elicited by pressing the thumb over the ball of the infant's foot and abruptly dorsiflexing the foot.

The abdominal and cremasteric reflexes are absent in the newborn but appear within the first 6 months of life. The *anal reflex*, however, is normally present in newborns. This is elicited by straightening and raising the lower legs with the baby in a supine position, scratching the perianal region with a pin and observing contracture of the external anal sphincter.

Infantile Automatisms

The infantile automatisms are reflex phenomena which are present at birth or appear shortly thereafter. Some remain only a few weeks while others persist well into the second year of life. The significance of these automatisms in a predictive-diagnostic sense is often debated. While it is agreed that some automatisms have prognostic value for central nervous system integrity, others seem to have only the characteristic of being interesting to recommend their testing. Each automatism will be listed here with the method of elicitation and the prognostic significance of its presence or absence. All are present at birth unless otherwise indicated. The time of disappearance will also be listed.

Blinking (Dazzle) Reflex—disappears after first year. The eyelids close in response to bright light.

Absence may indicate blindness.

Acoustic Blink (Cochleopalpebral) Reflex—disappearance time is variable. Both eyes blink in response to a sharp loud noise.

Absence may give indication of decreased hearing.

Palmar Grasp Reflex—disappears at 3 or 4 months.

With the baby's head positioned in the midline and the arms semiflexed, the examiner's index fingers are placed from the ulnar side into the baby's hands and pressed against the palmar surfaces. A positive response is one of flexion of all of the baby's fingers to grasp the examiner's forefingers. This method allows for comparison of both hands. If the reflex is absent or weak, it may be enhanced by offering the baby a bottle, since sucking facilitates grasping. The strength of the grasp is increased if the hand is flexed and decreased if it is extended.

Light stroking of the ulnar surface of the hand and fifth finger will produce extension of the thumb and other fingers (digital response reflex).

Rooting Reflex—disappears at 3 or 4 months. May be present longer during sleep.

With the baby's head positioned in the midline and his hands held against his anterior chest, the perioral skin at the corners of his mouth and at the midline of the upper and lower lips is stroked with the examiner's finger.

In response, the mouth will open and turn to the stimulated side. When the upper lip is stimulated, the head will retroflex and when the lower lip is stimulated, the jaw will drop. This response will also occur with stimulation of the infant's cheek at some distance from the corners of the mouth.

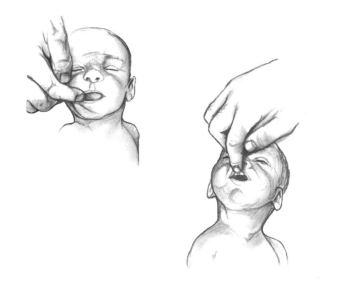

Trunk Incurvation (Galant's) Reflex—disappears at 2 months.

With the baby held horizontally and prone in one of the examiner's hands, the other is used to stimulate one side of the baby's back approximately 3 cm from the midline along a paravertebral line extending from the shoulder to the buttocks. This produces a curving of the trunk toward the stimulated side, with shoulders and pelvis moving in that direction.

Persistence of the grasp reflex beyond 4 months suggests cerebral dysfunction. It should be noted that babies normally hold their hands clenched during the first month of life. Persistence of the fisted hand beyond 2 months is also suggestive of central nervous system damage.

Absence of this reflex is indicative of severe generalized or central nervous system disease.

Transverse spinal cord lesions may be detected using this reflex.

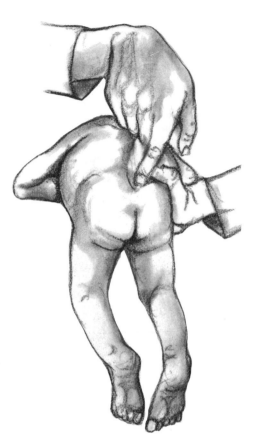

Vertical Suspension Positioning—disappears after 4 months.

While the baby is supported upright with the examiner's hands under the axillae, the head is maintained in the midline and the legs are flexed at the hips and knees.

Placing Response—is best after the first 4 days. Disappearance time is variable.

The examiner holds the baby upright by placing his hands under the baby's arms with the thumbs supporting the back of the head, and allows the dorsal surface of one foot to touch the undersurface of a table top. The procedure is demonstrated in the next four illustrations.

Care should be taken not to plantar flex the foot. The baby responds by flexing the hip and knee and placing the stimulated foot on the table top. This can then be repeated stimulating the other foot. With one foot placed on the table top, the opposite leg will step forward and a series of alternate stepping movements of both legs will occur as the baby is gently moved forward.

Fixed extension and adduction of the legs (*scissoring*) indicates spastic paraplegia or diplegia.

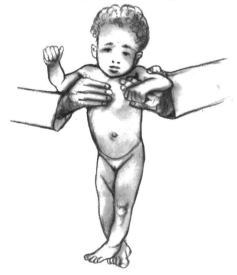

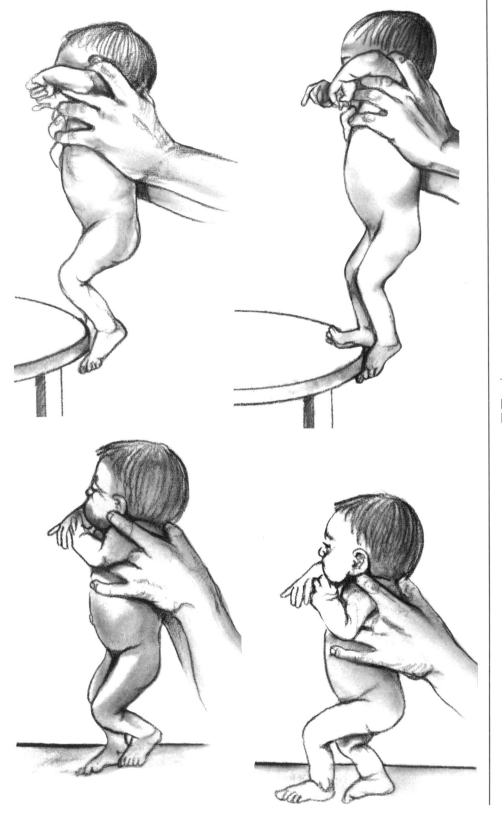

These responses are absent when paresis is present and in babies born by breech delivery.

Rotation Test—disappearance time is variable.

The baby is held under the axillae, at arms length facing the examiner and rotated in one direction and then the other. The head turns in the direction in which the baby is turned. If the head is restrained with the index and ring fingers, the eyes will turn in the direction in which the baby is turned (see figure on p. 389).

The head and eyes do not move, as noted, in the presence of vestibular dysfunction. Early detection of strabismus may be accomplished with this maneuver.

Tonic Neck Reflex—May be present at birth but usually appears at 2 months and disappears at 6 months.

With the baby in the supine position, as shown, the head is turned to one side with the jaw held over the shoulder. The arm and leg on the side to which the head is turned extend while the opposite arm and leg flex.

This reflex should not be entirely obligatory. When it is, it should be considered abnormal, at any age, and will persist beyond the time of expected disappearance in major cerebral damage.

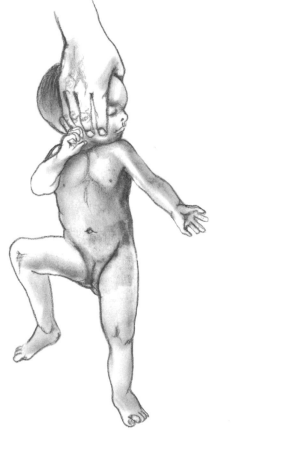

General—There are two mass reflexes which occur in the presence of normal subcortical mechanisms not yet under significant inhibitory control from higher cerebral centers. They are present at birth and disappear by the third month.

Their absence during the first 3 months of life indicates severe cerebral insult, injury to the upper cervical cord, advanced anterior horn cell disease or severe myopathy.

Perez Reflex—The baby is held in a suspended prone position in one of the examiner's hands. The thumb of the other hand is placed on the baby's sacrum and moved firmly toward the head along the entire length of the spine. A positive response is usually one of extension of the head and spine, flexion of the knees on the chest, a cry and emptying of the bladder.

The latter occurs with sufficient frequency to make this reflex useful in the collection of urine specimens from neonates.

Moro Response (*Startle Reflex*)—This response is elicited by any stimulus which suddenly moves the head in relation to the spine.

The methods of producing that movement include lifting the supine baby by the hands approximately 30 degrees from the examining table and allowing the head to fall back by releasing the hands quickly; holding the baby in the supine position, supporting the head, back and legs, suddenly lowering the entire body about 2 feet and stopping abruptly; holding the baby in the supine position supporting the back and pelvis with one hand and arm and the head with the other hand and allowing the head to drop several centimeters with a sudden, rapid, not too forceful movement (as shown in the two figures following); or producing a sudden loud noise, e.g., striking the examining table with the palms of the hands on either side of the baby's head.

The response itself is one in which the arms briskly abduct and extend with the hands open and fingers extended, the legs flex slightly and the hips abduct, but less so than the arms. The arms then return forward over the body in a clasping maneuver.

Persistence of the Moro response beyond 4 months may indicate neurologic disease; persistence beyond 6 months is almost conclusive evidence of such. An asymmetric response in the upper extremities suggests hemiparesis, injury to the brachial plexus or fracture of the clavicle or humerus. Low spinal injury and congenital dislocation of the hip may produce absence of the response in one or both legs.

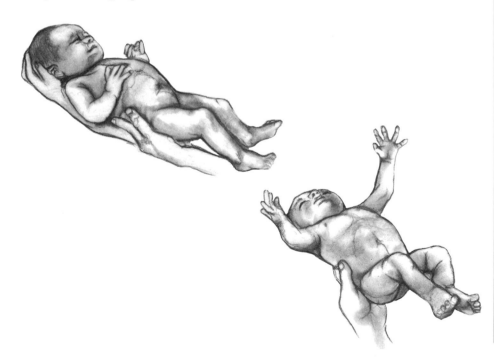

Neurologic screening to include assessment of positioning, spontaneous and induced movements, cry, knee and ankle jerk responses, and elicitation of the rooting, grasp, tonic neck, and Moro automatisms should be performed on all newborns. Babies showing abnormalities in these areas and those at risk should have complete neurologic assessments repeatedly.

Early and Late Childhood

Beyond infancy, when the infantile automatisms have disappeared, the neurologic examination is conducted in much the same manner as with the adult. Samples of handwriting and figure drawing by both hands are useful in detecting fine motor defects. Sensory testing for stereognosis, vibration, position, two-point discrimination, number identification and extinction are usually not testable in the child under 3 years of age and in many under 5 years. The gait should be observed with the child both walking and running. Asymmetric movements of the arms in walking or running may give indication of hemiparesis, as will unequal wear of the soles and heels on the child's shoes, although there are localized neurologic and orthopedic conditions that may produce unequal shoe wear.

The child should be observed rising from the floor from a supine position so that the examiner can note the manner in which the muscles of the neck, trunk, arms and legs are used to assume first the sitting position and then the standing position. (See figures on pp. 425 and 426.)

The following general findings in infancy should suggest to the examiner the presence of central nervous system disease:

1. Abnormal localized neurological findings
2. Failure to elicit expected responses
3. Asymmetry of normal responses
4. Late persistence of normal responses
5. Re-emergence of vanished responses
6. Developmental delays

Certain combinations of findings in infancy suggest specific diagnoses. The presence of the setting sun sign, opisthotonos and a disappearing or absent Moro response suggest *kernicterus.* In *congenital hemiplegia,* absent or diminished movement of the extremities involved plus abnormal posturing is seen rather than any changes in reflexes and muscle tone. *Bilateral cerebral palsy* produces hypotonia with normal or brisk reflexes, delay in reaching motor milestones and consistency in tonic neck patterns. The *spastic diplegias* produce variable dystonic spasms followed by hypertonus early in infancy and persistent clenched fists coupled with scissoring after the first few months. The athetoid and dystonic extrapyramidal group of diseases present with variable sets of signs.

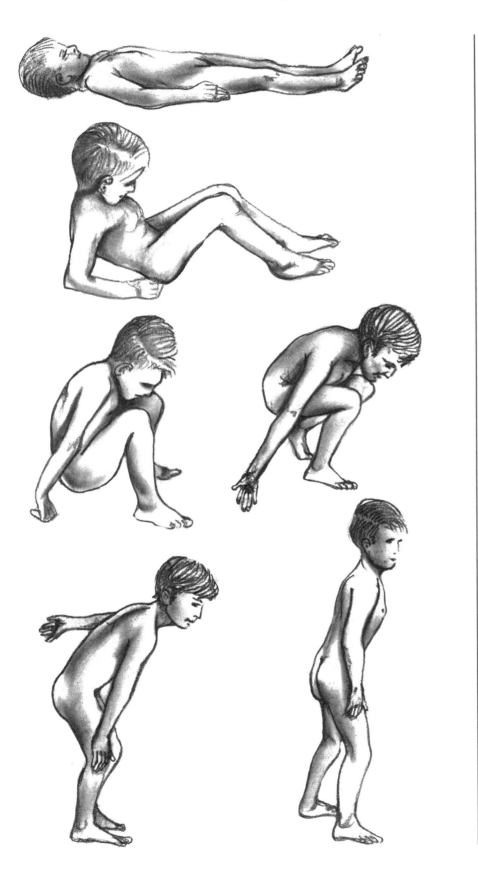

Evidence of neurologic deficits, muscular weaknesses and orthopedic defects may be detected here that would not be noted otherwise.

In certain forms of *muscular dystrophy* with pelvic girdle weaknesses, rising from a supine to a standing position is accomplished as shown below (*Gowers's sign*).

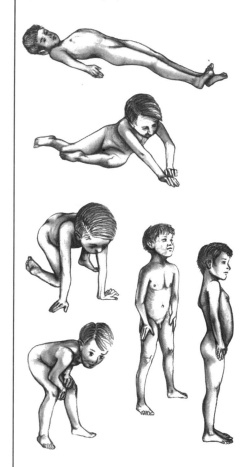

When nystagmus, unsteady gait or history of streptomycin therapy is present, vestibular function should be tested.

This is accomplished with the cold caloric test. Water at 65°F temperature squirted into the external auditory canal should produce nystagmus within 30 seconds.

The absence of nystagmus is indicative of drug toxicity, meningitis, brain tumor or labyrinthitis.

In essence the complete neurologic examination in infancy and childhood includes elements of all of the parts of the general physical examination as well as the specific components of the neurologic examination outlined here. The examiner is constantly assessing neurologic functioning throughout the course of every patient encounter. All of the observations made and impressions gained are used to determine the integrity of the central and peripheral nervous systems. This is equally true in the examination of adults.

BIBLIOGRAPHY

The references below have been selected for their usefulness to the student. Emphasis has been placed upon textbooks rather than original sources.

General References

ANATOMY AND PHYSIOLOGY

Guyton AC. *Textbook of Medical Physiology*. 5th Edition. Philadelphia: W.B. Saunders Co., 1976.

Basmajian JV. *Grant's Method of Anatomy*. 9th Edition. Baltimore: The Williams & Wilkins Co., 1975.

Grant JCB. *An Atlas of Anatomy*. 6th Edition. Baltimore: The Williams & Wilkins Co., 1972.

Gray H. *Anatomy of the Human Body*. 29th American Edition. Edited by CM Goss. Philadelphia: Lea and Febiger, 1973.

Morris Sir H. *Morris' Human Anatomy: A Complete Systematic Treatise*. 12th Edition. Edited by BJ Anson. New York: McGraw-Hill Book Co., 1966.

Anson BJ, McVay CB. *Surgical Anatomy*. 5th Edition. Philadelphia: W. B. Saunders Co., 1971.

PHYSICAL DIAGNOSIS—MEDICAL & SURGICAL

Burnside JW. *Adams' Physical Diagnosis. An Introduction to Clinical Medicine*. 15th Edition. Baltimore: The Williams & Wilkins Co., 1974.

DeGowin EL, DeGowin RL. *Bedside Diagnostic Examination*. 3rd Edition. New York: MacMillan Publishing Co., 1976.

Major's Physical Diagnosis. Edited by MH Delp and RT Manning. 8th Edition. Philadelphia: W. B. Saunders Co., 1975.

Hochstein E, Rubin AL. *Physical Diagnosis: A Textbook and Workbook in Methods of Clinical Examination*. New York: Blakiston Division, McGraw-Hill Book Co., 1964.

Judge RD, Zuidema GD. *Methods of Clinical Examination: A Physiologic Approach*. 3rd Edition. Boston: Little, Brown, and Co., 1974.

Kampmeier RH, Blake TM. *Physical Examination in Health and Disease*. 4th Edition. Philadelphia: F. A. Davis Co., 1970.

Macleod J. *Clinical Examination*. 4th Edition. Edinburgh: Churchill Livingstone, 1976.

Morgan WL Jr, Engel GL. *The Clinical Approach to the Patient*. Philadelphia: W. B. Saunders Co., 1969.

Prior JA, Silberstein JS. *Physical Diagnosis: The History and Examination of the Patient*. 5th Edition. St. Louis: The C.V. Mosby Co., 1977.

Walker HK, Hall WD, Hurst JW. *Clinical Methods. The History, Physical and Laboratory Examinations*. Boston: Butterworths, 1976.

Zatouroff M. *Color Atlas of Physical Signs in General Medicine*. Chicago: Year Book Medical Publishers, 1976.

Clain A. *Hamilton Bailey's Demonstrations of Physical Signs in Clinical Surgery*. 15th Edition. Baltimore: The Williams & Wilkins Co., 1973.

Dunphy JE, Botsford TW. *Physical Examination of the Surgical Patient: An Introduction to Clinical Surgery*. 4th Edition. Philadelphia: W.B. Saunders Co., 1975.

Walker WF. *Color Atlas of General Surgical Diagnosis*. Chicago: Year Book Medical Publishers, 1976.

MEDICINE, SURGERY AND PATHOPHYSIOLOGY

Beeson PB, McDermott W. *Textbook of Medicine*. 14th Edition. Philadelphia: W.B. Saunders Co., 1975.

Thorn GW, Adams RD, Braunwald E, Isselbacher KJ, Petersdorf RG. *Harrison's Principles of Internal Medicine*. 8th Edition. New York: McGraw-Hill Book Co., 1977.

Harvey AM, Johns RJ, Owens AH Jr, Ross RS. *The Principles and Practice of Medicine*. 19th Edition. New York: Appleton-Century-Crofts, 1976.

Schwartz SI. *Principles of Surgery*. 2nd Edition. New York: McGraw-Hill Book Co., 1974.

MacBryde CM, Blacklow RS. *Signs and Symptoms. Applied Pathologic Physiology and Clinical Interpretation*. 5th Edition. J.B. Lippincott Co., 1970.

Chapter 1. Interviewing and the Health History

Engel GL, Morgan WL Jr. *Interviewing the Patient*. Philadelphia: W.B. Saunders Co., 1973.

Enelow AJ, Swisher SN. *Interviewing and Patient Care*. New York: Oxford University Press, 1972.

Froelich RE, Bishop FM. *Clinical Interviewing Skills: A Programmed Manual for Data Gathering, Evaluation and Patient Management*. 3rd Edition. St. Louis: The C.V. Mosby Co., 1977.

Bernstein L, Bernstein RS, Dana RH. *Interviewing: A Guide for Health Professionals*. 2nd Edition. New York: Appleton-Century-Crofts, 1974.

Benjamin A. *The Helping Interview*. 2nd Edition. Boston: Houghton Mifflin Co., 1974.

Bird B. *Talking with Patients*. 2nd Edition. Philadelphia: J.B. Lippincott Co., 1973.

Knapp ML. *Nonverbal Communication in Human Interaction*. New York: Holt, Rinehart and Winston, 1972.

Freeman MG. Sexual history. In *Clinical Methods: The History, Physical and Laboratory Examinations*. Edited by HK Walker, WD Hale, JW Hurst. Boston: Butterworths, 1976, pp. 247-282.

Kübler-Ross E. *On Death and Dying*. New York: The Macmillan Co., 1969.

Sapira JD. Reassurance therapy. What to say to symptomatic patients with benign diseases. Ann Intern Med 77:603-604, 1972.

Feinstein AR. *Clinical Judgment*. Baltimore: The Williams & Wilkins Co., 1967.

Elling R, Whittemore R, Green M. Patient participation in a pediatric program. J Health Hum Behav 1:183-191, 1960.

Boyle WE. The pediatric history. In *Principles of Pediatrics: Health Care of the Young*. Edited by RA Hoekelman et al. New York: McGraw Hill Book Co., 1978, pp. 23-30.

Korsch BM, Freemon B, Negrete VF. Practical implications of doctor-patient interaction analysis for pediatric practice. Amer J Dis Child 121:110-114, 1971.

Starfield B, Borkowf S. Physicians' recognition of complaints made by parents about their children's health. Pediatrics 43:168-172, 1969.

Chapter 2: Recording the History

Hurst JW, Walker HK. *The Problem-Oriented System*. New York: Medcom Press, 1972.

Morgan WL Jr, Engel GL. *The Clinical Approach to the Patient*. Philadelphia: W.B. Saunders Co., 1969.

Chapter 5: The General Survey

Society of Actuaries. *Build and Blood Pressure Study*. Chicago, 1959.

Nichols GA, Kucha DH. Taking adult temperatures: oral measurements. Am J Nurs 72:1091-1093, 1972.

Nichols GA. Taking adult temperatures: rectal measurements. Am J Nurs 72:1092-1093, 1972.

Chapter 6: The Skin

Sauer GC. *Manual of Skin Diseases*. 3rd Edition. Philadelphia: J.B. Lippincott Co., 1973.

Fitzpatrick TB, et al. *Dermatology in General Medicine*. New York: McGraw-Hill Book Co., 1971.

Jeghers H, Edelstein LM. Pigmentation of the skin. In *Signs and Symptoms*. 5th Edition. Edited by CM MacBryde and RS Blacklow. Philadelphia: J.B. Lippincott Co., 1970.

Lipman BS, Massie E. Clubbed fingers and hypertrophic osteoarthropathy. In *Signs and*

Symptoms. 5th Edition, Edited by CM MacBryde and RS Blacklow. Philadelphia: J.B. Lippincott Co., 1970.

Bean WB. *Vascular Spiders and Related Lesions of the Skin.* Springfield, Ill.: Charles C Thomas, 1958.

Chapter 7: The Head and Neck

EYES

Havener, WH. *Synopsis of Ophthalmology.* 4th Edition. St. Louis: The C.V. Mosby Co., 1975.

Newell FW, Ernest JT. *Ophthalmology. Principles and Concepts.* 3rd Edition. St. Louis: The C.V. Mosby Co., 1974.

Vaughan D, Asbury T. *General Ophthalmology.* 8th Edition. Los Altos, Calif.: Lange Medical Publications, 1977.

Ballantyne AJ, Michaelson TC. *Textbook of the Fundus of the Eye.* 2nd Edition. Edinburgh: Churchill Livingstone, 1970.

Bedford MA. *Color Atlas of Ophthalmological Diagnosis.* Chicago: Year Book Medical Publishers, 1971.

Blodi FC, Allen L, Braley AE. *Stereoscopic Manual of the Ocular Fundus in Local and Systemic Disease.* St. Louis: The C.V. Mosby Co., 1964.

Arsham GM, Colenbrander A, Spivey BE. *Basic Instruction in Ophthalmoscopy.* Iowa City: The University of Iowa, 1971. (A teaching package of 80 slides, 2 audiotape cassettes and a study guide).

EARS, NOSE AND THROAT

DeWeese DD, Saunders WH. *Textbook of Otolaryngology.* 4th Edition. St. Louis: The C.V. Mosby Co., 1973.

Ballenger JJ. *Diseases of the Nose, Throat and Ear.* Philadelphia: Lea and Febiger, 1977.

Bull TR. *Color Atlas of E.N.T. Diagnosis.* Chicago: Year Book Medical Publishers, 1974.

MOUTH

Colby RA, Kerr DA, Robinson HBG. *Color Atlas of Oral Pathology.* 3rd Edition. Philadelphia: J.B. Lippincott Co., 1971.

Shafer WG. *A Textbook of Oral Pathology.* 3rd Edition. Philadelphia: W.B. Saunders Co., 1974.

NECK

Solnitzky OC, Jeghers H. Lymphadenopathy and disorders of the lymphatic system. In *Signs and Symptoms.* 5th Edition. Edited by CM MacBryde and RS Blacklow. Philadelphia: J.B. Lippincott Co., 1970.

Chapter 8: The Thorax and Lungs

Forgacs P. Crackles and wheezes. The Lancet 2:203-205, 1967.

Forgacs P. Lung sounds. Brit J Dis Chest 63:1-12, 1969.

Nath AR, Capel LH. Inspiratory crackles and mechanical events of breathing. Thorax 29:695-698, 1974.

Murphy RLH Jr, Holford SK, Knowler WC. Visual lung sound characterization by time-expanded wave-form analysis. New Eng J Med 296:968-971, 1977.

Capel LH. Lung sounds: a new approach. The Practitioner 219:633-639, 1977.

Pulmonary terms and symbols. A report of the ACCP-ATS Joint Committee on Pulmonary Nomenclature. Chest 67:583-593, 1975.

Norris GW, Landis HRM. *Diseases of the Chest and the Principles of Physical Diagnosis.* 5th Edition. Philadelphia: W.B. Saunders Co., 1933.

Chapter 9: The Heart

Hurst JW. *The Heart, Arteries and Veins.* 4th Edition. New York: McGraw-Hill Book Co., 1978.

Harvey AM, Johns RJ, Owens AH Jr, Ross RS. *The Principles and Practice of Medicine.* 19th Edition. New York: Appleton-Century-Crofts, 1976. Chapter 21, Clinical evaluation of the cardiovascular system, and Chapter 26, Cardiac murmurs and other manifestations of valvular and acyanotic congenital heart disease.

Hurst JW, Schlant RC. *Examination of the Heart. Part 3. Inspection and Palpation of the Anterior Chest.* Dallas, Texas: American Heart Association, 1972.

Leonard JJ, Kroetz FW, Leon DF, Shaver JA. *Examination of the Heart. Part 4. Auscultation.* Dallas, Texas: American Heart Association, 1974.

Chapter 10: Pressures and Pulses: Arterial and Venous

Kirkendall WM, Burton AC, Epstein FH, Freis ED. Recommendations for human blood pressure determination by sphygmomanometers. Circulation 36:980-988, 1967.

King GE. Taking the blood pressure. JAMA 209:1902-1904, 1969.

Moser M et al. Report of the Joint National Committee on Detection, Evaluation, and Treatment of High Blood Pressure. JAMA 237:255-261, 1977.

Thulin T, Andersson G, Scherstén B. Measurement of blood pressure—a routine test in need of standardization. Postgraduate Med J 51:390-395, 1975.

Marx HJ, Yu PN. Clinical examination of the arterial pulse. Progress in Cardiovasc Dis 10:207-235, 1967.

Fowler NO. *Examination of the Heart. Part 2. Inspection and Palpation of Venous and Arterial Pulses.* Dallas, Texas: American Heart Association, 1972.

Chapter 11: The Breasts and Axillae

Haagensen CD. *Diseases of the Breast.* 2nd Edition. Philadelphia: W.B. Saunders Co., 1974.

Haagensen CD. *Carcinoma of the Breast.* New York: American Cancer Society, 1958.

Leis HP. *Diagnosis and Treatment of Breast Lesions.* Flushing, N.Y.: Medical Examination Publishing Co., 1970.

Chapter 12: The Abdomen

Cope Z. *The Early Diagnosis of the Acute Abdomen.* 14th Edition. London: Oxford University Press, 1972.

Castell DO, O'Brien KD, Muench H, Chalmers TC. Estimation of liver size by percussion in normal individuals. Ann Intern Med 70:1183-1189, 1969.

Castell DO. The spleen percussion sign. A useful diagnostic technique. Ann Intern Med 67:1265-1267, 1967.

Sullivan S, Krasner N, Williams R. The clinical estimation of liver size: a comparison of techniques and an analysis of the source of error. Brit Med J 2:1042-1043, 1976.

Chapter 13: Male Genitalia and Hernias

Campbell MF, Harrison JH. *Urology.* 3rd Edition. Philadelphia: W.B. Saunders Co., 1970.

U.S. Dept. HEW. *Syphilis. A Synopsis.* Washington D.C.: U.S. Government Printing Office, 1968.

Wisdom A. *Color Atlas of Venereology.* Chicago: Year Book Medical Publishers, 1973.

Zimmerman LM, Anson BJ. *Anatomy and Surgery of Hernia.* 2nd Edition. Baltimore: The Williams & Wilkins Co., 1967.

Chapter 14: Female Genitalia

Novak ER, Jones GS, Jones HW Jr. *Novak's Textbook of Gynecology.* 9th Edition. Baltimore: The Williams & Wilkins Co., 1975.

Romney SL et al. *Gynecology and Obstetrics. The Health Care of Women.* New York: McGraw-Hill Book Co., 1975.

Pritchard JA, Macdonald PC. *Williams Obstetrics.* 15th Edition. New York: Appleton-Century-Crofts, 1976.

Wisdom A. *Color Atlas of Venereology.* Chicago: Year Book Medical Publishers, 1973.

Chapter 15: Anus and Rectum

Turell R. *Diseases of the Colon and Anorectum.* 2nd Edition. Philadelphia: W.B. Saunders Co., 1969.

Chapter 16: The Peripheral Vascular System

Allen EV. *Peripheral Vascular Diseases.* 4th Edition. By JF Fairbairn II, JL Juergens and JA Spittell Jr. Philadelphia: W.B. Saunders Co., 1972.

Solnitzky OC, Jeghers H. Lymphadenopathy and disorders of the lymphatic system. In *Signs and Symptoms.* 5th Edition. Edited by CM MacBryde and RS Blacklow. Philadelphia: J.B. Lippincott Co., 1970.

Chapter 17: The Musculoskeletal System

Beetham WP Jr, Polley HF, Slocumb CH, Weaver WF. *Physical Examination of the Joints.* Philadelphia: W.B. Saunders Co., 1965.

Mason M, Currey HLF. *Clinical Rheumatology.* Philadelphia: J.B. Lippincott Co., 1970.

Hollander JL. *Arthritis and Allied Conditions.* 8th Edition. Philadelphia: Lea and Febiger, 1972.

Raney RB Sr, Brashear HR Jr. *Shands' Handbook of Orthopaedic Surgery.* 9th Edition. St. Louis: The C.V. Mosby Co., 1978.

Moseley HF. *Shoulder Lesions.* 3rd Edition. Edinburgh: Churchill Livingstone, 1969.

American Academy of Orthopaedic Surgeons. *Joint Motion. Method of Measuring and Recording.* 1965.

Chapter 18: The Nervous System

Clark RG. *Manter and Gatz's Essentials of Clinical Neuroanatomy and Neurophysiology.* 5th Edition. Philadelphia: F.A. Davis Co., 1975.

Chusid JG. *Correlative Neuroanatomy and Functional Neurology.* 16th Edition. Los Altos, Calif.: Lange Medical Publications, 1976.

Haymaker W, Woodhall B. *Peripheral Nerve Injuries. Principles of Diagnosis.* 2nd Edition. Philadelphia: W.B. Saunders Co., 1953.

Curtis BA, Jacobson S, Marcus EM. *An Introduction to the Neurosciences.* Philadelphia: W.B. Saunders Co., 1972.

Alpers BJ, Mancall, EL. *Essentials of the Neurological Examination.* Philadelphia: F.A. Davis Co., 1971.

Van Allen MW. *Pictorial Manual of Neurological Tests.* Chicago: Year Book Medical Publishers, 1969.

Vick NA. *Grinker's Neurology.* 7th Edition. Springfield, Ill.: Charles C Thomas, 1976.

Thorn GW, Adams RD, Braunwald E, Isselbacher KG, Petersdorf RG. *Harrison's Principles of Internal Medicine.* 8th Edition. New York: McGraw-Hill Book Co., 1977, Sec. 3, Alterations of nervous function, pp. 69-157.

Plum F, Posner JB. *The Diagnosis of Stupor and Coma.* 2nd Edition. Philadelphia: F.A. Davis Co., 1972.

Darmody WR. *Management of the Unconscious Patient.* St. Louis: The C.V. Mosby Co., 1976.

Fahn S. Differential diagnosis of tremors. Med Clin N Amer 56(6):1363-1375, 1972.

Duvoisin R. Clinical diagnosis of the dyskinesias. Med Clin N Amer 56(6):1321-1341, 1972.

Chapter 19: Mental Status

Thaler O, Engel I, Goldstein R. Mental status examination. Unpublished. Dept. of Psychiatry, University of Rochester Medical Center.

Freedman AM, Kaplan HI, Sadock BJ. *Comprehensive Textbook of Psychiatry.* 2nd Edition. Baltimore: The Williams & Wilkins Co., 1975.

Kolb LC. *Modern Clinical Psychiatry.* 9th Edition. Philadelphia: W.B. Saunders Co., 1977.

Jacobs JW, Bernhard MR, Delgado A, Strain JJ. Screening for organic mental syndromes in the medically ill. Ann Intern Med 86:40-46, 1977.

Chapter 20: The Pediatric Physical Examination

Allen ED. Examination of the genital organs in the prepubescent and in the adolescent girl. Pediatr Clin N Am 2:19-34, 1955.

Barlow TG. Congenital dislocation of the hip, early diagnosis and treatment. Lond Clin Med J 5:47-58, 1964.

Barness LA. *Manual of Pediatric Physical Diagnosis.* Chicago: Year Book Medical Publishers, 1969.

Bigler JA. Interpretation of heart murmurs. Pediatr Clin N Am 2:441-448, 1955.

Bordley JE, Mardy WG, Hardy MP: Pediatric audiology. Pediatr Clin N Am 9:1147-1158, 1962.

Caceres CA, Perry W. *The Innocent Murmur: A Problem in Clinical Practice.* Boston: Little, Brown and Co., 1967.

Capraro VJ. Gynecological examination in children and adolescents. Pediatr Clin N Am 19:511-528, 1972.

Frankenburg W, Dodds J. *Denver Developmental Screening Text Manual.* Denver, University of Colorado Medical Center and Mead Johnson, 1968.

Gibson S. Eyes, hands and ears in the diagnosis of heart disease in children. Pediatr Clin N Am 1:3-12, 1954.

Goldring D, Wohltmann H. Flush method for blood pressure determinations in newborn infants. J Pediatr 40:285-289, 1952.

Gorman JJ, Cogan DG, Gellis SS. An apparatus for grading the visual acuity of infants on the basis of opticokinetic nystagmus. Pediatrics 19:1088-1092, 1957.

Graham BD. *Pediatric Examination in Physical Diagnosis.* Saint Louis, C.V. Mosby Co., 1969.

Hardy JB, Dougherty A, Hardy WG. Hearing responses and audiological screening in infants. J Pediatr 55:382-390, 1959.

Hoekelman RA et al (eds.). *Principles of Pediatrics: Health Care of the Young.* New York, McGraw-Hill, 1978.

Holt LB. *Pediatric Ophthalmology.* Philadelphia, Lea and Febiger, 1964.

Illingworth RS. *An Introduction to Developmental Assessment in the First Year.* London, National Spastics Society Medical Education and Information Unit, 1962.

Kempe CH, Silver HK, O'Brien D. *Current Pediatric Diagnosis and Treatment.* Los Altos, California, Lange Medical Publications, 1972.

Khermosh O, Lior G, Weissman SL. Tibial torsion in children. Clin Orthop 79:25-31, 1971.

Lowrey GH. *Pediatric Examination in Physical Diagnosis: A Physiologic Approach to the Clinical Examination.* Boston: Little, Brown & Co., 1968.

MacKeith RC. The theory and practice of reassurance. Guy's Hosp Gazette 74:138, 1960.

Paine RS. Neurological examination of infants and children. Pediatr Clin N Am 7:471-510, 1960.

Parmelee AH. Examination of the newborn infant. Pediatr Clin N Am 2:335-349, 1955.

Prechtl H, Beitema D. *The Neurological Examination of the Full Term Newborn Infant.* London, National Spastics Society Medical Education and Information Unit, 1964.

Spivek ML. Examination of the child. In *Practice of Pediatrics.* Edited by J Brennemann and I McQuarrie. Hagerstown, Md, WF Prior, 1970.

Tachdjian MO. Diagnosis and treatment of congenital deformities of the musculo-skeletal system in the newborn and the infant. Pediatr Clin N Am 14:307-348, 1968.

Thomas A, Chesni Y, Dargassies SS. *The Neurological Examination of the Infant.* London, National Spastics Society Medical Education and Information Unit, 1960.

Van Allen MW. *Pictorial Manual of Neurological Tests.* Chicago, Year Book Medical Publishers, 1969.

Wilbur HM. Teeth. Pediatr Clin N Am 8:91-95, 1961.

INDEX*

*Note: References to tables are listed in *italics*.